A LEGACY OF HEALING

THE ROLE OF NUTRITION, CHIROPRACTIC AND OTHER ALTERNATIVE THERAPIES IN SELF-HEALING

Dr. Christopher J. Amoruso, D.C., M.S., C.N.S.
and
Dr. Angelo C. Rose, D.C.

authorHOUSE®

AuthorHouse™
1663 Liberty Drive
Bloomington, IN 47403
www.authorhouse.com
Phone: 1 (800) 839-8640

© 2016 Dr. Angelo Rose; Dr. Christopher Amoruso. All rights reserved.

No part of this book may be reproduced, stored in a retrieval system, or transmitted by any means without the written permission of the author.

Published by AuthorHouse 11/10/2016

ISBN: 978-1-5246-4585-4 (sc)
ISBN: 978-1-5246-4586-1 (hc)
ISBN: 978-1-5246-4584-7 (e)

Library of Congress Control Number: 2016917824

Print information available on the last page.

Any people depicted in stock imagery provided by Thinkstock are models, and such images are being used for illustrative purposes only. Certain stock imagery © Thinkstock.

This book is printed on acid-free paper.

Because of the dynamic nature of the Internet, any web addresses or links contained in this book may have changed since publication and may no longer be valid. The views expressed in this work are solely those of the author and do not necessarily reflect the views of the publisher, and the publisher hereby disclaims any responsibility for them.

The following is an FDA mandated warning which I must provide to you:
This book is for educational purposes only. It is not intended as a substitute for the diagnosis, treatment, or advice of a qualified licensed medical professional. The facts presented in the following pages are offered for informational purposes only. Always consult a medical practitioner before embarking on any of the protocols in this book. Neither the author nor the publisher can be held responsible for any loss or claim arising out of the use, or misuse, of the suggestions made, or the failure to take medical advice.

DEDICATION

This book is dedicated first and foremost to the patients; people who, often through great personal hardship, suffering and personal sacrifice, have sought a better, more natural, holistic way of healing. It was my father's hope and dream that this book would reach more people searching for help than he was able to while in practice. Therefore, this book is also dedicated to his memory, and to his more than 50 years of hard work and constant study, all of which enabled this book to become a reality.

I also dedicate this book to my Lord and Savior, Jesus Christ. Working on this book has been a gift and I am continually humbled by Your wisdom and design.

Lastly, I dedicate this book to my family. I hope that this book will be as great a blessing for our family as my father's guidance has been for me.

ACKNOWLEDGEMENTS

First and foremost, I would like to thank God for blessing me with the experiences He has and for trusting and directing me to complete this book for my father; his were/are big shoes to fill. I am thankful for God's grace and for using me as a vessel for His healing. All Glory is His.

To my father, may God rest his soul. I am thankful for having been blessed to grow up with a father who had such a strong faith in the natural healing ability of the human body and its connection to our spirituality as human beings. I am also grateful for all of the wonderful things that he taught me and for the values he instilled within me, which have forever left an impression on me and have forged the man that I have become, as well as the man I hope to be. Most of all I thank him for teaching me to be a critical thinker, to not be afraid, but rather to question the world around me, to work hard, to think and to trust in God to illuminate the darkness.

My gratitude to my beautiful wife Rosanna as well as our three children, Isabella, Joseph and Angelo, for putting up with me through this daunting challenge, and for being patient whilst I spent much of my free time at the computer or buried behind books. Your support, love, and proofreading are as much a part of this book as anything else. I love you with all of my heart.

To Terry Eppridge without whom this book would not be. Her tireless efforts and patience are what made this book flow into a concise, accurate and organized work and made its eventual publication a reality. Her attention to detail and input are what made this book complete. I am forever grateful for her friendship and her work on this book. I also thank Marie-Celine Miranda for her experienced proofreader's eye.

I would also like to offer my most sincere gratitude and thanks to Dr. Chante Callis and Ms. Lauren Spooner whose work with proofreading and content were invaluable to the completion of this book.

To Sally Fallon-Morell whose work has inspired a revolution. Her writing and work as the co-founder of the Weston A. Price Foundation have helped countless people searching for traditional wisdom and healing, and have spurred a return to our traditional ways of eating and living. A special thanks to her for graciously allowing me to reprint the instructions for soaking/preparing foods and to disseminate the information to my readers.

To Dave Carlson for his artwork which makes ideas about the body come to life for the reader and makes explaining complex anatomy and its relationship to disease possible.

To Stephen Buhner, for permitting the reprint of some of his protocol for treating Lyme disease from his amazing book *Healing Lyme*. The importance of his work and knowledge in treatment/prevention of Lyme disease is immeasurable.

To Dr. Bruce West for kindly allowing us to reprint his Zypan Test.

To Backtalk Systems, who gave permission to reprint their intricate diagram of the spine and its extensive connections to the body. It is an image so essential for understanding Chiropractic's role in effecting change throughout the body.

To the Kansas Medical Clinic for the use of their diagram of the stomach and hiatal hernia thus giving our readers a better anatomical understanding of the digestive system.

To Foot Levelers for allowing the use of some of their images to portray just how important the feet are as the foundation of the spine and in our everyday health. Their well-crafted products served my father and his patients for much of his career and continue to serve my patients today.

To the doctors, researchers and writers from all walks of life who have contributed their talent and tireless works to the healing of human illness: Dr. Weston A. Price, Antoine Béchamp, Dr. Royal Lee, Dr. Francis Pottenger, Allan Savory, Dr. Stanislaw Burzynsky, Dr. Mary Enig, Dr. William Crook, Dr. Natasha Campbell-McBride, Dr. Thomas Cowan, Dr. Nicholas Gonzalez, and many, many others. You are truly the giants upon whose shoulders we stand. Thank you.

Lastly, but most importantly, thank you to every patient who trusted my father over his 50 years of practice, some of whom trust in me still today. And to the many who never met my father but who have trusted me to continue his work. It is from you that we learn and grow every day. Whether from success or failure, it is the many relationships we have developed over the years that have brought us to healing and led us closer to God, without whom we serve no purpose.

FOREWORD

This book by my father, Angelo C. Rose, is the culmination of a lifetime of work and practical experience as a holistic physician. (Amoruso is my father's correct family name — an interesting immigration story in itself.) Before his death, my father began writing this book so that his experience and wisdom in treating illnesses holistically could live on. My father was one of the Great Ones. You read and hear about people who embody selflessness and caring, wisdom and kindness. My father was one of those. He never pursued fame and was not greedy. He once told me that God took care of our family because he (and my mother, of course) always did the best they could to help others and to live honestly. At his funeral in March of 2007, a line of people an hour-and-a-half long waited to greet his casket, in an unspoken testament to the lives he touched. Some of the faces I recognized as current patients of mine whom I had inherited from him; some I knew as distant family or friends; and others were patients of his from before I was born, many of whom I had never met, and many of whom had not seen my father in decades. From different places, times, and with different experiences with my father, they shared a common thread — my father had touched their lives in a significant way, and they came to pay their respect to him. Each had a personal story to tell of how my father had helped them, or changed their lives. To this day I wonder how they received word of his passing. I remember thinking that if I could touch just a tenth of the people my father had touched, my life would be successful.

I grew up as the youngest of the six children of Felicia A. Maresca and Angelo Carlo Rose. Looking back, my childhood was quite normal by most standards. I always felt blessed and fortunate that my parents could provide us with a good home, quality education, and a loving family environment. My brothers and sisters were much older than I, so I would follow them around like a puppy looking to be included in all they did. We swam, played ball, had snowball fights, and ate dinner together as a general rule. We were raised as a God-fearing Roman Catholic family, though my father was far more spiritual in how he lived his life than he was a churchgoer. We neither attended Church regularly nor went around quoting scripture, yet God and His natural law were a part of the lessons our parents taught us. On a regular basis we received chiropractic adjustments especially if we were coming down with an ailment. We took vitamins regularly. When anyone in the family was hurt or sick, my father tended to it. He seemed to have all of the answers. It was so normal to me that I never really thought of our lives as being different until much later in life. Then I realized how different our upbringing had been.

For me, my father was my doctor. Growing up I never thought of that as special. It was cool to tell friends and to feel proud that my father held a respectable occupation and helped those who were sick. Like most children, I trusted my father, and did what he said to do, accepting it as the norm. As I grew older, I began to see that my father was governed by a set of rules very different from those of my friends' parents. He raised six children and influenced the upbringing of ten grandchildren according to a set of tenets which, at the time, many would have considered quackery. For example, as children, we were given enemas not aspirin to reduce a fever. When it came time for the schools to get everyone "up-to-date" on vaccines, "mysteriously" we were exempt.

The chasm between my upbringing and that of my friends began to widen. Naturally, I became inquisitive.

My first memory of this was when at a friend's house his mother offered me a glass of conventional pasteurized milk. I politely refused the drink. She asked, "Why not? Don't you know milk builds strong bones and teeth?" This is when it all hit home for me. Almost reflexively, I replied, "No, thank you, pasteurized milk is poison." Understandably, this created quite a stir at my friend's dinner table, one where milk was a regular fixture. I remember trying to explain how milk creates mucus in the body, and how milk is loaded with hormones and cows are given antibiotics and an unnatural diet. I also remember going home feeling very different.

A Legacy of Healing

I was not ashamed, but I became aware in that instant, almost like a bolt of lightning, just how different I was from everyone else.

A second experience which remains with me happened in my freshman year at Rutgers College during a measles outbreak. I received notice from the registrar's office that my vaccination records were not "complete." I was told that in order to remain in my classes, I would have to come down to the medical office to be vaccinated. When I told them I had never been vaccinated before, and did not plan on doing so, I was told I would have to leave school. I was not given options, nor was I treated with any kindness or respect. It was as though I suddenly became a *persona non grata*.

As you might imagine, I immediately became frightened and apprehensive. How would I get my course work done? Would I lose my semester and have to start over? What would happen to me? I would like to say that the college administration was helpful in clarifying things for me, but the opposite was true. I was shunned, made to feel like an outcast, and spoken down to by almost everyone I called upon seeking answers. I remember calling my father, asking him what to do. Then, the phone call came that opened my eyes to how things really worked.

One of the deans of the school explained to me "off the record," that they could not force me to leave school and to stand my ground. She explained that she was familiar with chiropractic, believed in the profession, had personal experience of it, and was a supporter. She was able to calm me down and lessen my worry about my academic life. We discussed how I should proceed and what I needed to do (my family used a religious exemption in the state of New Jersey to avoid all vaccinations). She also told me that if questioned, she would deny our conversation. Her words still ring in my ears twenty years later. Should you wonder, I never left school. No one in police gear or medical masks came to take me away. I finished my freshman year on the Dean's list and graduated three years later as though nothing had ever happened. But something important had happened in my life, and I would never be the same.

Twenty years and three degrees later I am the beneficiary of my father's pioneering and fearless efforts to help the sick. He thought outside of the box, and used traditional wisdom and critical thinking to bring about healing. I inherited my father's practice in 2005. He left big shoes to fill. I was blessed to work side-by-side with him, first as a son and student and then as a physician myself. I have been able to personally observe how natural healing methods worked for my entire family as I grew up. I have also heard countless stories from patients who were once under my father's care, people who were told there was nothing that could be done for them, women told they would not be able to conceive, patients suffering from Crohn's disease or from migraine headaches who had been placed on one drug after another. After years of suffering they found their way to my father. He was successful because he believed in what he was doing. At the very heart of that belief was his spiritual faith in our body's God-given ability to heal, a belief in the design of our Creator, a belief in the body's innate intelligence. This is the foundation of holistic healing no matter the specific field —whether chiropractic, nutrition, or naturopathic medicine.

Traditional cultures around the world understood the connectedness between body, spirit, and the world around us. This included food, drink, relationships, and the immediate environment. Today's culture has forgotten this approach. We look for pills to fix our problems. If we can't sleep, we pop sleeping pills; if we have a headache we take an aspirin. When more and more children are born with autism, learning and developmental problems and allergies, we look to Big Pharma for answers instead of Mother Nature. We take little time to make breakfast or sit together as a family at the dinner table and share our lives with each other. We have lost touch with our roots and with our humanity, playing instead on our iPads, following trends on Facebook and watching TV.

For the past twelve years I have had the privilege of continuing my father's practice in Bogota, New Jersey. When I first began practicing in 2002, my father worked side-by-side with me on patient after patient, teaching me how to think through diagnoses and identify dysfunction, passing on to me the wisdom his patients sought. After a few years he began slowly to withdraw from the practice in order to work on preparing this book. Late in 2006, after nearly completing the initial draft, he became ill, and was forced to stop his writing. Sadly, a few months later on March 23, 2007, he passed away. Since then I have worked tirelessly to document the sources of my father's techniques, the basis for his beliefs and to give explanations of his ideas, as well as polishing the rough edges of the writing he left behind.

It is my hope, as it was my father's, that this book will continue his legacy of healing for those who are ailing and unable to find help. I hope I have done an adequate job of transcribing his writings in a cohesive and organized manner, and have accurately filled in the holes my father left when he died. I have also provided resources and references of other wonderful healers and pioneers of traditional wisdom whenever possible, many of whom my father held in great esteem and spoke of often. For readers who knew my father, much of this book will bring him back to life. It will bring to mind his characteristic passion and caring, his strong opinions regarding health and our responsibilities to ourselves and each other. He was magnanimous. Above all, he embodied selflessness to a fault. It was this that led him to neglect his own health. But now he lives through me and through the words in these pages, through the countless hearts he touched and the lives he helped heal.

I am confident you will find this book as helpful as my father hoped it would be, and that this book will light the path for those of you who have found your health in darkness. It is my hope that this book will touch as many hearts and lives as possible. In the words of Andy Dufresne from the movie "Shawshank Redemption," "Hope is a good thing, maybe the best of things. And no good thing ever dies." I hope. . . .

Sincerely,

Dr. Christopher J. Amoruso, D.C., M.S., C.N.S.

FROM DR. ANGELO ROSE

To my patients and friends,

I am writing this book to help make life a little easier when illness strikes, to make coping with simple health problems and more serious ones a bit easier. For many conditions there are proven, time-tested remedies. We use these natural methods of healing, not to avoid the medical profession, but to avoid hindering the natural healing processes of the body. The use of medications like aspirin or antibiotics can be harmful. Reaching for drugs first may prolong recuperation time, weaken the immune system and create more serious problems. This book will empower you to accept responsibility for your own health. It is wise to keep in mind that when the body becomes "dis"-eased, it is not always a virus or bacteria that is to blame. Physical problems and body changes can be and often are normal — a baby running a fever, a clear runny nose, can be nothing more than a child teething; a ten-year old running a fever for a day with no other symptoms can be a simple growth spurt. This book is to serve as a guide to use common sense and to take advantage of God-given natural health.

When drugs, including antibiotics, are used, the body relinquishes its ability to work and is forced to react to that specific drug or antibiotic. For example, when a child has a fever and is given an antibiotic, the child's temperature may drop initially, but as soon as the effects of the antibiotic wear off, the temperature returns. This is a common occurrence which no honest doctor can deny.

For each different illness covered in this book, I show you the way to help yourself with simple treatment. For more complex issues, I offer you a framework from which to start your journey back to better health. In these cases you will need to work with someone familiar with alternative treatments and chiropractic. I guide you step by step in handling these problems. My motive is to prevent you from complicating a simple problem, not to keep you from consulting with your medical doctor. I hope you enjoy this book and put it to good use.

In good health,
Dr. Angelo. C. Rose, D.C.

TABLE OF CONTENTS

Introduction by Dr. Angelo C. Rose 1

SECTION I
INTRODUCTION
    The Politics of Corruption, Whom Do We Trust? 5
    A History Lesson: The Error of Our Ways 6
    Today's Agriculture: Cheap Food/Poor Health 7

SECTION II
THE HOLISTIC DOCTOR/PATIENT EXPERIENCE
    Physical Examination/Holistic Patient Assessment.................. 11

SECTION III
THE IMPORTANCE OF PROPER DIGESTION
AND THE FOOD WE EAT
    Intestinal Lining: Barrier Between Health/Sickness................. 17
    Food Quality.. 18
    Food Quantity 22
    Proper Food Combining 23
    The Importance of pH Balance 26
    General Dietary Guidelines for a Healthy Life 29
    A Word About Supplements 43

SECTION IV
THE HEAD
    Headaches: Different Types and Treatments........................... 47
        Crown Headache (Top of the Head) 47
        Temporal Headache (Side of the Head) 48
        Frontal Headache (Forehead).. 49
        Occipital Headache (Back of the Head) 51
        "Behind the Eyes" Headache (Lower Forehead).................. 52
        General Headache... 54
    Sinus Infections/Sinusitis and Allergies 55
    Conditions of the Ear... 61
        Middle Ear Infections/Otitis Media 61
        Earache (Middle Ear)... 65
        Tinnitus 65

Conditions of the Eye 67
    Conjunctivitis (Pink Eye) 67
    Styes 68
    Floaters and Glaucoma 69
Common Conditions of Mouth, Tongue, Throat 71
    Bruxism (Grinding of the Teeth) 71
    Bleeding Gums 72
    Thrush/Candidiasis (Yeast Infection) 72
    Conditions Affecting the Tongue 75
    Glossitis/Burning/Painful Tongue (Glossodynia) 75
    Angular Stomatitis 77
    Fissured/Cracked Tongue 78
    Geographic Tongue 78
    Sore Throat/Swollen Tonsils 78

SECTION V
CONDITIONS OF THE CHEST AND LUNGS

    Basics of Treating Lung Disorders and Congestion 83
    Chest Congestion Due to Bronchitis/Cold/Flu 84
    Germ Theory and Treatment for Common Cold/Flu 88

SECTION VI
CONDITIONS OF POOR DIGESTION/INTESTINAL TRACT

    Indigestion/Gastro-Esophageal Reflux Disease (GERD) 93
    Halitosis (Bad Breath) 99
    Flatulence (Gas in the Intestinal Tract) 100
    Irritable Bowel Syndrome (IBS)/Inflammatory Bowel
    Disease 102
    Constipation/Diarrhea 108
    Gallbladder Disease/Gallstones 109

SECTION VII
COMMON CONDITIONS OF THE JOINTS AND CONNECTIVE TISSUE

    Carpal Tunnel Syndrome (CTS) 114
    Sprains and Strains of the Knee 115
    Knee Pain and Other Knee Injuries 116
    Sprained Ankle Treatment 119
    Plantar Fasciitis 119
    Bursitis 122
    Lyme Disease 125
    Joint Pain in Young Children 132
    Joint Pain in Older Children 134
    Arthritis in the Adult 136
    Juvenile Arthritis 140
    Menopausal Arthritis 141

SECTION VIII
BACK/NECK PAIN/DEGENERATIVE DISC DISEASE/OSTEOPOROSIS

- Cervical Disc Syndrome 144
- Degenerative Disc Disease, Back Pain/Sciatica 150
- Osteoporosis/Arthritis and Calcium 156

SECTION IX
CONDITIONS OF THE MALE AND FEMALE REPRODUCTIVE TRACT

- Erectile Dysfunction (ED) 165
- Conditions of the Prostate 170
- Ovarian Cysts and Menopausal Symptoms 179
- Sexual and Reproductive Dysfunction 184
  - Painful Intercourse (Dyspareunia) 184
  - Menopausal Bleeding 187
  - Fibroids 189
  - Ovarian Cysts 191
  - Birth Control Pill 192
  - Feminine Hygiene 194

SECTION X
CONDITIONS OF THE URINARY TRACT

- Bladder and Urinary Tract Infections 195

SECTION XI
DISEASES OF THE CIRCULATORY SYSTEM

- Should Cholesterol Be Our Main Focus? 198
- Saturated Fat and Cholesterol – Real Facts about Fats 203
- Nutrition and Cardiovascular Disease 210
- Hypoglycemia 213
- Diabetes and Cardiovascular Diseases (CVD) 215
- Juvenile Diabetes 229
- Congestive Heart Failure 232
- Twelve Commandments for a Healthy Heart 237

SECTION XII
NEUROLOGIAL DISORDERS

- Multiple Sclerosis (MS) 238

SECTION XIII
DERMATOLOGICAL PROBLEMS

- Dryness and Cracking of Skin on Hands and Feet 241
- Fungus of Fingernails/Toenails 242
- Eczema 243
- Urticaria/Hives 245
- Skin Cancer/Sun Tanning 246
- Psoriasis 247
- Acne 250
- Boils 252

SECTION XIV
WOUND HEALING

- Cuts, Scrapes, Open Wounds, Bed Sores 253
- Burns 255
- Bruising 256

SECTION XV
PREGNANCY AND INFANT CARE

- Pregnancy and Prenatal Nutrition 258
  - Morning Sickness 262
  - Prenatal Nutrition 262
- Infant Care/Raising a Healthy Child 270
- Fevers in the Infant and Young Child 280
  - Fever Caused By Teething 281
- To Vaccinate or Not to Vaccinate? 283
- Dealing with Picky Eaters 288

SECTION XVI
ATTENTION DEFICIT HYPERACTIVITY DISORDER (ADHD) OPPOSITIONAL DEFIANT DISORDER (ODD)

- Attention Deficit Disorder ADD/ Attention Deficit Hyperactivity Disorder ADHD/ Oppositional Defiant Disorder ODD 291
- The 4 Rs Cleansing Protocol (Dysbiosis) 298
  - Treatment Using the 4 Rs Program for Intestinal Health .. 299

SECTION XVII
HOLISTIC TREATMENT OF CANCER

- Natural Treatment of Cancer 309
- Timeline of Suppression of Alternative Cancer Cures 313

SECTION XVIII
APPENDIX
    A. Important Protocols for Natural Healing 320
    B. Important Patient Self-Tests 338
    C. Recipes and Miscellaneous Information 344
    D. Important Resources 355
    E. Recommended Reading 359
    F. Appliances 362
    G. Charts and Illustrations 363
    H. Acronyms 369

Index 371

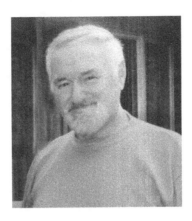

INTRODUCTION by Dr. Angelo C. Rose

The Beginnings: chiropractic and what it has meant for me, my family, and for the countless patients I have treated over the past 50 years.

Chiropractic has been a gift from God allowing me to give to others a wonderful, natural way of healing without the use of drugs and, more importantly, without causing more harm to the body. Natural healing comes only from within and it is my feeling that this is God's will. Only God can truly cure the body of any disease. Man can only assist this process by serving in the delivery of the natural course of healing.

But that's not where this story begins. To understand what chiropractic has meant for me, we have to go back to 1952. I was a freshman at William & Mary College on a scholarship for football. During one of the first games of the year, a scrimmage against Princeton, I was kicked in the face during a play where I was attempting to block a punt. In 1952 football players did not have the safer helmets we are all familiar with today. We had nothing more than a leather "helmet" with a chin strap. There was no facemask. What happened in the hours following my flying through the air to block that punt is mostly a blur. I can tell you, however, that by the time the play was over, I was blind. That's right, I couldn't see. I was taken to a doctor immediately, but there wasn't much they could do for me at that time. It wasn't long before I lost my scholarship to play football and was sent home with an uncertain future.

I spent the next 8 months or so learning Braille and being, as you might imagine, a little depressed. Then, one day, my mother came to me and said, "C'mon Angelo, we are going to the doctor." I was resistant because I had already succumbed to the idea that I would spend the rest of my life blind. But I was wrong. My mother took me to the office of a friend of my brother-in-law, a chiropractor in Jersey City, New Jersey not far from where we lived. All I really remember that day was that he laid me down on the table, looked at my x-rays, and performed an adjustment on my neck that I found very painful. I later came to learn that it was so painful because, as a result of my football injury, my skull had been moved completely out of its normal position with the very first bone of the spine (known as the Atlas or C1 vertebra). Apparently this was pinching the spinal cord where it exits the brain and creating a stasis of the cerebrospinal fluid in that region.

After the adjustment, I swore I would never go back to that doctor again. I was bitter, upset, and figured I was just wasting my time. But my mother didn't like that idea. She forced me to go back and allow this man a chance to help me. I'll spare you the unnecessary facts and just say that after a few treatments I began to see a hazy light when my eyes were open. I liken it to looking into the sun on a bright sunny day — you can't really see things clearly and defined, but you can see the light and its glare. It sounds hard to believe. Sometimes I have to pinch myself too. God had given me a second chance. He had shown me that the body can heal, it just needs to be given a fair chance. Needless to say, this ignited my interest in chiropractic which, at the time, was considered to be on an equal footing with witchcraft. I enrolled in the Chiropractic Institute in New York shortly thereafter.

When I graduated from chiropractic college, I took an oath to help as many people as I could in the most natural way possible. The philosophy of chiropractic is based on the body's own innate intelligence. This intelligence is based solely on natural processes and is ultimately derived from God. The simplest example I can give is this: if you cut your finger, over time the body heals, eventually forming a scar. How does the body know where the cut begins and ends? How does the body know when the finger is fully healed?

The answer is very simple, innate intelligence. This is accomplished without the use of drugs, medication, or surgery.

When my wife Felicia and I had the first of our six children, we decided to raise them naturally. Our first child was born in 1957, a baby boy we named Thomas. We had a natural delivery and my wife breast fed him for one year. Then he was taken off of the breast milk and we used fresh goat's milk and a natural diet consisting of organic fresh fruits, pastured meats and vegetables. We never needed a pediatrician because he was healthy and I would always check his spine. When he needed an adjustment, I gave him one. My wife and I went on to have a total of six children, four boys and two girls. Not one of our children was vaccinated or brought to a medical doctor for any treatment.

Chiropractic adjustments and a good, wholesome natural diet rich in fresh, organic fruits and vegetables were the foundation of their healthcare and the plan that my wife and I followed with our children throughout their lives. If we could not find organic fruits and vegetables, we would always wash them in either apple cider vinegar, Clorox bleach, or 35% food grade hydrogen peroxide (see Appendix C p. 351). This was done to oxygenate the food as well as to remove all chemicals and pesticides. Furthermore we made sure to keep the children away from all synthetic chemicals and unnatural foods.

When one of our children became ill for any reason, we treated the situation holistically. In other words, we allowed the body to heal itself, facilitating this healing by using a little common sense along with the natural remedies, procedures, and guidelines found throughout this book. Anyone can apply these principles to achieve better health and avoid the pitfalls of modern medication and surgery.

The proper approach to any condition starts with a thorough patient history. Diet must be questioned and reviewed; salivary pH must be checked; all medications and their side effects reviewed and documented. Food allergies must be considered, and when appropriate, tested for. All of this should be followed by a thorough physical examination of the abdomen, documenting where along the gastrointestinal tract the most sensitivity and inflammation exist.

Depending on the history and physical examination findings, some testing may of course be necessary. The first step in getting a patient back on the track toward health, however, is to identify their dietary shortcomings and to TEACH. In fact, the word doctor comes from the Latin "docere" meaning "to teach." Why this is almost NEVER mentioned or remembered is disturbing to me. So you must first sit down with a qualified professional (a knowledgeable chiropractor, medical doctor, naturopathic doctor, nutritionist, or dietician) who can go over your diet with you. You do not want someone who is going to teach you the dogma of the politically correct nutritionists and lobbyists. I recommend you contact the Weston A. Price Foundation at www.westonaprice.org for more information and try to work with a physician who is familiar with the foundation and their principles. Their website will help guide you.

Since every person is unique and their nutritional needs vary, it is impossible for me to give a diet that would be completely suitable for everyone/condition. Perhaps this is what is really wrong in medicine. Too often doctors (chiropractors and medical doctors) try to shoebox everyone with similar symptoms into the same treatment plan. This never works, and in fact, almost always produces bad results. People are unique with unique habits, experiences, stresses and lifestyles. They are not robots. Therefore I will discuss the main points you should know, and the rest is up to you and your physician.

SECTION I
INTRODUCTION

The Politics of Corruption, Whom Do We Trust?

Today the pharmaceutical and biotechnological industries have unprecedented power over the medical establishment and its principles of practice. Sadly, they also have a stranglehold on government. Their power also pervades the scholastic system, even esteemed universities like Harvard. Let me correct that, *especially* revered universities like Harvard. Take a walk on the Harvard campus and look at the names on some of the buildings. Donations come with a price, and the price is cooperation with the donor's agenda. The agenda of donor companies is to make money. This trickles down to the curriculum, what is taught, what products are endorsed and who are placed in positions of power. If you are skeptical, ponder this. On March 2, 2009 *The New York Times* published an article titled "Harvard Medical School in Ethics Quandry" by Duff Wilson, about a growing number of students concerned about the revolving door and conflicts of interest between Big Pharma and Harvard professors. The following is a summary of that article.

A Harvard Medical School student named Matt Zerden became concerned about the possible conflict of interest present between one of his professors and the pharmaceutical industry. Zerden's concern began when the professor, while lauding the benefits associated with cholesterol drugs, refused to address their dangerous side effects. Students who questioned this issue seemed to be belittled or treated with disdain. Zerden, doing his own diligent research, discovered that this professor was not only a full-time member of the Harvard Medical faculty, but was simultaneously being paid as a consultant to 10 drug companies, half of whom were makers of these very cholesterol drugs.

The information brought to light by Zerden's research began to grow into a movement at Harvard to push back against this corporate, higher education, conflict of interest. Soon, over 200 Harvard Medical School students and faculty had formed a coalition to expose and confront the influence of the pharmaceutical industry in the classroom and in research laboratories. The coalition's main concern was that money used to build Harvard's Medical School into a world-renowned facility was affecting its curriculum.

The article goes on to say that students expressed concern at the F grade received by Harvard from the American Medical Student Association, a national group that rates medical schools on how well they monitor and control monies received from industry and special interests.

Information on this kind of collusion should not surprise us. We need not look only at Harvard to realize that the corrupt tentacles of the pharmaceutical industry run deep in our society. An internet search of Cabinet members appointed by recent presidents reveals a revolving door in which high-ranking members of our governing institutions have held positions of authority on the boards of top pharmaceutical companies and vice versa. The influence of money and power in the field of medical education should give us reason to pause and to question the consequences of this conflict of interest for public health.

Books have been written on this topic. The information is there if one is willing to search for it.

A History Lesson: The Error of Our Ways

My point in the last segment was to expose a dangerous collusion. Information is only as good as its source. If the source is corrupt, then the information is of little or no value. We have to take responsibility for our health and for the direction we follow. We have to be critical thinkers, demand the right to obtain alternative care. Most importantly, we have to ask ourselves, "Are we really better off this way?" Our children are our future. If we don't have healthy children, the future is bleak.

Did you ever ask yourself why most insurance plans do not cover visits to alternative doctors for nutritional consultation and alternative therapies? Educating patients on healthy eating habits would cure many ills. Take gastroesophageal reflux disease, or GERD for example. With a willing patient and simple patient nutritional education on proper food combinations and supplementation, this problem can be cured. No need for costly endoscopies, CT scans or medical procedures including surgery on the stomach. Even the supplements needed, in most cases just two, are temporary.

A close look at those around us, family, friends, acquaintances, quickly shows the presence of many diseases and ailments. Both young and old as well as those in between are beset by poor health. Much of this is of our own doing. Supermarket shelves are laden with food products laced with harmful ingredients that prolong product life and shorten ours. The refining and processing of natural foods has created its own problems. The introduction of refined sugars and flours, canned goods, vegetable fats and polished rice have had a devastating effect on human health. Television advertising then entices us to take one drug after another in spite of harmful side effects.

Where did this deterioration of health begin? Weston A. Price, dentist and founder of the research section of the American Dental Association (ADA), answers this when he says, "Life in all of its fullness, is mother nature obeyed." We have become complicit in her destruction.

Today's Agriculture: Cheap Food – Poor Health

Although this topic is vast, I urge the reader to keep an open mind. It is not hard to understand that our fruits and vegetables are only as good as the soil from which they come. Where do soil nutrients come from? The produce we eat comes from the ground we cultivate. The healthier that ground, the healthier the plants which spring from it. There are many very informative books on this subject. One such book is *Soil, Grass and Cancer* by André Voisin. Although largely ignored by the mainstream agricultural community, the pioneering soil studies of André Voisin bring to light the complex relationship between soil quality, food composition and human health. Both a biochemist and a farmer, Voisin found, in his many years working his own farms, that "when the soil and grasses were cared for properly, the animals living upon that land would enjoy abundant health. And as a result, the people consuming these animals and their products would enjoy abundant health as well."

Author Joel Salatin in *Folks, This Ain't Normal* states that, "as our country grew at the turn of the 20th century, soil depletion, widening deserts, and burgeoning populations meant answers to soil fertility needed to be found, and fast." On p. 125 of his book, Salatin does an excellent job of summarizing the genesis of how we as a country lapsed from proper care of the soil and fled for greener pastures (pun intended):

> See, dear folks, those of us on the environmental side, the biological side, of agriculture are prone to point fingers at our grandparents and other ancestors and decry them as horrible people for spreading those bags of NPK (nitrogen, phosphorus and potassium) rather than making compost. But faced with the decision, most of us would have done the same thing. The truth is that when the starting gun went off in 1946 in a race to feed the world, in what would eventually become the chemical-based Green Revolution, the artificial chemical side had a two-lap head start. . . . By the 1920's and 1930s, people couldn't rid themselves of the manure fork fast enough . . . they were doing what they thought would be easier and better. But it wasn't normal in the great ecological balance sheet. (Ibid p. 128–129)

What Salatin is essentially pointing out is this: when we opted to move to chemical fertilizers and industrialization/mechanization of farming in order to feed an overpopulated earth, and feed it cheaply, we had to sacrifice something. And what we sacrificed was the soil quality, and therefore, the nutritional quality of what came from that soil. As a result, a decline in the health of the animals and humans that feed off of that soil was destined to follow. He adds, "If we step back and let nature teach us, we will learn all we need to know. The more we try to trick, shortcut, or adulterate these processes, the less productive and efficient nature will be."(Ibid p.135) This includes producing poorer quality, nutrient deficient food. Salatin states:

> After all, soil is fundamentally a living organism. It's a biological world down there under our feet. Yes you can fool things for a while, but eventually the balance sheet will bleed red. And the soil microbes, the actinomycetes (bacterial decomposers that give the soil an earthy odor), the azotobacter (microbes that grab atmospheric nitrogen and put it in the soil to feed plants), the mycorrhiza (fungi that build plant immunity), the earthworms will scream for — even demand — proper nutrition. (Ibid p. 130)

Our soil is our most precious commodity. Without healthy, organic soil, our food supply will quickly erode to nothing more than a cache of empty calories, devoid of trace minerals, vitamins and other nutrients known and unknown that our bodies depend on to be healthy. We would all do well to remember the Dust Bowl.

Essentially, not all apples are created equal. Or corn. Or cattle. The richer and healthier the soil, the richer and healthier the life which springs from it. Cheap food is really more expensive! The degenerative diseases and conditions that have become rampant are mortgaging our future, and the future of our children. The cheap food destroying the health of many is actually more expensive in the long run. Consider the long-term health care costs that lie in wait. It is also destroying one of America's greatest natural resources: her soil. To get our priorities straight, we need to think about the way we live.

In his book *Health at Gunpoint*, author James J. Gormley notes that "Agriculture has become a highly commercialized and politics-driven industry in which only a few have power and influence over everyone else." He goes on to point out that "in 2010 alone, the government spent $96.3 billion on subsidies and programs, most of which benefited the wealthiest large farms. When it comes to farming subsidies, health is frequently too expensive to take into account. Gormley goes on to point out that "the widespread availability of advanced farm equipment has allowed for improved productivity and efficiency while mechanization in combination with subsidies has resulted in over-farming, a problem that he feels has 'snowballed' out of control."(p. 45) The infamous Dust Bowl of the 1930's was caused by this same mentality of faster, cheaper production. As a result of the need for greater food supplies during World War I, farmers began to look for ways to till more land faster in order to keep up with demand. Fortunately for them, and unfortunately for the soil, this occurred at a point when the industrial revolution was providing advancements in machinery and equipment that allowed that very thing to happen. Damaged soil as a result of the over-farming combined with drought conditions led to the soil literally blowing away, turning some of our nation's most fertile lands into arid ones, and prompting Franklin D. Roosevelt to famously remark, "A nation that destroys its soil destroys itself."

In her book *Stolen Harvest*, Vandana Shiva notes that there is an intimate relationship between agriculture, animals and humans. And this relationship is reciprocal. You cannot affect one without affecting the other. Gormley adds that it is "this natural ecological chain that has been disrupted by soil erosion, which has become a problem in many areas of the United States. Not only is soil lost, but everything the soil contains, including earthworms, microorganisms, minerals, fungi, and organic materials that all work together to provide plants with necessary nutrients and environment. These microorganisms and nutrients strengthen plants and boost their natural resistance to disease and pests. They also provide other living creatures with the essential vitamins and minerals they need to stay healthy." (Gormley, p. 47) We are one of those creatures.

In conclusion, we must as a people, as human beings all inhabiting the same planet, come to terms with how we have treated the soil, and how we move forward. There are solutions. People like Allan Savory, Wendell Berry, Joel Salatin and others have already proven these solutions can work. But we must return to our roots, to our connection with Mother Nature.

SECTION II
THE HOLISTIC DOCTOR/PATIENT EXPERIENCE

Physical Examination/Holistic Patient Assessment

Great disparity exists in the experience of a patient visiting an allopathic physician for his/her condition versus that of visiting a holistic physician, because philosophically holistic care is not a symptom-based approach. On the contrary, holistic care is based on treating each person as unique. It's about restoring and creating balance.

In our office we use a reproducible framework that consists of five distinct examination areas for which we thoroughly assess our patients. Those five areas are: Pre-examination Surveys, Patient History-Lifestyle/Diet Assessment, Physical/Spinal/Structural Examination, Mental/Emotional/Spiritual-Stress Assessment and lastly Review of Findings. Every health problem is approached from this framework to find the areas of weakness in each category that have led to the loss of health. For example, some patients present with a very healthy diet, but overwhelming stress at work, a sedentary lifestyle, smoking, and lack of proper rest as the causative factors in their health problems. They may also have a history of structural problems like poor posture, *pes planus* (flat feet) and a history of motor vehicle accidents that have created imbalances. Whatever the area(s) of weakness, they must be addressed individually to restore the homeostasis and health of the whole person. This is not the traditional symptom-based approach of western medicine, where symptoms are treated with either drugs, surgery or chemotherapy/radiation. Holistic care must focus on the whole person. Symptoms are just one clue we use to trace the illness back to the cause of the dysfunction. To solve the individual's health problems, we must first get to know the person.

Before ever speaking to the patient, we begin by having them fill out a Systems Survey Form and a Toxicity Questionnaire designed by the nutritional stalwart Standard Process. The System Survey has 224 commonly found symptoms arranged into 9 groups, such as symptoms related to digestion or the liver and gallbladder.

These are not the only surveys available which offer insight into the origins of a patient's health concerns, but they are the ones I have chosen to use over the years and with which I have had great success. Assessing the surveys allows us to gain insight into the patient's nutritional needs and to pre-screen them for problems before we even speak to them. The Toxicity Questionnaire is designed to aid the practitioner in assessing a patient's potential need for a more detailed clinical purification program. Once these questionnaires have been filled out by the patient, they can be scored and interpreted by the clinician to give insight into which organ systems may be involved in the patient's dysfunction and to help build a foundation for beginning supplementation. A wise man once told me,"If you ask the patient the right questions, 90% of the time they will tell you what is wrong with them."

The Patient History-Lifestyle/Diet evaluation is made up of a thorough history of their current problem(s), their past history of illnesses, what they eat and drink, or do not eat and drink, what prescription medications they take, and whether or not they smoke, exercise, sit all day at work, and so on. For many of our patients, their health concern(s) and chief complaint(s) are often due to daily behavioral practices. Therefore, special attention is paid to a patient's diet and lifestyle habits. To do this more thoroughly, a patient may be asked to fill out a week-long food diary *before their first scheduled appointment*. Much helpful information can be gleaned this way. Much information is also brought to light in the history part of the examination where we get to speak one-on-one with the patient to find out their habits. Are they active and exercising? Do they skip breakfast or eat on the go often? Are they taking prescription medication(s) *that may be causing some of the symptoms for which they are seeking help*? Unfortunately this is far too common today as most Americans take prescription medications for one problem, only to end up with other problems as a result of their first medication.

The third evaluation area, the Physical/Structural/Spinal assessment, is central to the chiropractic profession. The first phase of this evaluation starts from the ground up, literally. We begin by performing a postural assessment of the patient beginning with the feet. Here we look for any foundational asymmetry in the arches of the feet. This will often show in the wearing pattern on the bottom of the patient's shoes, so we look there first. Since a detailed discussion of the biomechanics of the foot during gait cycle is beyond the scope of this book, I will focus on the main aspects of our concern. For more specific information on the phases of gait and the physics and biomechanics involved, consult Chapter 14 of *Joint Structure and Function*, by Cynthia C. Norkin and Pamela K. Levangie.

Typical signs of uneven wear will show on the heel especially, and can usually be easily recognized. It is also helpful to assess the Achilles tendon of both feet, noting whether the tendon is bowing laterally (outward, or also called Valgus), straight, or bowing medially (inward, or Varus). Examining the foot visually and making simple observations as to the structural alignment of the foot-ankle-knee complex gives information as to what will be occurring at the pelvic and spinal levels.

The most common structural foot deformity we see is called pes planus, or more simply flat feet. This can also be referred to by doctors as pronated. Some signs of this problem are callouses at the 2nd, 3rd and 4th metatarsal heads, a subluxated navicular bone, and valgus knees. A pronated foot will cause an internal rotation of the tibia and knee as well as a dropping of the pelvis on that side with a concomitant curvature of the spine with its apex on the contralateral (opposite) side. Essentially, one side of the lumbar vertebrae will become compressed while the other side is overstretched. Rotation of the lumbar vertebra will often occur as a result and this can lead to chronic back pain, weakness and recurring injury. This has far reaching implications for patients with degenerated discs and chronic low back pain. I explain to every patient with this condition that it is impossible to retain a chiropractic adjustment if your foundation (feet) are not balanced properly. As soon as a patient gets off the table and walks away, everything done to correct the spinal subluxations will begin to move back to the original malposition. Therefore it is crucial that every examination, especially in cases where the patient has chronic musculoskeletal complaints, begins with an examination of the feet. Everyone from children to the elderly and especially athletes will benefit from a balanced foundation beginning at the feet.

A Legacy of Healing

One word of caution regarding orthotics warrants mentioning here. Over the years I have seen many patients present to my office already wearing varying types of orthotics. Most of the orthotics coming from podiatrists are of the hard plastic type, and are simply a rigid "hump." In my experience these are the worst type of orthotic. The foot is a dynamic structure, with moving parts that expand and contract with the different movements of normal gait. They are not cement blocks meant to be held in a rigid position. Hard orthotics of this type not only prevent the foot from moving through its normal range of motion through the gait cycle, they also serve to transmit greater forces from the ground impact up through the leg to the pelvis and spine. Over time, this leads to greater wear and tear on the joints of the lower limbs as well as the pelvis and spine and is often detrimental to the patient. Orthotics should be supportive of the body's weight, yet flexible to allow normal movement of the different joints of the foot and ankle complex. They *should not be hyperflexible* like the popular Dr. Scholl's brand, for example. These do little more than provide cushioning as they are too flexible and collapse under the weight of the foot.

A second consideration is that most orthotics are cast while the patient is not weight-bearing. A patient's arch structure and movement will depend on ligament laxity, their weight, and prior injuries they have incurred. To get an accurate picture as to the extent of the arch collapse and asymmetry from right foot to left foot, the scan of the foot must be done in a weight-bearing position, which allows the clinician to measure the extent of the collapsed arches. This is why the V7 3-D Scanner by Foot Levelers is an ideal tool for the job.

After examining the feet visually we usually scan the patient's feet using the V7 3-D scanner. The scanner takes a three dimensional digital scan of the feet and assigns the patient a numerical pronation index. The index ranges from normal (0–34), mild (35–84), moderate (85–124) and severe (125 and above). This index represents the degree or severity of pronation of the feet and correlates with the need for orthotic support. Depending on the severity of foot pronation, we will often have Foot Levelers custom make orthotics for the patient. Orthotics made from the scan of the patient's feet serve to properly align the feet, knees, pelvis in the same manner that the foundation of a house supports the structures and rooms above. These supports can easily be worn in sneakers, most shoes and even in up to two inch high-heels. The more often they are worn by the patient, the more their feet and everything above are maintained in a balanced and aligned position. The Foot Levelers orthotics are one of the most efficient and effective tools I have used to ameliorate or even completely resolve low back pain, ankle pain/weakness, knee problems and more. I have worn the orthotics myself for over 25 years and have personally experienced their benefit.

Of significance here is the importance of the foundational support of the feet for young children. As mentioned, pedial foundation problems can lead to an imbalanced pelvis and spine. Scoliosis, or curvature of the spine in young children is a common consequence of this foundational problem. When children are screened for scoliosis, nurses and doctors almost never consider the feet as a factor. By evaluating the feet as the first phase of the physical exam, the doctor can glean valuable information that will help balance the pelvis and spine and prevent the future development of chronic musculoskeletal problems.

After evaluating the feet and the standing posture, we move to the examination of the spine. We identify subluxations, or more simply, malpositions of the vertebrae which result in an intereference with the communication between the spine and the brain, and from the spine outward to the organs and muscles. Since each vertebra has specific connections to specific organs and muscles, each subluxation lends clues to areas of the body which may not be functioning optimally (See diagram on p. 364 taken from *Backtalk Systems*) For example, a subluxation of the 6th thoracic vertebra tells us there is likely to be a stomach problem presenting in that patient. A problem involving the thyroid gland is likely to present with subluxations in the cervical and upper thoracic spine because the principal innervation of the thyroid gland is derived from the superior, middle, and inferior cervical sympathetic ganglia of the autonomic nervous system and parasympathetic fibers from the vagus nerves located in these areas. Therefore, the spine serves as a richly informative diagnostic tool when trying to identify areas of dysfunction as well as serving to help confirm a diagnosis.

After completing the examination of the spine, a thorough examination of the abdomen is completed, including palpation, visual inspection (for bloat or distension and ascites) and auscultation (listening to the lungs with a stethoscope). Areas of tenderness are noted and correlated with our history and other findings. For example, sensitivity and distension above the navel, just left of midline, in the area of the stomach, is highly suspicious for gastritis or GERD. If, in the history, our patient informed us that he/she has reflux or other gastric symptoms, then we begin to focus on the stomach as a possible culprit. We can correlate this with postural findings as well as spinal subluxation levels to rule out other differential diagnoses.

Neurological examination including Cranial Nerve Testing, deep tendon reflexes, and others are then performed to assess the status of the nervous system and higher cortical pathways.

Toward the end of the initial consultation, a decision is made as to the necessity of laboratory testing, including blood work, stool testing, nutritional/metabolic testing, etc. These tests, when applied judiciously and appropriately, can be invaluable in saving time and money as well as helping to choose the most efficacious treatment plan.

Once this examination is completed, a meeting with the patient to discuss the Review of Findings begins. In my experience, the Review of Findings is perhaps where the greatest divergence from western medicine exists. The overwhelming majority of my patients remark that very little was explained to them during their visit to conventional, allopathic doctors. They also comment that very little time was spent with them. Perhaps this has become an all-too-familiar pattern in western medicine. I am not saying that all doctors do this, or that it is only allopathic doctors who neglect a discussion of findings with their patients. I am stating what my patients tell me. I often ask whether their x-rays were explained to them or if they were given an explanation of what the diagnosis means. Unfortunately, the answer to these questions is often "no."

The word doctor has its roots in the Latin word for "teacher." The Review of Findings, in my opinion, is the most critical part of the interaction between doctor and patient. Here we lay out the explanation of the problem to the patient and our plan of attack for how to correct it. *This has to be clear and make sense to the patient or, in my opinion, we have failed them.* It is here that the doctor–patient relationship is forged, where confidence is established and trust is earned. When patients leave the office, their confidence and likelihood for success are intimately entwined in their understanding of the issues at hand and our plan for how to remediate the problem. It is our responsibility as physicians to uphold this standard. The rest is up to the patient. If they are willing to do the work, to learn and grow, and to walk hand-in-hand with us on this journey to wellness, there is no limit to what can be achieved.

SECTION III
THE IMPORTANCE OF PROPER DIGESTION AND THE FOOD WE EAT

Intestinal Lining: Barrier Between Health/Sickness

The human digestive system is so important that it has been called by some "the second brain." There is a wonderful book written by Michael D. Gershon, MD with this same title: *The Second Brain: Your Gut Has a Mind of Its Own*. Dr. Gershon discusses the enteric nervous system and how it functions, to a large degree, separate from our brain. Dr. Gershon notes that the majority of the body's serotonin is made not in our brains, but in our gut. This has tremendous ramifications for our health, including our mental functioning and well-being. My point is that we must first look to our gut when looking to address health and wellness in any other part of the body. Without proper digestive function, we cannot provide the body with the raw materials it needs to function efficiently. A large part of our body's health and well-being is predicated upon access to proper nutrition and complete and efficient digestion of whole foods. It is a mistake to assume that our modern day fast food/processed diet is sufficient to provide what we need for health.

This discussion is the most important part of this book because it provides the foundational concepts of the roots of diseases and other conditions. We as a society have lost touch with our bodies, and with that inner voice with which we should be in constant communication. We have also lost touch with where our food comes from, what is done to it, and what this means for our health.

We need to know what is in our food and what has been done to it, and to make healthy choices, thereby building a strong and healthy digestive system. This will help keep us free from the diseases of modern society, diseases that Weston Price found absent in traditional cultures not yet victims of a modern diet.

The main requirements for proper digestion and where most people go astray are explored below.

Food Quality

This is a very broad topic and only a few guides and encouragements can be given in the space of this segment. Your food is only as good as the soil it grows in. Plants receive all their nutrients from the soil. If that soil is deficient in iodine, you too will become deficient in iodine regardless of how much of that food you eat. Homeostatic soil organisms (HSO) are also crucial to the balance of the soil and health of the plant. Soil that is organically maintained, fertilized and cared for will produce food with a superior nutrient profile. This involves crop rotation, allowing the soil to rest, and proper animal husbandry. To learn more about growing food naturally and the superiority of organic farming, I recommend books by Joel Salatin, a farmer, author, scholar and activist dedicated to organic, sustainable farming and its benefits. Another source of information is the Weston A. Price Foundation. Visit their website at www.westonaprice.org. On the related topic of desertification, the research and work of Allan Savory is helpful. Type his name into the YouTube search window or type in desertification to watch his lectures to learn more.

If your food comes in a plastic package or a cardboard box, chances are it is dead food lacking the enzymes so vital to life. The first consideration to make when you think of the quality of your food is: Where did my food come from? What is it? Is it a fruit or vegetable or is it something that was processed, refined, sprayed, hybridized, radiated, genetically modified, degummed, chemically treated and put in a plastic bag or cardboard box? This may sound easy at first, but it can get confusing because of slick advertising and marketing. It can also be confusing because companies misleadingly use words like "All Natural" or "Organic" which seem, in and of themselves, to imply superiority. Do not be misled. Your first concern is to ask yourself this question, "Is the food I am eating in the form in which it would be found in nature?" A simple example is a stalk of broccoli, or a carrot. Those are whole foods. "Whole grain, American Heart Association approved, cholesterol-lowering" Cheerios are not. They are a recipe for diabetes, glorified junk food. Real cereal is an unprocessed grain (hence a seed) that must first be properly soaked and then cooked. The difference is one has been processed and refined, stripped of its nutrients, enzymes, and other nutritional components, known and unknown, marketed, commercialized and sold in a cardboard box stamped with a government badge. The end product is a dead psuedo-food enriched with synthetic vitamins. This is no comparison to what nature had originally supplied. It is dead food. No enzymes, no life. It won't even go bad, and if it does, it may take months or even years. It stays in your cupboard for weeks in its cardboard box ready to be eaten. No cooking, no inconvenience. Just add milk, ultrapasteurized and homogenized. But real cereal is a whole grain. Whether it is wheat, oat, or rice-based, the concept is the same. When you separate and remove the germ and the bran, and mill the product and package it, you no longer have a living, nourishing food. As Sally Fallon notes, ". . . refined carbohydrates are inimical to life because they are devoid of bodybuilding elements. Digestion of refined carbohydrates calls on the body's own store of vitamins, minerals and enzymes for proper metabolization" (Fallon S. Nourishing Traditions. Washington DC: NewTrends Publishing; 2001. 21).

Milk is another example of a good food altered by processing. As we find it in the stores, milk is not as beneficial as the advertising proclaims. Many people are allergic to milk, not because of the milk, but because of how it is processed and how the animals that produce it are cared for. Milk is pasteurized (and increasingly *ultrapasteurized* to even higher temperatures) and then homogenized. The heating and homogenization process create irreversible damage to enzymes, fats, proteins and vitamins that otherwise make raw milk a tremendously health-giving food (Schmid R. The untold story of milk, green pastures, contented cows and raw dairy foods. Washington DC: NewTrends Publishing, Inc. 2003. p. 261). Then there is the issue of how the cows were fed and treated. Were they restricted in a tight pen and forced to eat corn and soy instead of the grasses that nature intended? And was the animal given recombinant bovine somatotropin hormone to force it to produce more milk?

It comes down to simple chemistry. Also, it's not the *raw* milk that's dangerous. It's whether or not the animal is cared for properly and whether the milk itself is handled in a clean, hygienic manner. Raw milk is no more dangerous than any other food when it is handled or grown properly. When you investigate, you begin to realize that we have sacrificed our health in the name of profit, shelf-life and convenience. Milk is no exception. Pasteurization and homogenization of milk increase shelf life, improve the look (homogenization simply makes the milk uniform in color and consistency so that the cream will not rise to the top) and protect profits.

In 2006 when we had the contaminated spinach scare, it turned out that the spinach was probably contaminated with E. coli from *contaminated ground water the source of which was industrial cattle farming*. Manure lagoons used in industrial cattle farming contaminated the ground water and hence the spinach. Does that mean we should pasteurize, radiate, microwave, or use other technological processes to sterilize our food supply at the expense of all the nutrients that will be destroyed? Or are we missing the greater overall theme here? Weston A. Price was quoted as saying, "Life in all its fullness is Mother Nature obeyed." We need to take a second look at the industrial farming procedures we are using. Michael Pollan presents this case quite eloquently in his bestselling book *Omnivore's Dilemma*. Industrial farming procedures are not only affecting our health and contaminating our food, they are destroying the environment.

The topic of food quality isn't simple. We still have to consider whether our food was sprayed with herbicides, pesticides, and other chemicals; was the animal from which this product is derived given hormones, antibiotics, GMO feed from corn and soy? In light of these problems, buying organic seems wise.

Another tool helpful in educating people comes from Walter Crinnion's book *Clean, Green and Lean*. He shares with the reader the list of the dirty dozen regarding the most heavily sprayed fruits and vegetables that cannot be cleaned. For the most part, these fruits and vegetables should always be purchased organic.

Strawberries, peaches, apples, celery, sweet bell peppers, cherry tomatoes, spinach, cherries, imported grapes, tomatoes, cucumbers and nectarines

Visit www.ewg.org for the complete list and much more.

This list represents the fruits and vegetables we should always buy organic, because many of them cannot be sufficiently cleaned to remove the toxic pesticides and chemical residues. Crinnion also includes a list of the top 20 highest mercury-containing fish. This is helpful information to have when shopping or ordering out. Avoiding some of the more toxic fish is a great way to protect yourself from unnecessary exposure. For a more complete list, visit www.fda.gov/Food/FoodborneIllnessContaminants/Metals/ucm115644.htm.

Omega-3 Rich Fish to Eat
Alaskan salmon, halibut, tuna, cod, sardines, anchovies

Fish To Limit
Swordfish, shark, tilefish, king mackerel, white (albacore) tuna, warm water fish like orange roughy, shellfish like clams, lobsters, oysters, shrimp and scallops, fish whose color has been preserved with dyes, farmed fish (unless from responsible aqua-culturists)

The Weston A. Price Foundation offers invaluable information. Make a donation, whatever you can afford. Make use of their annually-printed Shopper's Guide, available for purchase on their website. It is a great tool if you are beginning to learn which food products to buy and which to avoid. Every patient that walks into my office gets a copy. Vote with your dollar. You can pay the farmer now for good quality, wholesome organic food - or pay the doctor later at the expense of your health. I also suggest joining the Environmental Working Group (EWG).

Food Quantity

Many Americans overeat, partly due to the fact that so much of the food common in the Standard American Diet (SAD) is loaded with empty calories. We are becoming a nation of dysglycemics, yo-yo-ing between hyperglycemia and hypoglycemia all day long. Our bodies receive signals to eat when we shouldn't be hungry. And when we eat, we eat too much. We even eat at the wrong times!

A great rule of thumb is this: practice leaving the table before you are full, not after you feel stuffed. Overall caloric restriction has been shown to be a very beneficial practice for almost every disease including cancer. The reason is simple. The body has to break down food completely, extract nutrients, and discard the waste efficiently to stay well. When we overeat, we overwhelm our digestive system and strain the enzyme system that functions to digest our food. Food then sits longer in our system and putrifies. This leads to a build-up of bacteria and their organic acid wastes. These bacteria are not out to harm us. They are actually trying to help us do what our body has failed to do on its own. They are part of nature's recycling system. Unfortunately, before long, we exhaust our nutrient-enzyme system, creating nutrient deficiencies and leaving behind partially digested food and the concomitant exposure to bacterial wastes and toxins.

The best thing is to practice self-restraint by eating smaller portions and doing simple exercises in moderation. For example, ask the waiter to leave the bread off the table when you dine out. Instead of two or three pieces, eat only one. Instead of having a whole dessert, share it. If you are going to have dessert, skip the bread and the pasta. Begin simply, work on one aspect of cutting back at a time. You may be used to having large sandwiches for lunch. Try removing the bread (or at least half) and having salad or some vegetables with your sandwich. Whatever you do, start cutting back on the overeating. A good rule of thumb is this: If you feel bloated, overly full or uncomfortable taking a deep breath, chances are you have overeaten. Most people overeat because of stress, anxiety or even boredom. So it is very important to stay active, keep busy and productive and avoid becoming a couch potato.

Proper Food Combining

Food combining is an important factor in improving digestion. Improper food combining can cause incomplete digestion and a slowing down of the bowel function. This has far-reaching consequences for overall health, especially when ignored for many years.

Here is the problem. Our ancestors ate what was in season, what they could hunt and preserve over long winters, and what they could gather or grow seasonally. The variety and combinations of foods were limited, and food was unprocessed in any way aside from fermentation which nature provided. Formerly, food combining was not an issue. But today we eat all types of processed foods, have poorer digestive function, and combine many varieties of foods/ingredients not meant to be eaten in combination.

Proper food combining is a critical part of aiding digestion. When practiced regularly, it will insure improved digestion and lessen the likelihood of digestive disorders. Here are a few rules of proper food combining, the purpose behind them and how they help us improve our digestion:

(Refer to chart on next page for more information)

Rule #1: ***Never eat protein*** (meat or animal product of any kind) ***with starchy vegetables.*** The reason is that starches require an alkaline environment for enzymes to break them down. In fact, starch digestion begins in the mouth with the release of the enzyme amylase. Proteins, however, require a highly acidic environment to be digested. A highly acidic environment deactivates starch enzymes. Therefore the two counter one another and lead to food sitting in the stomach too long. This creates a build-up of bacterial fermentation, leading to caustic organic acid production by the bacteria which then irritates the lining of the stomach and causes bloating.

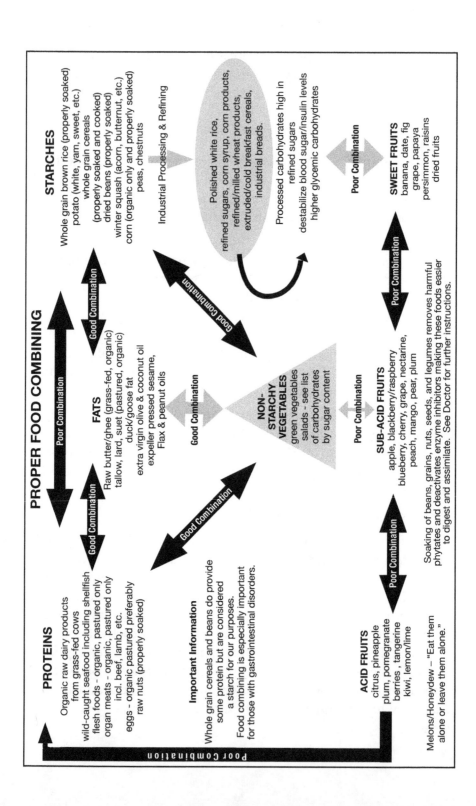

Rule #2: *Fruits are best eaten for breakfast alone or between meals.* Fruits are made from simple sugars. Therefore, they will digest rather quickly compared to other foods (approximately 30 minutes for most fruits to leave the stomach assuming they are ripe; bananas are an exception, they take about an hour). It is best to eat fruit in season and to eat one fruit at a time, waiting 30 minutes to one hour before having a different type of fruit. It is not a good idea to have a fruit salad. If you must, stay within one fruit category: acid fruits with other acid fruits; sub-acid with other sub-acid; or sweet with other sweet. Do not eat fruits and vegetables at the same meal, at the same time. Do not eat fruits with any kind of meat or animal product. If you want, you may combine acid fruits with soaked raw nuts or raw dairy (yogurt). Remember, organic is best.

Rule #3: *Never mix animal proteins at one meal.* Never mix shrimp and chicken or steak and fish. Doing so for most people places too great a demand on the stomach. Most patients I see already exhibit poor stomach function and insufficient hydrochloric acid production. Adding multiple proteins at one meal is often too great of a burden on the stomach. For more information on stomach acid and its importance to health as well as reflux disease (GERD), read *Why Stomach Acid Is Good for You,* by Jonathan V. Wright MD.

Rule #4: *Avoid eating meat and dairy together as much as possible.* This means trying to limit your cheeseburgers, or your cheesecake after eating meat. This refers mostly to processed dairy when combined with meat. It is also important to limit any sweets after eating meat. The combination leads to a slowing of digestion and a stagnation of the bowel.

Rule #5: *Eat melons alone or leave them alone.* Melons will ferment rapidly if kept in the stomach too long. Therefore, putting them into the stomach with other foods will slow digestion and lead to fermentation. It is best to *eat them 30 minutes or more before meals or between meals.*

Rule #6: *Never eat citrus fruits or fruit juices with cereals/grains.* This is a common American mistake at breakfast. The commercials practically beg you to have your orange juice with your cold cereal with milk. This is not a good combination for the digestive tract, nor is it a healthy breakfast to begin with. Cereals should be whole grains, soaked and cooked according to the traditional ways.

Our Paleo-ancestors did not have 24-hour 7-Elevens, Stop&Shops and other grocery stores at their disposal. Food was seasonal, dependent on the weather and the regional climate, and was often scarce. Even after the agricultural revolution when people settled down from their previous nomadic hunter/gatherer existence, only certain types of foods were available, *and they were always unprocessed*. The foods early peoples ate were the foods they could grow in season, gather or hunt. In the past, foods available at any one time were few in number and not complicated by processed and artificial components. The variety available today requires us to attend to the foods we combine at our meals.

The Importance of pH Balance

A discussion of the pH of the body requires definition and clarification. First of all, pH stands for "parts per Hydrogen" and it represents the acidity or alkalinity of an aqueous solution. More plainly put, it tells us the hydrogen ion concentration of any fluid. The pH scale is measured from 0 to 14 with 7 considered neutral like pure water. Anything with a pH lower than 7 is considered an acid, and anything above 7 is considered basic, or alkaline. The normal healthy blood pH, for example, is tightly regulated between 7.35 and 7.45. If the pH of the blood were to move outside of this range, the person would die. The normal pH of the urine is considered by most physicians to be from 6.5 to 8.0 in healthy people. I consider healthy salivary pH (or what I refer to as body pH) to be within the range of 6.8 to 7.2.

Discussion of how the body regulates pH is outside the scope of this book, but there are a few points I would like to make. First, the body produces most of its waste in the form of acids. In healthy individuals, these metabolic wastes are normally processed by the liver and kidneys and excreted through our urine, respiration and feces. Depending on the body's needs, it can adjust the pH of the blood accordingly to preserve health. However when the body becomes overburdened with wastes from processed foods and toxins, the pH of the body (and saliva) shifts to acidic. This common occurrence is due to the overconsumption of processed, nutrient-depleted foods and exposure to ubiquitous man-made toxins.

For a person to remain healthy, the intestinal tract must remain slightly acidic. Do not confuse this with salivary/body pH which is best maintained around neutral to slightly alkaline. A slightly acidic intestinal tract will ensure that most nutrients, like calcium for example, will be absorbed properly. One of the more popular bacteria residing in a healthy intestine is acidophilus. This bacterium received its name because it produces lactic acid as a by-product of its metabolism. Lactic acid helps to keep our intestinal tract slightly acidic (pH<7.0) and healthy. Just like keeping our home clean, our body wants to maintain a certain chemical balance in all areas for optimal health. In the intestinal tract, this involves processing food efficiently and maintaining a healthy bacterial population, while also removing wastes through regular bowel movements.

The importance of understanding pH balance cannot be overstated. All disease states including cancer thrive in an overly acidic body. Take the example of arthritis. The more acidic the body and therefore the blood become, the more the body will mobilize alkaline mineral stores from the bones and teeth to buffer this acidity and protect the body. Over time, the loss of alkaline minerals will result in osteopenia/osteoporosis and arthritic changes at the joints, as well as other health problems.

The main culprit in causing an acid overload is a highly processed, nutrient deficient diet. A book that outlines the effects of common foods on body pH is *Alkalize or Die* by James Baroody. It is important to understand how to maintain proper pH balance in order to maintain or even restore your health. There are many aspects to consider with regard to diet. Here is an overview of the main concepts that I have used to help my patients.

First, be sure to drink good, clean, pure water. I encourage my patients to utilize a reverse osmosis filter in their homes. There are many different types on the market for every budget. I recommend the Cuno Reverse Osmosis Water Purifier which can be purchased on-line for around $500. If you cannot afford a reverse osmosis purifier then I strongly suggest using a dechlorinator. Dechlorinators range in price from around $150 to $300 and are made by companies like Aquasana and RainShow'r. For those who can afford it, I recommend installing a reverse osmosis filter that will purify all of the water coming into your home (see Appendix F p. 362 for sources).

Second, eat a whole food diet rich in fresh, organic fruits, vegetables and salads. Fruits and vegetables, especially when consumed raw, are loaded with enzymes and nutrients which help to keep the body properly balanced and slightly alkaline. Lacto-fermented vegetables are also especially healthy, easy to digest, loaded with probiotic organisms and excellent in helping to alkalize the body. When eaten with acid-forming animal protein, this helps maintain a neutral to slightly alkaline pH. All animal products (meat, dairy, eggs, fish, etc) should be pastured/wild caught and organic. Do not overcook meats, as doing so denatures the protein structure rendering it toxic and unusable by the body. Medium rare is sufficient. Many people are wrongly concerned about cooking meat well to kill bacteria. However, bacteria grow only on the surface of meat and are rendered dead by medium-rare cooking. Ground meats, however, are a separate concern due to the mixing/grinding of the meat and should always be cooked well if purchased non-organic. Organic/pastured meats should not be a bigger concern as the animal was raised in a healthier and cleaner environment. Parasites/bacteria are a much bigger concern with concentrated animal feeding operation (CAFO) animal meats and therefore should be cooked more thoroughly.

All dairy products should be raw, organic, and from pastured animals grazing on grass. Once a product is pasteurized, the heat destroys the living enzymes, denatures proteins and some vitamins, and makes the food acid-forming and almost impossible to digest. This same concept applies to store-bought juices and other beverages. The pasteurization process destroys the enzymes and many delicate vitamins, making the food much more acidic and more problematic for the body. The truth is, the more a food is processed away from the way that it is found in nature, the more acid-forming and problematic for health it becomes. Artificially produced foods like sodas, sweets, most cakes, margarine, colorings, preservatives, and artificial flavors are all acid-forming junk for our bodies, and have no place in our diet. They destroy our health by forcing the body to use up vital nutrients in order to detoxify them and pass them out of our system.

One final important point with regard to maintaining a healthy pH involves our lifestyle habits. Sufficient rest is probably the most important of our lifestyle habits. Adequate rest provides our body with a chance to heal and repair. The average patient I see is mentally and emotionally stressed and gets far too little rest. Add cigarette smoking, lack of exercise and poor family structure and you have a recipe for acidic disaster. Remember, your body needs balance. Proper rest, aerobic activity, prayer or spiritual reflection and fun are all part of building a long, healthy, and prosperous life.

General Dietary Guidelines for a Healthy Life

Perhaps healthcare wouldn't be such a disaster if we were told the truth and used a little old-fashioned common sense when it comes to our food. Then we could spend our money on supporting the local farmer, enriching our health, and limiting the need for the doctor. A wise man once said, "You can pay the farmer now, or the doctor later." For good health it is preferable to pay the farmer for nutrient-dense, organic, pastured, traditional foods rather than to expect Advil, blood pressure medication, statins, and other drugs to magically provide one with gleaming health. We do not have a healthcare system in this country, we have a Sick-Care System. Do not misunderstand, medicine is necessary for emergencies, accidents, congenital problems, and for those who are careless about their lifestyle. In these and other more focused areas, medicine works wonders. The doctors providing this care are the best in the world. However, what I call our Sick-Care System is designed to bankrupt people's health through symptom care, collusion between the processed food industry and government, lobbyists, and the control exercised by chemical and agricultural giants like Monsanto, Tyson, and others.

People who want to medicate and who ignore the need to eat healthier, exercise, stop smoking, etc., should pay higher insurance premiums and deductibles. They may live as they see fit. But these adults are accountable for their health. They should not expect others to pay for the consequences of their lack of self-care. Those who want to live a balanced, drug-free life and age gracefully with independence, should demand better. Public health support should reward healthy practices, not harmful ones. When you buy car insurance, you earn a cheaper rate if you're a better driver. It's simple risk assessment. Life insurance is no different. Smokers, for example, pay higher premiums. And well they should. Their risk of illness is greater.

But our healthcare system is not transparent regarding our food and how it relates to our health. The agribusiness and chemical companies provide deceptive information. Additives and sweeteners cause addiction to products while providing long shelf-life, thus making food "convenient" and cheap, and maximizing company profits. Information linking foods, drugs, and chemicals to diseases and destruction of the soil and earth are concealed from the public. The Standard American Diet of processed grains and sugars, pesticides, artificial colorings and sweeteners then produces illness at increased rates.

Insurance premiums and hospital bills go up as people receive medications, surgery and treatment for illnesses that the very procedures of government and industry created. Controlling this information enables various industries to make cheaper, nutrient-poor foods and then market them to an overpopulated world as though they are health-giving and nourishing.

GMO labeling is a case in point. The legislation for this labeling used in standard law in places like China, Japan, Australia, Russia, New Zealand, and all 15 countries of the European Union was defeated in California in 2013 with money from Monsanto, the biggest agricultural and chemical company in the world. The overwhelming majority of Americans want GMO labeling. What intelligent consumer would not want to know what harmful ingredients may be in their food? The information regarding exactly what is in our food should be available to all of us, whenever we desire it, regardless of whether one is health-conscious or not. Doctors are required to obtain the informed consent of their patients. Should there not be informed consent regarding our food, too?

I would like to introduce my readers to the basic groundwork for healthy eating. Understand that I do not believe in a one-size-fits-all approach to eating. What is suitable for one person may not be suitable for someone else based on pre-existing health conditions, age, genetics, allergies, etc. A person with a gallbladder problem/disease, for example, will have to make adjustments that others will not have to make. However, these considerations aside, there are core characteristics to healthy eating that all should follow and learn. The best place to start in that regard is with the Healthy Eating Pyramid. I want to analyze it along with the most updated USDA Food Pyramid from 2013 for comparison. This way we can discuss the different aspects of the pyramids clearly, show how they differ, and how to implement the dietary principles we espouse.

In 2013 the U.S. Department of Agriculture released the NEW FOOD PYRAMID shown below. It breaks food categories into a spectrum to emphasize variety. Exercise was introduced as a component of the food pyramid, and 12 individualized intake profiles were added.

THE USDA NEW FOOD PYRAMID 2013

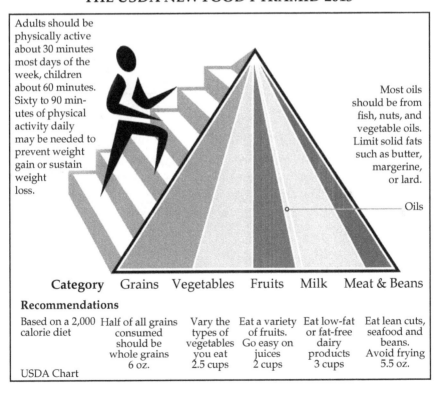

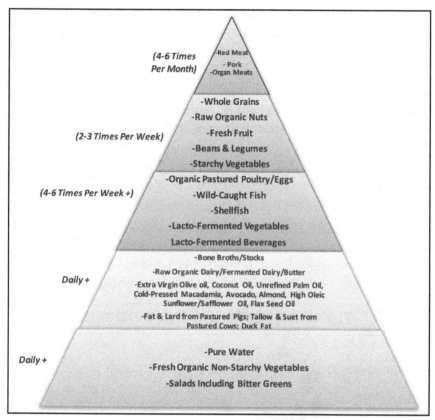

TRADITIONAL WISDOM FOOD PYRAMID

As you can see, the foundation of this pyramid is built on fresh, organic, non-starchy vegetables and leafy greens, as well as olive oil, coconut oil, raw butter and other raw organic dairy. For most people, limiting starchier vegetables and grains like potato, rice, beans, etc. is a good idea. This is because many patients consume too many refined sugars and starches, and not enough green/non-starchy vegetables. And so I recommend limiting the frequency of starchy vegetables as well as fruits. Though starchier vegetables and fruits are not unhealthy, they are not healthy for everyone. Since many people consume too much sugar, this simple adjustment can go a long way to improve digestion, health and even aid weight loss. Ultimately this must be decided on a case by case basis by a physician who is well-versed in nutrition. (Consult the list of fruits and vegetables based on carbohydrate content on pages 366-367 in Appendix G.)

Dr. Angelo Rose; Dr. Christopher Amoruso

I encourage patients to include in their diets lacto-fermented vegetables like sauerkraut as well as lacto-fermented beverages like kvass and kombucha. This helps take the place of soft drinks and pasteurized products which are devoid of enzymes and nutrients. Lacto-fermented foods/beverages are highly digestible, rich in enzymes, probiotics and nutrients, and are known to improve health. For learning how to make your own lacto-fermented foods/beverages consult *Real Food Fermentation* written by Alex Lewin. This culinary application is easier than you think, and is fun for the family. In fact, it is a great way to bring families together. Sally Fallon Morell's book *Nourishing Traditions* also has information on this topic and includes recipes.

The second level of our pyramid is built upon access to many of the good fats, including saturated fats, which were driven out of the American diet since the 1950's by so-called "fat experts". These "experts" were behind Ancel Keys when he popularized the cholesterol-diet-heart disease hypothesis after he manipulated the data in his Seven Countries Study. Keys later pointed out that the studies he initially did on rabbits were fatally flawed and the entire diet-cholesterol-heart hypothesis was "wrong all along, and we knew it," as Susan Schenck reminds us in her book *Beyond Broccoli*. For a further explanation of the history of the diet-heart-cholesterol hypothesis and how it pertains to the fats we should aim to include in our diet versus those we should avoid, see Section XI p. 198 of this book on cholesterol and heart disease.

Included in our list of good fats are any fat from organic, pastured animal meat including organ meats or wild-caught fish; extra-virgin cold-pressed olive, flax, palm and coconut oils; raw butter and raw ghee (aka clarified butter) from pastured (grass-fed) cows grazing on rapidly growing grasses in the spring and fall; and eggs from organic, pastured chickens. The following information helps to summarize fats and was taken from the Weston A. Price Foundation's website. I encourage my readers to join this non-profit foundation and explore the website for copious amounts of reliable information on almost every health topic:

Confused About Fats? The following nutrient-rich traditional fats have nourished healthy population groups for thousands of years.

For Cooking:
> Butter
> Tallow and suet from beef and lamb
> Lard from pigs
> Chicken, goose and duck fat
> Coconut, palm and palm kernel oils

For Salads:
> Extra virgin olive oil (also OK for cooking)
> Expeller-expressed sesame and peanut oils
> Expeller-expressed flax oil (in small amounts)

For Fat-Soluble Vitamins
> Fish liver oils such as cod liver oil (preferable to other fish oils, which do not provide fat-soluble vitamins, can cause an overdose of unsaturated fatty acids and usually come from farmed fish.)

The following newfangled fats are not recommended because they can cause cancer, heart disease, immune system dysfunction, sterility, learning disabilities, growth problems and osteoporosis:
> All hydrogenated and partially hydrogenated oils
> Industrially processed liquid oils such as soy, corn, safflower, cottonseed and canola
> Fats and oils (especially vegetable oils) heated to very high temperatures in processing and frying

Returning to the Pyramid we can see how the above recommendations regarding fats is at odds with the USDA's Food Pyramid. The USDA pyramid guides us to use only fats from vegetable oils, nuts and fish; to avoid saturated fats; and to limit solid fats like butter or lard. What they do not explain is that the vast majority of vegetable oils (soy, corn, canola, safflower, etc.) are damaged during processing and are often contaminated with harsh chemicals like hexane from the processing. To clarify this point, liquid oils are liquid at room temperature because they contain delicate double-bonds between their carbon atoms which prevents them from aligning into a more solid structure. If there is only one such double-bond, you have a monounsaturated fat; if there are two or more, you have a polyunsaturated fat. Both types of fats in their natural, unprocessed state are needed by our bodies. However, in the industrial production of these oils in order to extract them from their source (corn from the germ of a corn kernel, soy oil from soybean, etc.) harsh chemicals like hexane and 2-methylpentane are used. Residues of these chemicals are often left behind in the oil itself. Furthermore, according to Wikipedia, "After extraction, the corn oil is then refined by degumming and/or alkali treatment, both of which remove phosphatides. Alkali treatment also neutralizes free fatty acids and removes color (bleaching). Final steps in refining include winterization (the removal of waxes), and deodorization by steam distillation of the oil at 232–260°C (450–500°F) under a high vacuum."

This processing, along with the heat involved in distillation, damages the delicate carbon-carbon double-bonds of the fats (predominately polyunsaturated), destroys vital nutrients like vitamins and enzymes, and leaves us with a product which is devoid of the life-giving properties nature endowed it with. This is true for all liquid oils processed in this manner (soy, safflower, cottonseed, canola, etc). Liquid oils are delicate and must be handled that way or their nutritional components will be destroyed, making them unhealthy to consume. Unfortunately, because this processing is cheaper than unrefined, extra virgin, expeller pressed methods, these oils are touted as beneficial and are ubiquitous in most fried and processed foods. The appropriate government agencies frequently do not disclose these facts to the public.

The only place in the pyramids where there is agreement about fats is in the avoidance of margarine and man-made trans-fat. When it comes to dairy, the USDA tells us to use fat-free or low-fat dairy but says nothing about it being the number one food allergy, nor do they mention the nutritional superiority of grass-fed, non-pasteurized/non-homogenized fresh full-fat raw milk. Unless a patient has a preexisting gallbladder problem, I advise using raw grass-fed full-fat dairy.

The third level of the pyramid includes eggs, chicken, and pork from pastured, organic sources as well as wild-caught fish and shellfish. Why pastured sources? Simply because that is the way nature intended these animals to be and because factory animals (CAFO — Concentrated Animal Feeding Operation) are fed corn and soy which, unless organic, are genetically modified and nutritionally inferior. In addition, animals not raised organically are often given antibiotics and hormones, and live in squalid conditions. Furthermore, corn and soy are not the native diet of these animals (chickens and pigs are omnivores, meaning they eat both animal/insect and vegetable) and this affects their health as well as their nutrient profile. When you eat an animal you are eating what it ate. Chris Masterjohn has begun some groundbreaking research on this subject, and has published an interesting article entitled "Fatty Acid Analysis of Grass-fed and Grain-Fed Beef Tallow" in the Winter 2013 issue of *Wise Traditions*, Volume 14, No 4. His research shows that the diet of the animal can drastically impact the profile of the fatty acids found in the animal, as well as the ratio between the omega-3 and omega-6 forms of these fatty acids found in the animal.

Also to be avoided are farmed fish, especially salmon, so prevalent in restaurants and stores. Choose only wild-caught Alaskan salmon (which is either King, red or silver) and never purchase Atlantic salmon as it is always farmed. Walter Crinnion remarks that "farmed Atlantic salmon is just about the most toxic food you can eat."(Crinnion W. Clean, green and lean; get rid of the toxins that make you fat. Hoboken, New Jersey : John Wiley, Inc.; 2010. p. 63)

Concerning pork, it should always be marinated in an acidic medium for several hours to several days to help pre-digest the protein and ensure proper digestion of the meat. I typically recommend lemon juice or raw organic apple cider vinegar for this purpose. Interesting research is being done on how this acid marinating can help make pork more digestible. Research published by the Weston A. Price Foundation shows that in people eating unmarinated pork, red blood cells tend to behave abnormally and clump together. This is not a good thing with regard to clot formation, vascular flow and cardiovascular disease. However, when the pork is properly marinated and prepared, the red blood cells of the tested subjects behaved normally and did not clump together. For further information visit the Weston A. Price Foundation's website.

Perhaps the most glaring discrepancy between the pyramids involves grains. Grains can be just as confusing to the average American as fats are. Most of my patients think they are doing well when they are buying whole grain bread at the supermarket. They have no idea about how most wheat is bromated, bleached, and has added harmful ingredients like high fructose corn syrup (HFCS), vital gluten and hydrogenated oils. The commercial wheat we know today is highly hybridized and has added gluten content to impart more favorable baking attributes to bread and dough. The consumer is usually unaware that improperly prepared or processed whole wheat products can cause mineral deficiencies (via the action of phytates) and intestinal distress (via glutenins and gliadins). They are also unaware of the digestive advantages and nutritional superiority of sprouted and sourdough-leavened techniques in bread-making. Corn, like wheat, is a grain and a world staple. At present, roughly 95% of corn is genetically modified to produce its own pesticide and to withstand the death causing effects of spraying with Round-Up, a Monsanto product. Only organic corn on the cob should be purchased. It then should be soaked in an acidic medium before cooking and eating.

These facts are important considering that the USDA recommends making grains like wheat and corn the staple of your diet, rating them even more important than vegetables. They advise daily consumption of 6 ounces per day with only half being from whole grains. What this amounts to is a diet loaded with whole grain, cold, extruded breakfast cereals, whole wheat bagels, breads, wraps, pasta, and muffins. Even more worrisome, many of these products are made with rancid vegetable oils, including hydrogenated oils, "enriched" with synthetic vitamins, and refined sugars (the next time you buy whole wheat bread at the supermarket, read the label). That translates to an epidemic of diabetes, osteoporosis, cancer and many other degenerative conditions. Dr. William Davis, author of the best-selling book *Wheat Belly* was on the Dr. Oz program during the summer of 2013 explaining this very fact about wheat (the most common grain used along with corn). If you have diabetes or want to understand the truth about wheat in greater detail, read his book.

Our pyramid, however, recommends using far less grain in the diet, the majority coming from whole grains that have been soaked and properly prepared before eating. We stress the importance of using whole grains that have been prepared by soaking, sprouting or sour leavening to neutralize phytic acid and other anti-nutrients.

A Legacy of Healing

One example of this is preparing steel-cut oatmeal rather than cold, extruded breakfast cereals. We also encourage our patients to use breads sparingly, and to purchase only breads that are sprouted or sourdough-leavened and free of preservatives, high fructose corn syrup, soy, hydrogenated oils, etc. Bread should always be consumed with ample raw butter from pastured cows to improve its digestibility and to slow the digestion of the carbohydrate. On this topic, I recommend *Nourishing Traditions*, by Sally Fallon. She gives instructions for soaking grains to make them more digestible and facilitating the removal of anti-nutrients and enzyme-inhibitors. She includes recipes and ideas for making your own granola as well as the names of companies that sell organic soaked and sprouted grains on the internet. One that I use is "To Your Health Sprouted Flour Company" in Fitzpatrick, Alabama (see Appendix D Resources p. 357). You can purchase many kinds of grains including gluten-free types in whole form or already ground for you and done in a delicate, low-temperature manner so as to preserve the enzymes and nutrition of the grain. I use the Jupiter grain mill made by the German company *Schnitzer Getreidemuhlen* to freshly grind my grain at home (Appendix D Resources p. 357).

Another glaring difference between the two pyramids involves dairy. The USDA recommends that everyone drink three cups a day of low-fat and fat-free dairy. *But not just any dairy.* Conventional CAFO dairy products made from cows that were raised shoulder to shoulder with other cows, standing in their own feces, and given RBST (recombinant bovine somatotropic hormone). These hormones force the cattle to produce more milk than nature intended. In addition, the animals are given antibiotics to ward off infections developed from being confined, mistreated and forced to eat GMO corn and soy they would otherwise not eat. Have you ever questioned the source of the virulent strains of E. coli reported in the news? Their origin is the stomachs of cows denied the diet and conditions nature intended for them. If you are wise enough to buy organic milk you still have to clear the pasteurization/homogenization hurdle that the USDA would rather you not know about. They attest that it is to protect you from the dangers of unsafe raw milk. Yet no mother I know of pasteurizes her breast milk before feeding her infant child. The truth is, pasteurization largely wipes out numerous protective factors, deactivating the various leukocytes, antibodies, enzymes and binding proteins, while reducing the activity of medium-chain fatty acids, lysozymes, oligosachharides, hormones, growth factors and beneficial bacteria. (Schmid R. The untold story of milk p.101) Actually, we are not lactose intolerant, we are pasteurization intolerant.

Milk homogenization became widespread in America in the 1930s and nearly universal in the 1940s — the same decades during which the incidence of atherosclerotic heart disease began to climb. (Enig MG. Milk homogenization and heart disease. Wise Traditions 2003 Summer;4(2):) Homogenization is done so that the cream will not rise to the top; fat is less dense than the liquid portion of milk, thus the milk will stay uniform (homogenous-hence homogenization). This damages the delicate fats found in the milk. When milk is homogenized, it passes through a fine filter at pressures equal to 4,000 pounds per square inch, and in so doing, the fat globules (liposomes) are made smaller (micronized) by a factor of ten times or more. As a result, the fat molecules become evenly dispersed within the liquid milk and will no longer rise to the top. During homogenization there is a tremendous increase in surface area on the fat globules. The original fat globule membrane is lost and a new one is formed that incorporates a much greater portion of casein and whey proteins. This may account for the increased allergenicity of modern processed milk.

I warn my patients to avoid conventional pasteurized/homogenized dairy. Milk is our biggest allergy food. It causes an overproduction of mucous when consumed. Removal of dairy clears up recurring ear infections in children, eczema in children and adults, and many gastrointestinal problems as well. People say, "You need to drink milk for strong bones." However, pasteurization renders the calcium in conventional milk nearly impossible to absorb as the process destroys the phosphatase enzyme needed by the body to absorb the calcium in milk. Many patients find this hard to believe because of advertising and marketing.

For these reasons I recommend only raw, organic dairy from clean, healthy Jersey and Guernsey breed cows. This includes yogurt, cheese, kefir and butter. Chris Masterjohn, author of *The Biochemical Magic of Raw Milk: Glutathione*, remarks that "one of the many benefits of raw milk may be its ability to promote the production of a wonderful little compound called 'glutathione'. This tiny compound consists of just three amino acids, but it is the master antioxidant and detoxifier of the cell." (Wise Traditions, Winter 2010.11(4)70.) Masterjohn notes that excessive heating of milk (pasteurization and ultra-high temperature pasteurization) denatures (destroys the structure of) crucial whey proteins that serve to boost glutathione levels in our liver.

Unfortunately, in many states the sale of raw milk is illegal. A food consumed for thousands of years is illegal to market. For more information on the real history of milk and details beyond the scope of this book read *The Untold Story of Milk* by Ron Schmid, ND. Refer to Appendix D p. 355, A Campaign for Real Milk, for resources to learn more and to find fresh raw milk in your area.

At the very top of my pyramid I have included organ meats and red meat from organic, pastured animals for two very important reasons. First, organ meat and red meat are "a rich source of nutrients that protect the heart and nervous system; these include all of the fat soluble vitamins and co-factors, vitamins B12 and B6, zinc, phosphorus, carnitine, coenzyme-Q_{10} and more." (Weston A. Price Foundation) We need to consume these foods in some amount regularly to obtain nutrients that are not available through other sources. Second, I understand that many people, either for moral, ethical or nutritional reasons have come to believe that eating meat is wrong. I direct those of you who are confused about vegetarianism/veganism and the facts about red meat to two books written by lifelong vegans Susan Schenck, and Lierre Keith respectively, called *Beyond Broccoli* and *The Vegetarian Myth*. These books explain the rationale behind vegan diets as well as the importance of eating animal foods. If you limit the amount of red meat or organ meat you consume, be sure to compensate by including raw butter, seafood including shellfish, eggs and other pastured, organic animal products. Those who wish to eat meat more frequently should do so, being sure it is from organic, pastured sources. I recommend eating meat that is medium rare or rare so as not to damage its delicate amino acid profile. One caveat with meat is this: since there is a fairly large epidemic of poor stomach function in this country (hypochlorhydria — see Section VI in this book on indigestion and

GERD) it is very important to work with a doctor familiar with digestive enzymes before consuming larger portions of red meats. This is to ensure the full digestion and breakdown of meat into the individual amino acids. Due to poor stomach function, many people are unable to digest meat. If ignored this can lead to other health problems. Keep in mind, meat should never be combined with starches at a meal. Please refer to Proper Food Combining on p. 23 for a detailed explanation.

Regarding general dietary guidelines, one last consideration is the importance of including bone broths in the diet. "Meat and fish stocks are used almost universally in traditional cuisines, but the use of homemade meat broths to produce nourishing soups and sauces has nearly disappeared from American culinary tradition" writes Sally Fallon in her classic work *Nourishing Traditions*, p.116. Especially rich in gelatin, minerals, cartilage, marrow, and vegetables, meat stock is extremely nutritious, as well as very easy to digest. Gelatin acts first and foremost as an aid to digestion and has been used successfully in the treatment of many intestinal disorders, including hyperacidity, colitis and Crohn's disease. Fallon notes, "The wise food provider, who uses gelatin-rich broth on a daily or frequent basis, provides continuous protection from many health problems." (Ibid p. 117) *Nourishing Traditions* also contains recipes for making different types of stocks including beef, fish, and chicken. Homemade stocks should be the cornerstone of everyone's diet and are preferable to those ready-made broths purchased in supermarkets. The latter often contain MSG and sodium and may be made with questionable ingredients. Below is a summary of the important facts to remember when it comes to our own individual food pyramid. I encourage all of my patients to do their best to satisfy as many of the criteria as possible. The pyramid is flexible, so work to achieve the main points and consult with a qualified professional familiar with these principles and those of the Weston A. Price Foundation to tailor the pyramid to your specific needs. Life is balance. No one is perfect, but if you have more pros on your side than cons, chances are you will stay healthy and vibrant.

1. Make non-starchy green vegetables and salads a cornerstones of your diet while enjoying starchier vegetables from time to time but

not in excess. This is a sensible and important recommendation, as most Americans consume excessive carbohydrates on a daily basis.

2. Choose from organic, pastured meats including beef, chicken, duck, pork, turkey, as well as wild-caught fish including shellfish and organic eggs from free-range chickens. Remember, the health of the animal you eat is only as good as the diet that animal had and the environment in which it lived. Always choose organic, and if possible, choose pastured and for fish always buy wild-caught.

3. Include organic, pastured organ meats like liver and tripe in your diet as much as you can. Liver is rich in fat soluble vitamins and other nutrients which are difficult to get from other sources.

4. Include organic, sprouted or soaked whole grains in your diet. DO NOT consume processed grains like those found in bagels, cold extruded breakfast cereals, flour products, etc. Reject store-bought "whole grains" that are junk food in disguise. Read the labels and, when in doubt, use your Weston A. Price Shopper's Guide.

5. Soak all grains, seeds, raw nuts, legumes and beans to eliminate phytate, enzyme-inhibitors and anti-nutrients thus improving their digestibility and increasing vitamin and mineral content.

6. Use fresh herbs from your own garden. Plant basil, mint, parsley, oregano, and others and learn to include them in your cooking. If you don't have room for a garden, use planters and place them near a window or on your balcony.

7. Use only unprocessed/unrefined sea salts — Celtic brand or Himalayan — and use it generously.

8. Make bone broths and stocks on a weekly basis and consume them liberally. Drink the broth as a tea or use for cooking/sautéing and making soups. If you don't have time to prepare broth at home, I recommend ordering from U.S. Wellness. Their website is www.grasslandbeef.com.

9. Try to incorporate lacto-fermented vegetables like sauerkraut in your diet. Better yet, learn to make them at home. It's easy as well as spiritually rewarding. Be aware of store-bought brands that add vinegar, sugar and other ingredients.

10. The diets of healthy primitive and non-industrialized peoples contain no refined or denatured foods such as refined sugar or corn syrup, white flour, canned foods, pasteurized, homogenized, skim or low-fat milk, refined or hydrogenated vegetable oils, protein powders, artificial vitamins or toxic additives and colorings. (Weston A. Price Foundation)

11. Never consume pasteurized/homogenized conventional dairy from CAFOs. Instead join a local Co-op or cow-share and enjoy fresh, organic, pastured dairy products Emphasize those that are fermented like raw yogurt and kefir. Refer to the Weston A. Price Foundation to find a cow-share or co-op near you.

12. Avoid fats from industrially processed oils like canola, corn, soy, cottonseed, sunflower, and others. These oils are often in baked and packaged products like cookies, potato chips, bars, bagels, muffins, etc. Read the labels.

13. Never consume hydrogenated or partially hydrogenated oil of any kind and always avoid industrial trans-fats. New phone apps exist to help you identify these foods. One is from the Environmental Working Group and is called "Food Scores". The Weston A. Price Foundation (WAPF) also has an app called "Find Real Food."

14. Drink pure water every day in between your meals. Invest in a reverse osmosis filter or carbon based filter which eliminates volatile organic compounds, chlorine, and fluoride. Excellent filters can be purchased at www.radiantlifecatalog.com.

A Word About Supplements

A warning about supplements. This industry can be just as unscrupulous as the pharmaceutical industry as regards quality, honesty in product claims, and efficacy. This may be influenced by the fact that many of the bigger name brand vitamin companies are owned by pharmaceutical companies. For example, the well known Centrum® vitamin line is owned by Pfizer. This cheap multivitamin contains, among other things, calcium carbonate, better known as chalk. Research proves that calcium carbonate is nearly impossible for the body to use. In addition, Centrum® contains FD and C Yellow #6 Aluminum Lake, hydrogenated palm oil, polyethylene glycol, sodium benzoate (a dangerous preservative), sucrose, and titanium dioxide. Titanium dioxide is a nanoparticle used in sunscreens and, according to the Canadian Center for Occupational Health and Safety, may be a human carcinogen. Polyethylene glycol is made from ethylene glycol, better known as antifreeze.

This issue was presented in an article published by the Associated Press and reported on the Fox News website on June 10, 2009. The article, entitled "Many Vitamins, Supplements Made by Big Pharmaceutical Companies," states:

> The Pharma giant Wyeth, (acquired by Pfizer) for example, makes Centrum® and other supplements, and Bayer HealthCare of aspirin fame makes the One-A-Day line. Unilever, Novartis, GlaxoSmithKline and other big pharmaceutical firms also make or sell supplements. "They're moving into more and more of these products," said Steven Mister, president of the trade group, Council for Responsible Nutrition. However, size does not guarantee quality. Big companies are more likely to seek out bulk ingredient suppliers in less developed countries, said Jana Hildreth of the Analytical Research Collective, a group of scientists advocating better supplement testing. "They're going to demand lower prices, and with the prices they demand comes lower quality. You basically get what you pay for," she said.

I contend that these companies are well aware of the fact that cheap, fractionated, man-made vitamins cannot be adequately utilized by our bodies, nor do they have the efficacy we would hope for. Consumers can choose medications instead. This way, the pharmaceutical companies are capturing the market at both ends, thus pleasing their stockholders.

A recent study in the *Annals of Internal Medicine* 2013 painted a less than pleasant picture of vitamin supplementation. The first article reported the effects of vitamin supplements for disease prevention in adults who had no nutritional deficiency. The second evaluated the efficacy of multivitamins in preventing cognitive decline in men over 65. The third measured the effects of a high-dose multivitamin on people with a previous cardiac event. The study concluded that there were no benefits from the supplements in these populations. (Guallar E, et al. Ann Internal Med. 2013;159(12):850–51) The methodology of this study has numerous flaws. Among them is the fact that the authors cannot possibly take into account every lifestyle factor, such as diet, exercise, stress level, drug interactions, etc.

My point is this. Have the authors of the studies or the readers of their reports considered the quality of the vitamins used in the study? As a chemistry major in college, I know that minute differences in the position of atoms, charges, or three-dimensional structure/arrangement can make a difference when it comes to how things work in our body. Take for example, reverse T3, the faulty hormone made by the thyroid gland as a result of high cortisol levels and adrenal fatigue. By simply removing the wrong iodine atom from the hormone, it is rendered ineffective in the body, much the same way a key that is made with the teeth in reverse order would not open the intended lock. It's like your right hand and your left hand — they may look the same, but in three-dimensional space they are different. You cannot superimpose them. A right-hand glove will not work on your left hand. This happens quite often with synthetic, or man-made supplements. Chemistry cannot replicate identically what nature has designed. On the atomic level or elsewhere, something will be missing or different. It is questionable whether the lifeforce of food can be created in a lab from synthetic materials.

For our bodies to be nourished, our food, our supplements must be of good quality. Supplements should be taken only from whole-food sources, unprocessed and unaltered. Ron Schmid, ND notes that "one of the significant factors in choosing a supplement is the source of the nutrients it contains. . . . Vitamins, for example, may either be extracted from foods, synthesized in biochemical or biological processes, or grown within single-celled organisms."(Schmid R. Making sense of nutritional supplements. Pottenger P, J Health and Healing. 2013 Fall;36(3):12.) He further states that "even small amounts of the synthetic forms of fat-soluble vitamins may be toxic." (Ibid p. 12) This toxicity does not occur when we eat a healthy diet of whole-food, or ingest unprocessed supplements free from fillers and other additives.

Vitamin E is an example. Most cheap brands of vitamins use the synthetic form of one of the vitamin E factors, identified as "dl-alpha tocopherol." The "l" is the tip-off about the molecule's stereochemistry (a fancy word for its three-dimensional structure and spatial arrangements of molecules), and tells us it is synthetic. Real vitamin E from food, as found in wheat germ oil for example, consists of four different tocopherols, α (alpha), β (beta), δ (delta), and γ (gamma) as well as the trace mineral selenium, and four compounds known as tocotrienols. All these parts were put there by nature to function harmoniously together. When we take fractionated portions of vitamins without their complementary parts, we ingest a substance that can create a dangerous imbalance in our body.

When it comes to vitamins, herbs, or any other supplement, the primary concern should always be the quality and source of the product. Supplements should be just that, "supplements" for our food, which, for one reason or another, may not be providing all of the nutrition our lives demand. The first priority should be to eat a nutritious, unprocessed, traditional diet. To eat the SAD (Standard American Diet) and take a One-a-day, or a Centrum®, is a mistake. A recent editorial taken from the Price Pottenger *Journal of Health and Healing* (Vol. 36, no.3) from the fall of 2013 states:

> Does this mean one can eat the SAD, consume a few supplements, and live a healthy life? Not at all. This diet is deficient in healthy animal proteins and fats, as well as many other important nutrients, and high in toxins, sugars, refined grains, and overcooked, overprocessed foods. Eating a diet according to Dr. Price's principles is essential to attaining optimal health.

In conclusion, it is important to choose high-quality, unprocessed vitamins when supplementing your diet. Ideally, one should work with a qualified professional familiar with the Weston Price Foundation's principles, and knowledgeable in using whole-food vitamins and supplements. Using Standard Process vitamins with my family and in my practice, I have seen first-hand what quality nutritional supplementation can do to restore the health of the sick. Standard Process founder, Dr. Royal Lee, believed in whole-food nutrition. He stressed the importance of preserving the enzymatic activity and complete structure of whole-food supplements and espoused this philosophy in all of the products he made. There are many other companies that hold to this higher standard when making their products. Green Pasture™ Products is one. I have provided a list of good sources in Appendix D p. 355 of this book. To quote Dr. Lee, "One of the biggest tragedies of human civilization is the precedence of chemical therapy over nutrition. It's a substitution of artificial therapy over natural, of poisons over food, in which we are feeding poisons in trying to correct the reactions of starvation."

SECTION IV
THE HEAD

Headaches: Different Types and Treatments

Many doctors treat headaches with medication, frequently unsuccessfully. The headaches, at times relieved temporarily with medication, will usually come back. In this approach the medication is never treating the real cause of the headache. Actually the headache is telling the doctor the location of its root cause. This is a shift in the typical paradigm whereby all headaches are a problem inside of the head and are treated with analgesics (pain killers).

Crown Headache (Top of the Head)

I refer to a headache on the top of the head as a crown headache. Nine times out of ten, it is related to a problem within the uterus or ovaries and is caused by an increase in the pressure in the cerebrospinal fluid surrounding the brain. This increased pressure is caused by irritation of the sacral region of the spine from which the uterus and ovaries receive their innervation. The parasympathetic innervation to the uterus is derived from pelvic splanchnic nerves at the 2nd, 3rd, and 4th sacral levels, and the ovaries receive their innervation from these same parasympathetic fibers. The chiropractic treatment for this type of headache centers around adjusting the sacral region of the spine accordingly, including soft tissue in the area of the sacrum and gluteal muscles. A very effective home remedy for this is the use of the herbs Evening Primrose Oil or Black Cohosh, and compounds isolated from soy known as Isoflavones. Dietary considerations are often necessary to treat the cause and prevent the reoccurrence of these types of headaches and one should consult a qualified nutritional counselor. The treatment should include reducing refined sugars, xenoestrogens, Birth Control Pills (BCPs), and treating specific nutrient deficiencies. Further testing may be necessary, including salivary hormone panels to identify any areas of deficiency or imbalance. Diagnos-Techs can be used for salivary testing (see Appendix D p. 357 #16 for information). These imbalances can then be corrected with further diet and supplement changes.

Temporal Headache (Side of the Head)

A second type of headache is the temporal headache. Covering an area near the temples roughly the size of a golf ball, this type of headache is usually associated with the kidneys. As a chiropractor, I initially look to the spine. Most patients with this type of headache will also have a problem in the lower thoracic and sacral regions of the spine. Sensory input from the kidney travels to the T10-11 levels of the spinal cord and is sensed in the corresponding dermatome. "The nerve supply of the kidney and its ureter is provided by the renal plexus, a variable network of autonomic nerve fibers and ganglia. The renal plexus is a branch of the celiac plexus. It is largely supplied by sympathetic fibers from the least thoracic and first lumbar splanchnic nerves."(Marieb EN, Hoehn K. Human anatomy & physiology. 4th ed. Menlo Park CA: Benjamin/Cummings Science Publ; 1998. p. 968) Thus, pain in the flank region may be referred from corresponding kidney. With a patient complaining of this type of headache, I give a chiropractic adjustment to the thoraco-lumbar junction as well as the sacral region of the spine and some simple home remedies as noted below.

The first remedy is to make fresh parsley tea (see p. 320 for directions) and drink three cups per day. A second treatment is the herb Fever Few taken at a dosage of two times per day for three days and then once a day for one week thereafter. In more severe cases, a more thorough kidney detoxification may be necessary. See Andreas Moritz's book *The Miracle Liver and Gallbladder Flush* for full details on the protocol regarding kidney detoxification.

Nutritional support for the kidneys is very important. For this we use several Standard Process products, including Renatrophin®, Renafood® and Arginex®. These products are crucial not only in rebuilding the kidneys at the cellular level, but in aiding in detoxification and nutritional support. Anyone with kidney trouble should work with a qualified practitioner, using chiropractic adjustment to the areas of the spine mentioned above, as well as lifestyle and diet changes. For specific dietary changes, see Section III The Importance of Proper Digestion.

Frontal Headache (Forehead)

The third type of headache is the frontal, referring to the forehead region. This type of headache is related to a poorly functioning stomach, most often associated with a lack of proper hydrochloric acid production (also known as hypochlorhydria). Roughly 95% of these cases are due to this lack of hydrochloric acid (HCL) production. The remainder of cases are due to its overproduction. One must perform the Zypan Test (see Appendix B p. 343 for instructions) in order to determine whether the cause is overproduction of HCL or lack of sufficient HCL. Hydrochloric acid is necessary not only to properly begin digestion of food, but also to destroy/neutralize bacteria that may be ingested with a meal.

A condition known as gastritis (inflammation of the stomach lining) can precipitate a frontal headache. The inflammation and damage associated with gastritis prevents the stomach cells, called parietal cells, from being able to properly produce HCL. As a result, food, especially protein, is difficult to digest. This results in the overgrowth of bacteria that would otherwise be neutralized by the HCL. The bacteria begin to break down the proteins which the stomach was unable to digest. They then proliferate, feeding on the undigested food in the stomach, and producing organic acid waste products as they feed. Most of these acids, like butyric acid and proprionate are very caustic to the lining of the stomach.

In this way, the organic acids further compromise the stomach and can lead to gastroesophageal reflux disease (GERD). As the bacterial organic acids build up, they cause the muscular layer of the stomach to spasm, pinching the stomach into an hourglass shape. This results in forcing the stomach contents up into the esophagus and throat. A very common and well-known bacteria, Helicobacter pylori, or H. pylori for short, is often blamed for causing GERD. From a holistic standpoint, it is more important to isolate what has led to the malfunction of the stomach rather than blame the bacteria as the cause. In most cases, a diet rich in processed foods and caustic, artificial, man-made chemicals causes the initial damage to the stomach. Although this is a topic for a different discussion, it bears stating that seeking the advice of a qualified nutritionist is important. *Why Stomach Acid Is Good for You* by Jonathan V. Wright, MD is a helpful resource.

Chiropractically speaking, we expect to find a subluxated vertebra in the upper thoracic region of the spine, *(subluxation refers to the malposition of a vertebral bone which causes irritation to the spinal cord and nervous system. The subluxation is what a chiropractic adjustment serves to correct)* specifically sympathetic innervations being derived from preganglionic fibers arising predominantly from T6 to T8 spinal nerves. Parasympathetic supply is from cranial nerve X, known as the Vagus nerve. Think of it as you would the wiring from the switch on your bedroom wall, traveling up the wall and through the ceiling to the light itself. Without these pathways remaining intact, the light would not receive its message and turn on and off when the switch is operated. The chiropractor must treat this subluxated region and change the patient's diet in order to correct the digestive problem and to prevent its reoccurence.

Nutritionally, the first line of defense in resolving this problem is using a good digestive enzyme (with or without hydrochloric acid depending on the result of the Zypan Test. (Refer to Appendix B p.343 for further information.) Second, it is important to use the herb Licorice Root (also referred to as DGL, or deglycerized licorice) to help heal the damage that has been done to the lining of the stomach. DGL comes in both capsules and in chewable lozenges. The herb should be standardized and taken in the dosage of two lozenges, chewed or sucked on, 10 minutes prior to each meal. For a specific dietary approach for stomach problems, including gastritis and GERD, read Section VI p. 93.

Occipital Headache (Back of the Head)

The fourth category of headache is the occipital, named after the occipital bone of the skull located in the back of the head where the neck begins. This type of headache is usually caused by poor bowel habits such as constipation, gas and bloating. Upon patient examination, we find very tight muscles in the lower thoracic and lumbar spine corresponding to the spinal region which innervates much of the intestinal tract. Abdominal examination reveals food backed-up in the intestines, and tenderness, especially in the area of the ileocecal valve. This is the most common area of trouble because it is the location of a very important valve that connects the last part of the small intestine (ileum) with the first part of the large intestine (cecum). This valve, known as the ileocecal valve, will often become irritated or dysfunctional from poor diet or other problems, causing blockage.

Treating this area with a special reflex treatment and a chiropractic adjustment takes time. However, once this area is relieved of the irritation and blockage, there is a significant change in the body. To treat this area properly, several protocols must be followed. First, the patient must be given intestinal flora (also referred to as Acidophilus, or Probiotics) which are the different types of beneficial bacteria in the intestines. These bacteria live in symbiosis with us. We provide them with a home, and they help us digest our food, ward off harmful bacteria and yeast, and provide us with certain vitamins that we would not otherwise be able to absorb. Second, the patient must take Standard Process Lactic Acid Yeast™. It helps acidify the intestinal tract and provide a beneficial growth environment for the helpful bacteria like acidophilus. Ultimately, this will restore a proper environment to the intestinal tract.

If constipation is not fully relieved with this protocol, there are several other products useful in restoring proper functioning. Swiss

Kriss, Smooth Move tea, and licorice root all help to achieve proper functioning. They do not have to be taken long term and can be discontinued once normal peristalsis and bowel movements return.

Finally, diet must be changed to one with properly prepared complex carbohydrates and lacto-fermented vegetables rich in fiber and nutrients. A diet rich in processed, simple sugars can lead to a build-up of yeast and other harmful microorganisms which create gas, bloating and a slowing of the peristaltic movements of the intestinal tract. Constipating foods like dairy, banana and breads must temporarily be avoided. Furthermore, developing the habit of drinking more water regularly is crucial to restoring a healthy bowel. Specifics on proper diet are in Section III, The Importance of Digestion and the Food We Eat.

"Behind the Eyes" Headache (Lower Forehead)

The fifth category of headache is the lower forehead region, also described as the "behind the eyes" headache. This is known as the sinus headache and is associated with an overproduction/build-up of mucus. It usually begins with stomach and intestinal trouble because of irritation to the intestinal tract or stomach created by processed food or poor combinations of food (see Section III p. 23 on Proper Food Combining for an in-depth discussion).

The stomach and intestinal tract are made up of a specialized mucous lining which serves to protect the tract walls. The mucus, produced by special cells called goblet cells, is meant to prevent damage to the lining of the stomach and intestine as well as to trap bacteria and other harmful pathogens. This is the same mucous lining that covers the walls of our sinuses, throat and lungs.

When this region is irritated, whether from caustic processed foods or the ingestion of poorly combined foods (or any of a myriad of things that can upset the lining of the intestinal tract and stomach), the goblet cells will begin to produce more mucus as a protective mechanism. Constant irritation will lead to the overproduction of mucus which ultimately makes its way up to the sinuses creating congestion. Be attentive the next time you overeat or eat a meal having an excessive amount of processed dairy. You may find that shortly thereafter your sinuses become stuffy. You may not have the headache, but the irritation is there.

Allergies to certain foods can trigger this mucus build-up as well, and will often result in headaches. These headaches are cleared up by getting the patient away from the most irritating foods. The most common allergy-causing foods are conventional dairy, wheat, corn, soy, and even improperly prepared nuts. However, with so many chemicals and artificial ingredients added to our foods, there can be many other triggers. It may be necessary to have the patient follow an elimination diet to identify the true culprit. With today's Standard American Diet so full of processed foods, man-made additives and toxins, this can be a daunting task.

Once the dietary habits of the individual have improved and the common irritants have been removed, one must concentrate on cleaning the sinuses. With a few simple procedures, you can remove the swelling and inflammation of the sinuses that cause these headaches. The following are two very successful procedures.

1. A mixture of one part Glycothymoline (a mouth wash) and 10 parts filtered/purified water. Put this mixture into a Birmingham nasal douche. Lie on your bed or a bench flat on your back with your head hanging over the bed and your nostrils pointing up toward the ceiling. Place the douche into the nostril on one side while holding the spout. Release the spout. This allows the solution to go up into the sinus and will destroy the bacteria that have accumulated in the sinus cavities. Repeat this procedure three times on each nostril. Then put a light coating of castor oil on the sinus areas of your face (in between the eyebrows, just under both eyes, and over the eyebrows). Do this every night.

2. A second product helpful for cleaning the sinuses is Xlear (pronounced Clear). You can use this product by pointing your head toward the floor and spraying the solution up the nostrils toward the top of the head. Repeat this three times on each side and continue to repeat during the day until you have complete relief. If the spray goes into your throat you are doing it wrong. You can also substitute Argentyn 23 Nasal Spray, made by Natural Immunogenics, for the Xclear. (See Appendix D p. 357 for information on Argentyn 23.)

General Headache

The sixth and final type of headache is the general type. The general headache will often be described as occurring all around or throughout the head, and usually manifests as a pounding sensation. In my clinical experience, this is due to a toxic overload, or what many alternative-minded physicians will call autointoxication. Autointoxication is a condition in which there is a fundamental breakdown in the body's organs of cleansing and elimination (the kidneys, liver, intestines, etc.). This leads to the body's inability to remove toxins that originated either in the environment, through the diet, or from metabolism. As a result, many of these toxins are reabsorbed into the bloodstream or are deposited and stored in the fat of the body.

Treatment for this type of headache is a diet exclusively of liquids and vegetable juice, especially lacto-fermented vegetable juice, as well as salads. To be successful in treating the general headache, you must detoxify the colon and thereby assist in detoxification of the kidneys and liver. This is done by taking an enema, or colonic. Many are unfamiliar with the great health benefits of using this technique. See Appendix A p. 321 for instructions on the procedure.

Once this enema protocol is completed, a strict focus on dietary changes must be made. The diet should temporarily be changed to a higher carbohydrate type consisting of whole foods. Breakfast should be ripe fruits spread out throughout the morning. You may eat a different type every 45 minutes to an hour, but do not mix fruit types at any one time. Lunch should consist of a starch meal including either a sweet potato, brown or wild rice, or lentils combined with two green vegetables. All legumes, beans, grains, nuts and seeds should be soaked to remove antinutrients and enable proper digestion (see Appendix C p. 344-46 for soaking instructions). Dinner is to consist of a small salad of mixed greens. Make your own dressing from olive oil, flaxseed oil, unpasteurized organic apple cider vinegar, fresh lemon, Celtic sea salt, mashed avocado (optional) and fresh cracked pepper. With the salad have two steamed or lightly sautéed green vegetables and a 6-8 ounce piece of protein (either fish, chicken, turkey, or lamb). Nuts may be taken as a snack but they must be soaked first and then dried in an oven on low temperature or in a dehydrator (see Appendix C p. 344 for soaking instructions). Nuts must be organic and purchased in sealed packages, NOT from open bins.

Sinus Infections/Sinusitis and Allergies

The next topic is irritation and inflammation of the sinuses of the face. There are two sinuses on either side of the face just above the eyebrows in the lower center of the forehead known as the frontal sinuses; two more located just below the eyes at the cheekbones known as the maxillary; between the eyes at the nasal bridge are the ethmoid sinuses; and finally in the bones behind the nasal cavity are the sphenoid sinuses. The sinuses are lined with a soft, pink tissue known as mucosa. Normally, they are empty except for a thin layer of mucus. Most of the sinuses drain their contents into the nose via a small channel called the middle meatus. It is believed that the purpose of these sinuses is to warm and humidify the air we breathe as well as to function as part of the immune system.

What happens in the case of sinus problems is clear to anyone who has experienced a sinus infection. Inflammation causes mucous build-up, obstructing breathing and creating a pressure within the sinuses that often creates headaches and discomfort. Not only is the person unable to breathe through the nose, they may also find themselves so uncomfortable that they cannot carry out their normal responsibilities. Conventional medicine blames this inflammation and build-up of mucus on either a bacteria or virus, or perhaps an allergen, like pollen or ragweed. Although this may appear on the surface to be true, in most cases the bacteria/virus is merely a symptom of a deeper problem.

In my years of clinical experience, it was people with poor digestive function who had the most sinus trouble. My personal hypothesis on the connection is this: offensive foods or bacteria cause the stomach and intestines to produce more mucus as a protective mechanism. Since the lining or mucosa of the intestinal tract is continuous and very similar in nature to that of the sinuses, anything causing a stimulation of this protective mechanism will also stimulate mucous production in the sinuses. Food that can damage or weaken digestion, also weakens our immune system since most of our immune system is located throughout the digestive tract. With a weakened immune system, any bacteria, virus or yeast will have an easier time finding a place to thrive and cause problems. Our sinuses, being warm and moist, are a great place to start!

The same principle may be true of allergy sufferers. An underlying digestive problem is frequently accompanied by a specific food allergy. When the underlying digestive problems are addressed, the sinus problems and allergies soon disappear or are greatly diminished. Our immune system is now able to handle the viruses and bacteria we are exposed to since a large part of our immune system is spread throughout our digestive tract.

To determine if a food allergy is involved, there are several options. We can carry out kinesiologic testing using specific foods. This can be done by a doctor trained in kinesiology and is highly accurate. A second option is salivary testing that can be done by certain labs. They can test for specific foods allergies to the most common foods: cow's milk, soy, wheat/gluten and corn. They can even test for the most common intestinal parasites through taking a stool sample. These tests are often covered by insurance and are not cost-prohibitive to carry out. For a list of recommended labs see Appendix D p. 355-58.

The most simple, cost-effective way to test for a food allergy is to perform an Elimination Diet. This is done by removing the most commonly offensive foods one by one for a minimum of two weeks while monitoring the changes. Once an offensive food is eliminated, symptoms subside greatly indicating the allergy. After the initial two week period, the food can be slowly reintroduced again, one food at a time, watching for symptoms. It is wise to start with the reintroduction of conventional, pasteurized dairy first (including yogurt, cheeses, etc) as this is the single most common allergy causing food. Then proceed to wheat, corn and soy as these are next in the line of offensive foods, and watch for any symptoms or changes in how you feel.

The normal intestinal environment, or flora, is made up of billions of bacteria from many different genera and species. These bacteria live in a symbiotic relationship with us, providing us with a variety of nutrients while we provide them with a place to live. However, when the environment of the intestinal tract is altered or interfered with, pathogenic (disease causing) bacteria and yeast can take over. This condition, dysbiosis, can be caused by the overuse of antibiotics and other medications. These drugs destroy the normal, healthy intestinal environment and give pathogenic bacteria and yeast a stronghold. People who have recurring sinusitis typically test positive for candidiasis (yeast infections). If this is suspected we do a test called D-arabinitol through a simple urine collection. If concomitant gastrointestinal symptoms are a factor, a stool test may be used as well. We usually use Genova Diagnostics Labs for their high quality, accurate, and technologically advanced methods.

Treatment for conditions related to sinusitis has two parts. First, we treat the source of the problem: the environment and health of the intestinal tract. Second, we treat the sinuses directly to address the symptoms and provide relief. The diet should eliminate all the more common offensive mucus-forming foods. The most problematic foods in order of importance are pasteurized/homogenized dairy (including yogurt, cheese, etc.), wheat and wheat products (think pasta, cakes, cookies, cereals), soy and soy-based products, processed corn and corn products, and conventional (non-organic, CAFO) meats that are high in fat and must also be eliminated temporarily. These foods are not unhealthy in themselves. In fact, the opposite is true. The problem is often how the food is processed (e.g. pasteurization, hybridization, bleaching, milling, etc.) or in some cases how the animals were fed or treated. For more on this discussion, see the later in this section on food processing.

To treat the sinuses, do the following:

1. Use warm compresses over the sinus areas.
2. Use Argentyn 23 Silver Hydrosol Nasal Spray – This product is sold only through professionals and is amazingly effective and safe. To learn where to purchase Argentyn 23 and how to locate physicians in your area who sell it contact Natural Immunogenics Corp. or visit their website at www.natural-immunogenics.com (see Appendix D p. 357 #15).

3. Douche the sinuses with a good quality douche bulb or Neti Pot. One can easily be purchased at most pharmacies. Use a solution of Glycothymoline (a bottle can be purchased for around $10 on www.amazon.com) and water. The appropriate mixture is 10 parts water to one part Glycothymoline. Mix ten ounces of water with one ounce of Glycothymoline and place this mixture in the Neti Pot. Follow the directions that come with the Neti Pot to proceed. This douching can be repeated 2–3 times on each side. Repeat twice a day if necessary until complete relief is achieved. You may also use Argentyn 23 Silver Hydrosol to spray/wash out the sinuses.

4. Castor oil, preferably expeller pressed, unrefined, can be purchased in Whole Foods, at most quality health food stores, or on the internet. A good brand is sold by Heritage Store and can be purchased at www.heritagestore.com. A light coating of the castor oil can be spread onto the skin over the sinus areas before bed each night. This will facilitate circulation throughout the sinuses, helping to keep them clear.

Allergies/Food Sensitivities

Most people become sensitized to pollen, dust, certain food(s) and more. As a result, the body has an immune reaction to that allergen/irritant. Conventional medicine tells us that these food allergies are generally genetic and there is nothing we can do to eliminate them. Conventional patients are often given allergy shots (which contain mercury) or are prescribed harmful allergy medications laden with side effects. A good example of a food allergy is lactose intolerance. African Americans and Asians, due to their genetic makeup, are more likely to have a problem with lactose, the disachharide sugar (two sugars linked together) in milk and other dairy. What is not explained is that raw milk normally contains the lactase enzyme that allows for the easy digestion of this disaccharide. During pasteurization, this enzyme, along with many other nutrients, is destroyed. Actually, the patient is pasteurization intolerant, not lactose intolerant. For readers interested in a more in-depth discussion of this topic, Ron Schmid gives a detailed explanation of this in his book *The Untold Story of Milk*.

Dr. Angelo Rose; Dr. Christopher Amoruso

The one thing that conventional medicine does not test for when treating allergies is the pH of the body. A normal salivary pH reading stays between 6.6 and 7.2. Our pH is a reflection of the inner chemistry of our body. Just as a pool's pH balance must be maintained in order to keep the pool running properly, so our body's pH must be maintained to keep our body running healthfully. In fact, our blood's pH must be regulated within four hundredths of a percentage to sustain life. Most waste products produced by our metabolism and digestion are acidic in nature. If our body builds up too much waste which it cannot remove, whether from poor diet, lack of rest, smoking, etc., then our body is likely to become too acidic.

I have found that patients function best with a pH between 6.8 and 7.0. This is the range at which the body functions best and healing is promoted. Stray anywhere outside of this range and the body will begin to experience inflammation, immune system dysfunction, and illness. My protocol in cases where a patient's pH is too acidic is to put them on an alkaline diet. When this type of diet is maintained, pH will slowly normalize and, in 95% of the cases they will no longer suffer with these allergies. In fact, they will often notice other improvements as well – joint pains diminish, energy increases, and the immune system strengthens.

Looking at the body with regard to balancing the pH, you may wonder how or why allergies can be affected. Different foods are digested in different ways. If there is not an adequate amount of gastric juice and enzymes produced in the stomach and intestines, incomplete breakdown of food results. These partially digested foods begin to ferment and, as a result, yeast and bacteria build up. The combination of fermenting waste and bacteria/yeast irritate and inflame the lining of the digestive tract. Constipation, diarrhea and even mucous stools can result. Ultimately, this alters the body chemistry as nutrients are lost and wastes are reabsorbed through the digestive tract as a result of improper bowel elimination.

What commonly results are sensitivities to acid foods such as grains, nuts, oranges, or even cheese/dairy. In some cases, it is due to the way the foods have been processed. Milling, hydrogenation, genetic modification, bleaching, and bromating deplete vital enzymes and nutrients and can create foreign compounds that our body must now deal with. For example, pasteurization of dairy destroys certain enzymes necessary for its proper digestion. One such enzyme in milk is phosphatase, which is required for the proper absorption of calcium. Damaging these enzymes and other nutrients makes the food more difficult to digest and therefore more irritating to our system.

In other cases, improper preparation of foods makes them difficult to digest. Nuts, seeds, beans, legumes and grains should all be naturally fermented, sprouted or soaked to make their nutrients available for digestion and to remove phytate and enzyme inhibitors (Weston Price Foundation). Improperly prepared foods are difficult to digest. As a result, allergies may develop, especially if the digestive system is already weakened. Most people are unaware of these facts and continue to eat the offending foods. As a person consumes these foods on a regular basis, mucus is produced in the digestive tract as a protective mechanism. This can lead to sinus congestion, swelling, headaches and other allergy symptoms. In rare cases, a person may find that a food they once could eat now causes their throat to itch or swell. Others develop acid rashes or eczema on their skin. Each case is different, though the mechanisms are similar. In the overwhelming majority of allergy cases, poor food choices and poor food combinations are the cause.

One final topic to consider in allergy cases involves food additives. Man-made food additives and preservatives can often result in allergies and health problems. One such additive that causes problems is aspartame. There are many others. Taking a good history including a food diary is necessary to properly rule out allergic reactions to food additives and preservatives. In some cases, testing may be necessary.

To properly treat these cases, I first put the patient on the appropriate diet to adjust the body's pH. I also make use of the elimination diet, removing the most common allergy-causing foods including dairy, wheat, corn, soy and nuts. In some cases I will do stool analysis and IgG4/IgE allergy testing using Genova Diagnostics Labs. Identifying and removing allergy-causing foods allows the digestive system a chance to heal and also removes a big part of what is causing the problem. As the patient's health progresses, these foods can be reintroduced in moderation and monitored for allergies. For these patients, chiropractic adjustment must be centered around the mid-thoracic region from T4–T9 as these relate to the digestive tract. Also, C4 and C6 in the cervical spine must be adjusted to alleviate any subluxation in this region which is intimately connected to the sinuses. Reflexology can be used to treat all of the necessary digestive zones involved.

A helpful remedy in working with allergies is the use of organic apple cider vinegar. Two teaspoons can be mixed into 8 ounces of warm water with ½ tsp of raw, local honey and sipped with each meal (see Appendix A p. 321). This will help improve digestion and alkalize the body's pH at the same time. Furthermore, raw honey (must be unheated, unrefined, unfiltered and unprocessed) has been used for a long time to treat allergies with great success. We can also make use of natural homeopathic remedies like *Euphrasia officianalis, Urtica doica, Hydrastis canadensis* and others. They are often combined in a formula to help with nasal congestion. Work with a professional for the appropriate choices and dosage.

Conditions of the Ear

Middle Ear Infections/Otitis Media

Most ear problems develop as a direct result of sinus infections or from problems in the throat. The reason for this requires a simple lesson in anatomy (illustration on p. 63). The eustachian tube, also known as the phayrngotympanic or auditory tube, is a canal that connects the middle ear to the back of the throat (pharynx). It is lined with mucus, just like the nose and throat. It helps to clear fluids out of the middle ear and maintain a proper pressure balance between the inner and outer ear. Colds and allergies can cause irritation of the eustachian tube and cause the mucosal lining of this passageway to become swollen and filled with fluid. If the eustachian tube becomes blocked, fluid can easily build up in the middle ear. This creates the perfect environment for bacteria and viruses (like the virus that causes the common cold) to create an infection which in turn causes the ear drum to swell and bulge.

What causes the eustachian tube to become blocked or inflamed and lead to an ear infection? Simply stated, the eustachian tube can be blocked from mucus build-up in the throat (also swelling from the adenoids, which are tiny lymphatic glands high in the back of the throat) and/or from a post-nasal drip related to a pre-existing sinus condition. Infection results from the simple anatomical proximity and connection between the eustachian tube and the back of the pharynx. Bacteria from irritated, congested sinuses travel into the eustachian tube via transport from the nasopharynx when we sniff and swallow or have a post-nasal drip. In this way bacteria and viruses easily spread up the tube and create an infection site in the middle ear. But what causes this mucus build-up in the sinuses in the first place? Typically, irritation to the digestive tract from poor eating habits, food additives and artificial flavors, etc., cause an increase in the production of mucus to protect the lining of the stomach and intestinal wall. When this irritation becomes chronic, overproduction of mucus in the membranes of the sinuses and lungs can occur. This commonly happens when an allergy-causing food like pasteurized milk in infant formulas is consumed regularly.

Symptoms that commonly accompany this type of problem are lung and sinus congestion, dizziness, constant sniffling/runny or encrusted nose, acute pain in the ear (may be worse lying down), fever, and trouble hearing. In some children too young to speak and tell us where they have pain, the only symptom may be a constant tugging on the ear or a refusal to drink from the bottle as swallowing will increase the pain. It is very common for children and infants drinking cow's milk or milk-/soy-based formulas from a bottle, especially while lying down, to develop an ear infection.

Since we have previously discussed how conventional pasteurized cow's milk, wheat, most starches and soy products are common mucus producers, it isn't hard to understand how these foods can create or contribute to an ear infection. Once the mucus begins to build up and block the eustachian tube and clog the lymphatic drainage of the area, the middle ear is prone to infection by bacteria and viruses. (See diagram on p. 63.) It is crucial for children and adults alike to avoid all conventional pasteurized dairy products,

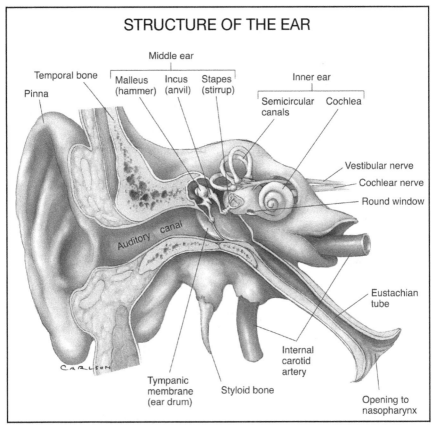

EarAnatomy ©Dave Carlson

as well as conventional wheat, soy and corn (a good idea for most of us anyway). It may also be necessary to remove eggs, beans and other starches (especially the root vegetables like potato, parsnips, squash, etc.). This should be determined by a qualified physician. Remember, always treat the gut first!

The chiropractic and natural treatment for this condition is centered around proper diet, chiropractic manipulation of the cervical spine and soft tissue techniques to increase lymphatic drainage in the area of the ear. In doing so, we facilitate the lymphatics in all of the cervical area to drain the waste accumulating from the infection and enable the immune system to restore a healthy environment and eliminate the bacteria and viruses. Soft tissue work will include stretching and adjusting the ear itself to facilitate better blood flow and therefore healing. Not all chiropractors are familiar with this technique, so one may need to ask.

Treatment also consists of several natural protocols available in our own kitchen or from a nearby health food store.

First, use sweet oil (refined olive oil) drops in the ear. At bedtime, place two drops of sweet oil into the affected ear while in a side-lying position (affected ear facing up). Place a small cotton ball in the ear. In the morning remove the cotton. Repeat as needed.

Second, fresh oregano can be used as follows:

Place one heaping tablepoon of oregano into one quart boiling water. Remove from the stove immediately after adding the oregano and cover, allowing it to steep (approximately 3–5 minutes).

Allow to cool to tepid temperature so that it will not burn you.

While lying on your side with the involved ear facing upward, place oregano tea into ear until ear is approximately half full. Place a piece of cotton in the ear and stay in that position for approximately 15 minutes. Repeat twice a day.

Third, a protocol involving castor oil will help. Take a small amount of castor oil on your finger and coat the area around the ear, front and back. Do this at night before bed and again in the morning (see Appendix D p. 356 for information on The Heritage Company for high quality castor oil).

Finally, one can use homeopathic cell salts to aid the immune system in reestablishing balance. Using tissue cell salts #4 (Ferrum Phosphate) and #12 (Silica), take 4 tablets of each cell salt three times per day under the tongue, waiting 5 minutes in between each cell salt. Take until the condition has resolved. Tissue cell salts are available at most health food stores.

During any problems with the ear, it is also very important to remember to keep the nose and sinuses as open and clear as possible. It may be necessary to use the Netti Pot and, as previously noted, to remove all dairy, wheat products, refined sugars, corn and soy. (See list of sugars in Appendix C p. 354-55 under the heading *The Forgettable 40.*)

Earache

Earaches can be very painful. The following are natural treatments that I have used over the years with great success:

1. A combination of Garlic, Mullein and St John's Wort in liquid drops. Work with your practitioner for dosages.
2. Olive Leaf Extract, used to fight infection. Can be purchased in capsules and taken as directed.
3. Onion Poultice: cut a large onion in half and place it into the oven and heat it until it is half cooked. Remove from the oven and place onion into a white athletic sock (you may also use gauze). Place this against the ear when it is nice and warm. Be careful not to burn yourself! This will have a drawing effect on the pressure that builds in the ear during an earache.
4. Place a few drops of warm olive oil into the ear.
5. Make a paste with onion powder and warm water. Place it around the outside of the ear surrounding the opening of the canal. This will relieve the pain.
6. Argentyn 23 Colloidal Silver Nasal Spray (Appendix D p. 357#15) – Follow the directions on bottle, spraying the sinuses repeatedly throughout the day, or as directed by your physician.
7. Blue Ice™ Fermented Cod Liver Oil – Give 1 tsp per day to help support the immune system.

Tinnitus

Tinnitus is the perception of sound within the human ear in the absence of a corresponding external sound. More commonly, it is referred to as "ringing in the ears." It can be a slight annoyance for some and a debilitating problem for others. It is believed that the ringing is caused by an overproduction of endolymph fluid which can cause dizziness as well as the ringing noise. In my practice, I came to find that tinnitus is most commonly caused by longstanding sinus problems, taking aspirin which can cause the eardrum to inflame, side effects from other medications, and arthritic changes inside the ear. The cure for tinnitus has eluded the medical profession for many years.

The first step in treatment of tinnitus is to eliminate the possibility that it is a medication causing the problem. I make use of WebMD's database on side effects to check each medication that the patient is on. Second, you must perform a proper examination of the ear to check for excess wax and/or ear drum inflammation. An inflamed eardrum will appear bulging and shiny whereas a healthy drum appears flat and pearly white in color. If this is found, the patient's sinuses must be cleared before any improvement of the tinnitus can be seen. For treatment protocols, refer to page 55 of this section on sinus conditions.

Treatment protocol

Innervation of the external ear is provided by Cranial Nerves V (Trigeminal Nerve), VII (Facial Nerve), IX (Glossopharyngeal Nerve) and X (Vagus Nerve). The nerve supply of the inner ear is provided by Cranial Nerve VIII (Vestibulocochlear Nerve). Therefore, chiropractic treatment must address the upper cervical spine, especially the Atlas (C1) and Axis (C2). This will help facilitate better movement of the cerebrospinal fluid and better drainage of the lymphatics in the neck. Lymphatic drainage to the sinuses/cervical region plays an important role in the treatment because it is believed that overproduction of the endolymph in the ear results in a degeneration in the tiny hairs that transmit sound vibrations within the inner ear. Therefore, soft tissue work to the ear, cervical spine and manual sinus drainage are crucial in the treatment of tinnitus. See the previous section on the ear and the sinuses for these protocols.

Finally, my nutritional approach to treating tinnitus is aimed at improving tissue oxygenation. The supplements are as follows:

1. Co-Enzyme Q10 – 100 mg per day. Preferably taken in the ubiquinol form. Do not purchase the powdered form.
2. Active vitamin A (Retinol) – Best taken from fermented, high-vitamin cod liver oil. Dosages vary from a scant ¼ tsp per day for children to two tablespoons per day for adults. Consult with a qualified practitioner for specifics.
3. Argentyn 23 Silver Hydrosol (see Appendix D p. 357 #15) – This is a liquid and can be taken by adding drops directly to

the mouth sublingually. Consult with a physician for more information.
4. Flaxseed Oil – Take two tablespoons per day. Use either Barlean's or Udo's oil. Both are available in most health food stores.
5. Magnesium – Preferably in the lactate form (Standard Process). Take the equivalent of 750–1,000 mg per day. Magnesium has been shown to help prevent damage to the hair cells in the inner ear.
6. Manganese – 10–20 mg per day. Deficiency of this important trace mineral has been linked to tinnitus.
7. EDTA (Ethylene Diamine Tetraacetic Acid) – consult with a knowledgeable physician.

Conditions of the Eye

Conjunctivitis (Pink Eye)

The eye can become infected from any problem that originates in the nasal passages. It is a good idea to check the nose in many cases of eye problems. For conjunctivitis many doctors will immediately administer antibiotics, while others take a more holistic view. In my experience, a natural holistic approach produces excellent results. We must first appreciate that the eye is constantly bathing in a fluid that keeps it moist and clean. This fluid, in part, is drained through the sinuses in the corner of the eye adjacent to the nose.

First the nose and sinuses must be rinsed according to the protocols outlined in the previous section. This is accomplished using a Neti Pot and Glycothymoline as described. Then, the eye must be washed out with a solution of one teaspoon of pure witch hazel mixed into 8 ounces of ice cold pure filtered water (do not use tap water). Put this mixture into an eye cup (you may also use a shot glass if you do not have an eye cup) and flush out the eye by holding the cup to your eye, tipping your head back, and allowing the mixture to wash into the open eye. Try to keep your eye open so that the mixture comes into contact with the eye. If you have difficulty keeping your eye open, try blinking into the cup a few times. This will ensure that some of the fluid comes into contact with the eye as needed. Flush out each eye as described 3 times. Repeat in the morning, afternoon and evening. At night, coat the upper and lower lids and across the bridge of the nose with castor oil. This is done to bring blood to the area. Castor oil has a wonderful ability to dilate the blood vessels under the skin and thereby help improve circulation and drainage. Use only cold-pressed extra virgin unrefined castor oil. This protocol may also be used for any hemorrhages of the eye where a blood vessel breaks (as often occurs if the eye is hit or during colds and infections).

The most important vitamins for overall eye health are the bioflavonoids (also known as vitamin P), vitamin A (cod liver oil), and vitamin E all from natural, whole food sources. (See p. 29 on General Nutritional Guidelines in Section III for more information). Vitamin E should be sourced from wheat germ oil or other natural, whole food sources to contain all of the mixed tocopherols, selenium and the tocotrienol compounds. I recommend Standard Process Cataplex® E at a dose of six per day (two with each meal). Vitamin A is best utilized in its active retinol form found in pure, fermented high vitamin cod liver oil (see Appendix D p. 355 #4 for more information on where to purchase). Take 2-3 capsules with food in the warmer months, and up to 6 per day in the winter months. As for vitamins C and P (bioflavonoids), I recommend Standard Process Cataplex® A-C-P or Cyruta®. Both are excellent sources of the C and P family in their whole food form. Take 3-6 per day with food. You may also use the Synergy Company's Pure Radiance Vitamin C as it is a high quality whole food supplement made from different organic berries/fruits like Camu camu. Dosages for Pure Radiance C will vary according to your needs, but generally I recommend anywhere from ½ teaspoon a day as maintenance up to several tablespoons per day.

Styes

A second, very common condition of the eye is known as a stye. A stye may also be confused with a similar condition known as chalazion. Styes are infections in the eye that form lumps along the edge or periphery of the eyelid (upper or lower). They appear as small, red lumps that may be painful or annoying. If the stye forms on the inside of the eyelid, it is called a hordeolum. A chalazion is a slightly larger lump in the eyelid that is usually not painful. These two conditions can often occur in patients who have experienced inflammation of the eyelid, a condition known as blepharitis.

The treatment for these conditions is as follows. Using a plain black, Lipton tea bag or chamomile tea, place the tea bag in warm water just long enough to warm the tea bag so that it will not burn you. Place the warm tea bag on the eye over the affected area for 20–30 minutes. Repeat this three times per day. At bed time, place a coating of castor oil over the area of the stye on the lid of the eye. Repeat until the stye is gone. This normally takes only a few days.

Floaters and Glaucoma

Eye floaters are black or grey spots which can spontaneously appear in your vision field. Eye floaters may look like black or gray specks, strings or cobwebs that drift about when you move your eyes. The Mayo Clinic's website states that "most eye floaters are caused by age-related changes that occur as the jelly-like substance (vitreous) inside your eyes becomes more liquid. When this happens, microscopic fibers within the vitreous tend to clump together and can cast tiny shadows on your retina, which you may see as eye floaters." They explain further, "over time, the vitreous changes in consistency and partially liquefies — a process that causes it to shrink and pull away from the interior surface of the eyeball. As the vitreous shrinks and sags, it clumps up and gets stringy. Bits of this debris block some of the light passing through the eye, casting tiny shadows on your retina."

Conventional medical treatment for floaters usually involves one of two options for the patient. The first is to wait and/or learn to live with the floaters. Over time, they can settle out of the visual field or the patient can learn to ignore them to a significant enough degree as to be able to live without much of a problem. When this isn't the case, conventional medicine usually recommends vitrectomy, or removal of the gel-like vitreous liquid. In its place a synthetic solution is pumped to help the eye maintain its shape. Eventually the eye will make new vitreous fluid to replace the solution, but this does not necessarily stop new floaters from forming. Furthermore, there are risks with the surgery including bleeding and retinal tears.

Floaters may also result from having previous eye surgery, trauma, diabetic retinopathy, and even from glaucoma. Glaucoma is an increase in the intraocular pressure (pressure within the eye) which, in most cases, occurs slowly over time. In my experience and opinion, many floaters that persist for longer periods of time without disappearing are caused by glaucoma. In many cases, if this condition is not addressed promptly, it can lead to blindness. Important to note is that certain medications, especially corticosteroids like prednisone, are known to cause glaucoma. Conventional treatment for glaucoma usually first involves eye drops to reduce formation of fluid in the front of the eye. These eye drops can often have side effects which affect the heart and lungs and are therefore, in my opinion, not the best option in most cases. A second option is laser surgeries which all attempt to force the fluid to flow better through the eye.

There are many natural things which I have used over the years to treat glaucoma and floaters successfully. I have typically treated glaucoma nutritionally by changing the diet first. Glaucoma is typically associated with the SAD of processed carbohydrates and refined sugars. This is why diabetics have a greater risk for developing both floaters and glaucoma. Sadly, this fact is almost never considered as part of a conservative and natural treatment plan. Therefore, in my office, changing the diet is the first step in attempting to correct these two problems of the eye. The patient must be counseled to avoid high glycemic foods which consist of essentially all processed carbohydrates and many higher-starch vegetables and fruits. Removing all fluids (including juices and alcohol) except for purified water is also essential. For the specifics consult this book's Section XI p. 215 on diabetes.

Supplementation for the eye begins with a high quality cod liver oil. For this I recommend Green Pasture™ Blue Ice™ Fermented Cod Liver Oil at a dose ranging from 1 teaspoon per day up to two tablespoon per day. High-quality cod liver oil like this is rich in vitamin A, omega-3 fatty acids and myriad other compounds crucial to reducing inflammation and restoring function to the eye.

Secondly, to lower the pressure in the eye, we use A-C Carbamide® made by Standard Process. This supplement consists of natural compounds which work together to act as a natural diuretic and promote healthy fluid balance, a key to resolving glaucoma and therefore floaters. We also use Oculotrophin PMG® as well as Iplex® by Standard Process. Oculotrophin provides the eye with all of the nucleoprotein-mineral extracts the eye cells need for growth and differentiation. Iplex®, a product which helps support normal eye function, especially the vascular, cellular and connective tissue of the eye, is also very helpful. Dosages are based on individual needs, but are typically 3–9 Oculotrophin PMG® per day; 3–6 Iplex per day; 6 capsules per day of AC Carbamide®.

Common Conditions of Mouth, Tongue, Throat

Bruxism (Grinding of the Teeth)

Bruxism, a condition related to a calcium and pantothenic acid (vitamin B5) deficiency, can cause loosening of the teeth and receding gums. A warning sign is sensitivity to hot and cold foods and drink. It is usually necessary in the short term to supplement the patient with 500 mgs of vitamin B5 two times per day or in the form of a B-100 complex taken with food. The calcium, preferably calcium lactate, must be taken with a full glass of water on an empty stomach. In general, patients with B-vitamin deficiency will benefit from taking a urine organic acids test using the Genova Diagnostics Lab. The test is easy to do, affordable and can be completed with a kit in the privacy of your own home.

There are several other vitamins that are very helpful in the event of bone loss. Standard Process has two vitamins called Biost® and Biodent® that restore bone. I have seen cases where teeth that were once loose became firm and hard again. Although not a dentist, I have had many patients ask me about this problem. Trying the aforementioned suggestions, most of my patients have achieved amazing results with their teeth. It is important to remember that nothing takes the place of a good diet.

For a complete treatment to strengthen the teeth and overall oral health, you must examine the gut and digestive function. We do this through the Genova Diagnostics Lab by using a stool test known as the GI Effects Complete Stool Profile. This test is informative because it tells us whether the patient has the proper probiotic bacteria in their intestinal tract as well as many other important markers of digestive function. This includes a measurement of pancreatic and biliary function, screening for gluten sensitivity as well as testing for yeast, pathogenic bacteria, and even parasites. Based on the results, the physician can make specific adjustments to your diet and supplement recommendations. Once the health of the gut is improved, the teeth will also improve.

Bleeding Gums

Bleeding of the gums is a very serious problem and should be addressed expeditiously. First consult with your holistic physician to determine if you have a digestive or intestinal problem. This may require stool testing and/or a 4 Rs protocol to treat the underlying cause of poor digestion. Digestive disorders almost always precede bleeding of the gums and a more serious condition called pyorrhea. If pyorrhea is not treated immediately it will almost certainly lead to loss of teeth and can even spread infection via the circulation in the gums to other parts of the body including the heart and brain. Furthermore, since bleeding of the gums usually signifies a vitamin C and vitamin P (Bioflavonoid) deficiency, there are cardiovascular ramifications as well.

Once the underlying digestive disorder is under control, the following supplements must be implemented:

1. Natural vitamin C including the vitamin P factors (the Bioflavonoids) – We use Cataplex® C by Standard Process at a dose of six per day or Pure Radiance Vitamin C by The Synergy Company at dose of six per day.
2. Bio Dent® by Standard Process – three tablets per day
3. Biost® by Standard Process – three per day
4. Cataplex® ACP by Standard Process – three per day

Thrush/Candidiasis

Candidiasis, a very common ailment, is usually accompanied by a thick, white coating on the tongue known as thrush. This is indicative of a predominance of yeast in the body and may be accompanied by the following symptoms: fatigue, inability to focus or concentrate, anxiety, depression, urinary symptoms, mood swings and more. A good book on this subject is *The Yeast Connection*, by William G. Crook, MD or *The Yeast Syndrome* by John Trowbridge, MD. They include all of the specific information you will need regarding changing your diet and, when combined with the information below, will help you conquer this difficult and stubborn problem.

To confirm the diagnosis of candidiasis clinically, we can test for the presence of yeast in the system by performing a special stool test. This test can be ordered by your physician through special labs that do this type of testing. The lab sends you a kit with all of the directions and tools you will need to take the sample needed to evaluate your condition. This sample is then sent back to the lab for testing. One lab that does this testing is DiagnosTechs Lab in Kent, WA (www.diagnostechs.com). The test is very affordable and can be helpful in confirming a diagnosis when symptoms are unclear.

Why is candidiasis such a common problem? The overuse of antibiotics is partially to blame. Many doctors do not explain to their patients that antibiotic usage not only kills bad bacteria, it also destroys the good, the very same bacteria that we depend on to protect our intestinal mucosa (lining) and keep our digestive tract healthy. Furthermore, use of antibiotics opens up the door to yeast and other opportunistic pathogens, some of which are resistant to that specific antibiotic. Antibiotics are designed to work against bacteria. Yeast and viruses are not bacteria and are not affected by antibiotics. Frequently, a patient will take an antibiotic for one problem, and end up with another.

The first line of defense with candidiasis is proper diet. Some foods which are excellent at killing off yeast are garlic, broccoli, cabbage, onions, plain raw yogurt, turnips and most other green vegetables. Reduce the intake of yeast-laden foods such as industrially prepared pickles, ketchup, baked goods, cakes, fruits — especially raisins, figs, apricots, other dried fruits, juices, processed white sugar, and honey. For detailed information and a complete list of allowable foods and supplements, see the two books mentioned earlier.

After eliminating dietary sources of yeast, it is wise to enlist the help of some natural remedies. Yeast can be very difficult to remove from the body as they are known to use their hyphae (somewhat like legs) to burrow into the walls of the intestine and anchor themselves. The first approach I use is administering an escalating dosage of MMS also known as chlorine dioxide (for information on how to order and use, see Appendix D p. 357 #14). Chlorine dioxide is powerful against viruses and is a potent antibiotic as well as fungicide (kills yeast and fungi as well). It comes in a liquid which must be activated. To do this, we use a liquid solution of citric acid (the very same citric acid found in lemons and other citrus fruits) mixed with the MMS to form active chlorine dioxide. Once the liquid chlorine dioxide is activated, it can be added to water and taken internally twice per day. Then, successively add one more drop each day or two until you reach 15 drops. Once you reach the 15 drop dosage, you stay at this dosage for one week before tapering back down to a maintenance dose of 4 drops twice per day.

A second powerful antifungal product that can be used to fight candidiasis is the herb pau d'arco, named after the South American tree from which it is extracted. It contains, among other things, selenium which is one of our body's natural defenses against yeast infections both internally (vaginal or intestinal/systemic) and topically (athlete's foot, etc.). I recommend using the herb to make a tea. This herbal tea is perhaps the most widely used method of taking this herb. Taheebo tea, another name for pau d'arco, may be found in most health food stores as well as on the internet. To prepare the pau d'arco tea, mix 3–6 tablespoons of the inner bark tea with one quart of cold, distilled water in a teapot. Use a glass or stainless steel teapot, not one of aluminum, tin, or other type. If using tea bags, you may follow their ratios instead of measuring by tablespoons. Allow the herbal tea to reach a boil, and then let it slow boil for 20 minutes or longer. This allows the beneficial compounds such as lapacho to be disseminated. Once 20 minutes of slow boiling have passed, the compounds have been released into the tea drink, and it is ready to be removed from the heat.

There is one more antifungal product which bears mentioning that I have used with some success to treat candidiasis. It is known as caprylic acid and is available in most health food stores and can be taken orally to treat internal yeast infections. It is sometimes sold as a product known as Yeast Fighters. It should be taken 2–3 times per day while following the anti-yeast diet previously described. Some other products I have used over the years with success are

OrthoMolecular's Candicid Forte and GI Microbe-X by Designs for Health, and Lauricidin, a concentrated form of lauric acid, a fat extracted from coconut.

Conditions Affecting the Tongue

Glossitis/Burning/Painful Tongue (Glossodynia)

Burning, painful tongue, another common condition of the mouth, can be treated successfully without medication. This condition is usually caused by a poor digestive system with resultant vitamin deficiency, and one has to look specifically at the stomach to get to its cause. In many cases where a patient presents with a painful, burning tongue, the stomach is unable to digest food properly. This leads to a failure to produce proper digestive enzymes and therefore a failure to break down food completely. As a result, malabsorption of certain B vitamins, particularly vitamin B3 (niacin) occurs. The tongue will often appear reddened and the patient will complain of burning/pain on the surface of the tongue. Swelling and redness start at the tip and lateral margins of the tongue and progress to cover the entire surface. (Wild D. The skin, tongue, and nails speak. Loveland CO: Unique Perspective Press; 2012. p. 36–37.) Interestingly, a vitamin B-3 deficiency can also appear as fissures (cracking) on the lips.

The diet for this condition should consist not only of foods rich in B vitamins, it should also be based on more easily digested whole foods while avoiding processed, refined foods like white flour, sugar, and alcohol. In the initial phases, the diet should be shifted to 90% whole fruits and vegetables, beans/legumes and brown/wild rice (soaked according to the directions in Appendix C p. 344). As far as supplementation to help aid this condition, I use Standard Process Cataplex® B and Cataplex® G. These two whole food vitamins will provide the niacin as well as the complete B complex necessary to support the healing of this condition. Later on, as digestion improves, organic liver can be added as it is a tremendously rich source of B vitamin and iron.

Chiropractic treatment for this condition should be focused on the region of the spine which innervates the stomach and upper gastrointestinal tract. The region that corresponds to this area of the digestive tract is the 4th through 6th thoracic vertebrae (see Vertebral Subluxation and Nerve Chart in Appendix G p. 364). Chiropractic adjustment must treat and correct the misaligned (subluxated) vertebrae in this area. Almost without exception, the patient will feel great sensitivity and pain when these three vertebrae are palpated. This is caused by the stomach, irritated and inflamed, constantly sending a noxious signal to that region of the spine. When this noxious signal is constant over a long period of time, the spine and the muscles surrounding that area become contracted and irritated. This causes the vertebrae to shift out of position relative to the vertebrae above and below. When this misalignment is corrected, the nervous system is better able to communicate back and forth from the brain to the stomach and vice versa. With this help the body can use its own innate intelligence to begin the healing process. The best solution to this condition is to correct the dietary problems that created the stomach inflammation in the first place.

A final important consideration in the treatment of this condition is the use of Bennett Technique, a form of reflexology performed on the abdomen that helps the nervous system in healing the irritated areas of the gastrointestinal tract. It relaxes the muscular wall of the intestine as well as the gallbladder and facilitates proper movement of the bowel. If the bowels are not normalized (2–3 bowel movements per day) further supplementation with magnesium or other natural laxatives as well as enemas may temporarily be needed. Consult your physician for further information.

A very similar condition to the burning, painful tongue is the brown coated tongue. This indicates a specific problem with the gallbladder, an important organ responsible for proper digestion of fats, removal of wastes, and many other functions. It must be treated with proper diet and chiropractic treatment. The first step is to change the diet as follows: reduce the "bad" fat intake from fried foods, conventional pasteurized dairy, and processed vegetable oils as well as refined sugars as these are the most offensive to the gallbladder. The second step is to cleanse the gallbladder naturally using a combination of 2 ounces of extra virgin, cold-pressed olive oil with 2 ounces of freshly squeezed lemon juice. Mix the two and just before bed, drink the 4 ounce mixture. Then lie on your right side for 15 minutes, with your right knee bent up toward your chest and with a hot water bottle covering your lower right rib cage (at the side of your body where your ribs end). Finally, you must go right to sleep after following this procedure. In the morning, you may notice you have a loose bowel movement. Take note that you may see small, round and oval pea-shaped stones floating in the toilet. They are usually green or tan in color and gelatinous in texture. These gallstones, or "sand", are responsible for clogging the bile ducts and create inflammation in the gallbladder, thus preventing proper movement of bile from the liver and gallbladder into the intestinal tract. This procedure should be repeated two nights in a row for a proper cleansing to treat this condition. In fact, it is a good idea to perform this cleansing a few times per year to cleanse the gallbladder and promote healthy digestion. For a more thorough cleansing of the gallbladder, read *The Miracle Gallbladder and Liver Flush* by Andreas Moritz.

One last note of importance : with vitamin B-12 deficiency, a patient may present with a swollen and painful tongue similar to what was described above, but with a glossy appearance. Regardless, the treatment consists of improving the digestion of the patient with supplemental vitamin B-complex, and avoidance of refined/processed foods and alcohol, all of which deplete B vitamins.

Angular Stomatitis

Angular stomatitis, inflammation and cracking at the angles of the mouth, is a common condition resulting from the SAD. The patient will often complain of concomitant sore throat or even atrophy of the taste buds. (Wild p. 34–35) This is another clear sign of B vitamin deficiency like glossodynia, but in this case it is specifically related to vitamin B-2 (riboflavin). The tongue is often involved and will present with a purplish or magenta color. (Ibid p. 34)

Treatment for this is identical to the treatment of glossodynia in the previous section. I am not in favor of using synthetic vitamins, therefore riboflavin alone is not prescribed. Use Cataplex® B and Cataplex® G by Standard Process to provide the entire B Complex family and make the necessary dietary changes. It is also wise to increase ones intake of whole foods rich in riboflavin and other B-vitamins, such as freshly ground liver, soaked whole grains, and raw dairy. For more imformation, see Section III p. 29 on general dietary guidelines.

Fissured/Cracked Tongue

A fissured/cracked tongue signals a long-standing B-complex deficiency as well as more serious stomach and intestinal issues. This situation often involves gastritis and/or ulcers, whether gastric or peptic. Any patient presenting with this type of tongue should be given a thorough history and a physical examination including abdominal exam. Subluxation of the mid-thoracic verterbrae (T4–T6) will often be present, and must be addressed and corrected with chiropractic treatment. Furthermore, the patient must be counseled on dietary changes specifically to relieve the digestive tract. The specific protocol for this ailment is found in Section VI p. 93 on GERD and Indigestion as well as in Section III, The Importance of Proper Digestion.

Geographic Tongue

In geographic tongue, the surface of the tongue appears with alternating patches of white and red resembling the land masses of a map. (Ibid p. 56) Geographic tongue almost always indicates candidiasis, a systemic yeast. For treatment information, refer to p. 72 on Thrush/Candidiasis as well as Section III. Work with a practitioner familiar with the 4 Rs approach to cleansing the gut and consult Natasha Campbell McBride's book *The Gut and Psychology Syndrome*.

Sore Throat/Swollen Tonsils

When we become ill, our instinct to run to our medical doctors for antibiotics indicates we may have forgotten how to think for ourselves, neglecting to apply a little common sense and old-fashioned know-how. Nowhere is this more true than in cases of strep/sore throats which are often, but not always, accompanied by a cold or flu, and even swollen tonsils. Sore throats can be caused by several different factors. Most commonly it is a postnasal drip that spreads bacteria to the posterior pharynx (throat). In this case the patient may experience on and off bouts of soreness with seemingly no cause. Secondly, a sore throat can be caused by a general immune system weakness with a concomitant vitamin/mineral deficiency.

My philosophy is this: our body is well-equipped with an immune system chock-full of specialized cells and lymphatic glands designed to deal with bacterial and viral invaders. These lymphatic glands are spread throughout the body, including the neck and throat. In the throat, we call these glands tonsils and adenoids but they are merely branches of our immune system in place to eradicate cellular waste and foreign invaders. The crucial point is that western medicine blames the bacterium for the infection. The villain is a bacterium in the genus Streptococcus (hence the expression "strep throat"). It is my contention that bacteria are NOT the true causative agent as we have been led to believe.

When our bodies are deprived of the proper balance of nutrients found in a truly unprocessed, whole food diet, our immune system suffers. Modern processing of food, as well as all of the colorings and preservatives conspire to deplete important nutrients our immune system needs, overwhelming our body's detoxification pathways. Add to this the stress of modern living, mental/emotional stress, smoking, alcohol, lack of proper rest, and it should not be difficult to see how our bodies can become run-down. Ultimately this leads to a toxic overload of waste, a build-up that burdens our immune system. Remember, our cells produce waste of their own on a daily basis which must be handled by our immune cells. Eventually the immune system reaches a breaking point where it can no longer keep up with the burden being presented to it. The result is that any opportunistic bacterium, whether from outside sources or those already present in the body, or any virus, is free to take over and shift the balance of power toward illness. This can happen in any tissue in the body.

Are invading bacteria and viruses really to blame? In my opinion, no. In most cases, a healthy immune system would easily handle the situation and keep them at bay. In fact, many researchers and alternative doctors will tell you that bacteria and viruses are merely trying to help break down and deal with the waste that our immune system can no longer handle. They are a last-ditch effort to clean up the waste our body isn't handling on its own. When this waste is constantly burdening our depleted body, there are consequences–the symptoms of a sore throat, muscle spasms of the neck and upper back, headache and so on. The next time you blame a fellow worker or family member for passing you their cold, consider looking inward at your own habits and how you are treating your body.

We return to the sore throat situation. What can we do to address this problem without using potentially harmful antibiotics and medications? That depends on how run-down the patient is.

Generally speaking, here is what one must know/do:

1. Gargle using a mixture of 2 oz. of 3% hydrogen peroxide (any pharmacy) and 2 oz. of filtered or spring water. Take small sips, one at a time until all 4 oz. are gone. Tilting your head back, try to gargle as long as you can with each mouthful. Spit out and repeat until all 4 oz. are gone. Do not worry if you accidentally drink a little, it will not hurt you. Do this 2 or 3 times per day. You may also substitute fresh pineapple juice for the hydrogen peroxide as the enzymes in the pineapple juice are excellent for killing the bacteria.

2. Herbal Throat Spray Phytosynergist by Standard Process/ Mediherb. This spray is excellent for soothing the throat and supporting the immune system. Use 4 sprays into the mouth every 2 hours until relief is established. For children, use 1–2 sprays.

3. Argentyn 23 Silver Hydrosol throat spray by Natural Immunogenics Corp (see Appendix D #15 for information on ordering). This is quite effective and can be taken under the tongue as well as gargled with.

4. Zinc Chelate Lozenges. This form of zinc is necessary for proper immune system function. Take 2–3 lozenges per day until relief is established. You may also use Elderberry Lozenges which can be found in most health foods stores.

5. Glycothymoline. Mix one part glycothymoline to 10 parts water and use as a gargle. You may also sniff the mixture up the nasal passages and into the throat. This will act as an antibiotic without the side effects. Glycothymoline is available online through The Heritage Store (see Appendix D p. 358 #21).

6. Simplify the diet. Most importantly, eliminate all of the common food allergens like pasteurized/homogenized dairy and soy, soda, white flour, and other processed foods. Eat only green non-starchy vegetables, especially lacto-fermented vegetables as well as fresh bone broth soups and pastured meats. Follow the dietary guidelines in Section III. *Nourishing Traditions* by Sally Fallon contains instructions for making bone-broth soups.
7. High Vitamin Fermented Cod Liver Oil. Two teaspoons a day or 6–8 capsules for adults. For children, see dosages listed in Appendix A p. 320. We prefer Green Pasture™ Cod Liver Oil products.
8. In more severe cases, support the immune system with Congaplex®, Immuplex®, and Thymex® (all made by Standard Process). For more on how to treat colds and the flu, refer to our protocols in the next section, Section V page 88.

Chiropractic treatment protocol

9. The final step in treating this condition is some soft tissue stretching and a good chiropractic adjustment, specifically to the cervical spine. Soft tissue work to stretch and pump the lymphatic glands and muscles of the neck will aid the body in removing the waste that has accumulated in the area. Many chiropractors, massage therapists, and physical therapists will know how to do this. This will aid the struggling immune system and hasten recovery.

Finally, I would like to consider the topic of swollen tonsils. I have treated many children and adults where the tonsils were so swollen and large they nearly occluded the throat, and in many cases were even pustulated. Most doctors would prescribe antibiotics, and, if the situation recurred, which it almost always does since the patient's immune system and nutrition are ignored, the tonsils are surgically removed. However, when using the steps above to treat the throat, support the immune system, and improve the diet, even the worst case of swollen tonsils can be remedied. The key is a manual draining of the lymphatics of the neck (described in step 9 above) *and a manual draining of the tonsils themselves*. Physicians, take note that we actually go in with our fingers and manually drain the tonsils.

Chiropractic treatment protocol

1. First, with the patient seated, we perform soft tissue stretching to the entire neck, including the sternocleidomastoid muscles (SCM), trapezeii and suboccipitals as described above in #9.

2. Using a sterile glove, and with the patient seated comfortably and back supported, the tonsils must be drained manually with the index finger of the doctor. Spray the finger with a copious amount of Argentyn 23 (a potent natural antibiotic) so that when contacting the tonsil, the Argentyn will be spread into the tonsil directly. To begin, the doctor uses his opposite hand to steady the head of the patient. A tongue depressor may be needed in order to control the tongue if the patient tends to gag easily. The index finger is gently flexed and is pressed against the tonsil in a pumping manner with light to moderate pressure in a medial to lateral direction. Give the patient a break periodically, switching from right side to left, making sure to pump each tonsil several times. Be prepared to have the patient spit out each time into a sink or basin, and provide tissues or a paper towel as well. Do not be worried or surprised to see some blood and/or puss on the finger or when the patient spits out. This is evidence that the tonsil was infected and is congested. Extracting blood and pus from the infected tonsils is actually the goal of the treatment. We are assisting the body in removing the dead tissue which it has accumulated. Having fresh spring water for the patient to drink is helpful as well as comforting.

3. Lastly, after pumping the tonsils several times, for maximum benefit have the patient gargle with a small amount of Argentyn 23 Silver Hydrosol, spitting out after each gargle. Repeat this several times during and after the treatment. It is a very simple procedure and one that can go a long way in saving the patient from unnecessary antibiotics and possibly surgery.

Surgery to remove the tonsils is not a simpler and easier way to deal with the problem. Tonsillectomy comes with its risks. In December of 2013, Jahi McMath, a young California girl went into a coma after "routine" tonsillectomy surgery. The surgery, ironically done as a treatment for sleep apnea from which Jahi suffered, ended in death. This young death is a tragic reminder of the risks that come with surgery.

SECTION V
CONDITIONS OF THE CHEST AND LUNGS

Basics of Treating Lung Disorders and Congestion

Congestion of the lungs is a problem commonly misunderstood. Nearly all allopathic physicians treat lung conditions with antibiotics, anti-inflammatories, bronchodilators and mucus-blocking drugs like Mucinex. Very seldom does the physician ever address the digestive tract and the diet. One should begin with a very light diet, eliminating the more common mucus-forming foods which are conventional pasteurized dairy of any kind (including cheese, yogurt), wheat and other starches.

The use of eucalyptus oil on the chest will help to keep the airways open as the vapors are inhaled upon evaporating from the chest. You can also take cotton balls soaked in eucalyptus oil and place them in a plastic Ziploc bag. Simply open the bag every 20 minutes or so and breathe in deeply through the nose, inhaling the vapors. I advise my patients to place a few drops of the oil on their pillows before bed so as to inhale the vapors throughout the night.

It is also important to keep blood coming toward the lungs to facilitate the removal of toxins thus clearing the lungs. To do this, keep on your chest a hot water bottle filled with hot water from the sink (NOT boiling water) for a half hour. Repeat three times a day. Be sure to take the air out of the bottle before sealing the cap and keep a light tee shirt on so that the bottle does not burn your chest.

This procedure should be followed along with performing an enema two times per day, even if you are not constipated. Taking an enema is an excellent way to reduce a fever as well as to help relieve the body of toxins that are not being cleared effectively via the bowel. Sterile water can be made for the enema by boiling water, then covering it and allowing it to cool to room temperature. You may also use organic coffee which is excellent in acidifying the intestine and helping the liver detoxify the body's waste. Refer to the Appendix A p. 321-22 for complete instructions on taking an enema.

Supplementation is also crucial in treating congestion of the lungs. The main way that this is accomplished is simply by supporting the immune system. We do NOT seek to "suppress a cough" or use aspirin to lower a fever. We support the immune system with the following vitamins and nutrients:

1. Argentyn 23 Silver Hydrosol – take as directed on the bottle.
2. Congaplex® by Standard Process – take two capsules every 2 hours at the first sign of a cold/congestion for 48–72 hours. Then reduce to four to six per day prophylactically.
3. Blue Ice™ Fermented Cod Liver Oil – take four to six capsules a day with food until the congestion/cold resolves. Then take 2–3 capsules a day prophylactically. If using the liquid, take one teaspoon 3 times a day for the first 48–72 hours, then decrease to 1 teaspoon a day.
4. Zinc Liver Chelate™ by Standard Process – take two tablets a day.
5. Immuplex® by Standard Process – take three to six a day if you are chronically immune compromised.
6. Broncafect® by Medi Herbs – two tablets 2–4 times a day
7. Andrographis by Medi Herbs – one tablet 2–4 times per day

Chest Congestion Due to Bronchitis/Cold/Flu

True influenza is an infectious disease transmitted through the air in infected secretions (i.e., mucus), caused by an RNA virus in the Orthomyxovirus class of viruses. There are three subtypes of viruses in this class, called A, B, and C with the subtype A associated with the most severe symptoms (Cowan TS. Preventing and treating the flu. Wise Traditions. Weston A. Price Foundation. 2013 Spring; 50). There are two important aspects of these facts that most people ignore. First, since the causative agent in the flu is a virus, antibiotics are useless. Some doctors will argue that giving antibiotics in cases of the flu is important to protect against the possibility of a secondary infection. The flu vaccine itself poses some dangers. Dr. Cowan notes that some of these dangers include: "leaving us with chronic inflammation as our bodies struggle to clear these inflammatory toxins, such as mercury, formaldehyde, and dead viruses, and an increased susceptibility to chronic disease."(Ibid p. 51) He concludes that, "In all, flu vaccines have too many problems to recommend them against an illness that should be fairly straightforward to overcome."(Ibid p. 51)

In *A Shot Never Worth Taking: The Flu Vaccine* published by the International Medical Council on Vaccination, Kelly Brogan, MD writes of the flu vaccine:

> The Cochrane Database — an objective, gold-standard assess-ment of available evidence has plainly stated, in two studies, that there is no data to support efficacy in children under two, and in adults. Even the former Chief Vaccine Officer at the FDA states: "There is no evidence that any influenza vaccine thus far developed is effective in preventing or mitigating any attack of influenza."

Liking the idea of being protected from the flu does not equate to being protected. See more at http://www.vaccinationcouncil.org/2013/11/27/a-shot-never-worth-taking-the-flu-vaccine-by-kelly-brogan-md/#sthash.GWkPFXBT.dpuf

Regarding the flu, and any other condition involving mucous build-up, begin by reducing the mucus-forming foods such as conventional pasteurized/homogenized dairy of all types, wheat and flour products including pasta, cakes, and cookies, and all refined sugars. Dr. Cowan agrees, noting that "as far as flu prevention, the best approach is, of course, a nourishing traditional diet with an emphasis on good fats, lacto-fermented foods and a gelatin rich bone broth."(Ibid p. 51) For more specifics, refer to Section III of this book, The Importance of Proper Digestion.

Once the dietary approach is corrected, one must focus on cleaning out the intestines. They must be thoroughly cleaned using hydrocolonic therapy done by a professional, or by an enema administered at home. See Appendix A p. 321-22 for the procedure.

The following list of home remedies can be of use to open the airways and facilitate removal of congestion:

1. Bring two quarts of water to a boil. Add two tablespoons of cayenne pepper and one heaping teaspoon of Vicks® VapoRub®. Stir this mixture, cover, remove from the stove. Next, get a stool

or small chair. Sit in the chair while placing the pot on the stool or small chair in front of you. Be sure to use a hot plate so that you do not burn the surface of the stool or chair. The patient sits with his/her head approximately 12–18 inches above the mixture. A towel is draped over the entire head and mixture to create a tent so that the vapors can be inhaled. Remove the cover from the pot and begin inhaling through the nose with deep breaths. The patient stays under the tent for 5–7 minutes constantly taking deep breaths. This can be repeated 2–3 times per day. You may also do this same procedure using thyme essential oil drops or eucalyptus oil. **Note**: you do not have to replace the water each time. Simply reheat and add a little more Vicks®.

2. Drink a glass of hot water with the juice of ½ lemon, one tablespoon of whiskey and ½ teaspoon of raw, unheated, unfiltered honey (see Appendix D p. 358 #22 for recommended brands). This drink is called a hot toddy and can be taken 2–3 times per day.

3. Keep your feet warm by taking a teaspoon of Vaseline® mixed with a teaspoon of cayenne pepper and rubbing it into the soles of your feet. Then put on a pair of socks.

4. Mustard Plaster for the chest: Place one heaping tablespoon of Colman's Mustard Powder and 3 tablespoons of flour into a cup. Add white vinegar slowly, mixing until the consistency is that of pancake batter. Then place the ingredients onto a piece of cloth 5 inches wide x 10 inches long covering only one half of the cloth. Fold the unused portion of the cloth over the other half containing the mixture. Place directly on bare chest for approximately 30 minutes, covering with a dry towel. The mustard plaster will produce heat that will draw blood to the chest area and will help clear the congestion. This may be repeated two times each day for three days. The mustard plaster can also be placed on the back in between the shoulder blades. **Caution:** This mixture may become very hot. The patient is cautioned to remove the plaster if it becomes too hot. If any redness or burning occurs, coat the area with a small amount of raw honey or USF Ointment® made by Standard Process.

An important side note on the use of heating pads. They should not be used for this procedure. Putting any electrical device on the body can interrupt the body's own electrical/magnetic field and therefore its nerve energy. As a result, free radicals, precursors to cancer, can build up causing further cellular breakdown. My advice is to avoid using electrical heating pads or electric blankets.

The chiropractic treatment for chest congestion must also address areas of the spine, innervating the lungs as well as affecting the immune system. The main area of the spine involved regarding the lungs is the upper thoracic region including T1–T4 (at the base of your neck where your back begins). The adjustment should seek to remove any subluxations in this area and restore proper positioning of the spine. This includes soft tissue work to the trapezius muscles and stretching under the scapulae to release the rhomboid muscles. This will enable better lung expansion and augment oxygenation of the lungs. In our office we also teach the patient how to breathe properly, or diaphragmatically. Most people are accessory breathers, lifting the ribs to obtain oxygen.

Another technique to ameliorate the relief of chest congestion is percussion of the lungs. This is done with both hands of the doctor in a slightly "cupped" or flexed position so as to form a cup shape. The patient is to lie down on their stomach while the hands are used to gently percuss, or "bang" on the back from the top of the back to just below the shoulder blades. This is done in a gentle but firm manner, somewhat like the action of playing the drums. It can be done multiple times throughout the day to help break up the congestion.

One other technique to treat lung congestion is resuscitation. This is done with the patient lying on his back. The doctor takes both hands, placed with palms at the level of the chest, and applies a steady, firm pressure downward while vibrating the hands as the patient breathes out through the mouth. At the bottom of the movement, the doctor quickly releases the pressure of his hands as the patient inhales rapidly through the mouth. This helps force extra air into the lungs as well as remove dead air trapped in the bottom of the lungs. This action is repeated 3–4 times. Caution: Be careful with elderly and more delicate patients when applying pressure down onto the chest. Do not press overly hard. You do not want to break or sprain the patient's ribs. The objective is simply to help push all of the air out of the lungs as the patient is exhaling.

The purpose of resuscitation is to force oxygen into the lungs, expanding them. The reason is that when the lungs become overburdened with mucus and fluid, oxygen levels drop and the body suffers. The lungs are now no longer able to expand and pull in air the way they normally would. When congested and irritated, the lungs fill with more mucus and fluid causing less air to enter through normal breathing. As a result, the lungs fill with dead air, which is oxygen-deficient and high in carbon dioxide waste. This reduces the volume of oxygen (VO2) in the blood and organs where it is vitally needed. In consequence, the entire body suffers and disease states can thrive.

If a cough is present, I recommend that a patient not attempt to suppress it. A cough is the body's way of attempting to clear an irritant from the lungs and hence from the body. Generally we work to support the immune system and facilitate the removal of these irritants rather than suppress the cough. If you are in a situation that demands relief from a cough, I suggest trying this natural cough syrup:

> One medium size onion finely chopped and placed into a glass (use food processor if you have access to one)
>
> Four tablespoons of filtered or spring water poured over the onion
>
> Two heaping teaspoons of brown sugar poured onto the mixture
>
> Cover the glass with plastic wrap and allow it to sit for one hour or overnight. Then, take one tablespoon of this mixture at least 4 times a day, after breakfast, lunch, dinner and at bedtime.

Note: Information on specific supplements I recommend for the flu is in the next segment on the common cold/flu.

Germ Theory and Treatment for Common Cold/Flu

There are over 200 viruses blamed for the common cold. To find the source and to treat the cold or flu I think we need first look at the condition of our immune system. Since most of our immune system is seated in the digestive tract, it is here that we should first look for the origin of our health problems. When the body's digestive tract becomes inundated with toxins, incompletely digested foods, chemical additives and processed foods devoid of nutrition and irritating to the intestinal lining, waste builds up until our body can no longer process it and remove it. Constipation ensues, absorption of wastes backward into the bloodstream begins, and pathogenic bacteria and viruses multiply as the environment becomes more toxic. If one is healthy to begin with and the immune system is strong, then those viruses and bacteria will not find an environment where they can thrive and cause sickness. This requires a nutrient dense, unprocessed diet, proper rest, a good mental attitude, regular aerobic exercise and a deeper understanding of our spirituality and connection to nature. I believe that this is the way nature intended it.

Pathogenic bacteria and viruses are a natural reaction to the change in environment from one of health to one of abuse, and a change in the immune system from one that is strong to one that is weak. This theory was initially proposed by biologist and chemist Antoine Béchamp (1816-1908) in his book *Microzyme Theory*. He states: "germs are not the cause, but the result of the disease." Christopher Bird, in *The Galileo of the Microscope: The Life and Trials of Gaston Naessens*," p. 41, tells us that Gaston Naessens confirmed Béchamp's findings nearly 100 years later when he developed advancements in optics resulting in a more powerful microscope. "With his exceptional instrument, Naessens, as we shall call him, went on to discover in the blood of animals and humans – a hitherto unknown, ultra-microscopic, sub-cellular, living and reproducing microscopic form, which he christened a somatid ('tiny body'). And, strangely enough, it was seen by Naessens to develop in a pleomorphic, or "form-changing" cycle, the first three stages of which – somatid, spore, and double spore – are perfectly normal in healthy organisms, in fact crucial to their existence."(Ibid p. 30) "Naessens went on to discover that if, and when, the immune system of an animal, or human being, becomes weakened or destabilized, the normal three-stage cycle goes through thirteen more successive growth stages to make up a total of sixteen separate forms, each evolving into the next."(Ibid p. 35) And as this life cycle progresses (as a result of a weakened immune system), so does the disease progress.

The somatids and other stages Naessens discovered, and which Béchamp had first alluded to nearly a century earlier, are merely the body's reaction to stresses: poor eating habits, lack of rest, stress, processed foods, medications and antibiotics. The list of stressors is endless. I cannot scientifically prove this theory, but my long experience has shown evidence of its validity. In addition, pioneers of a theory known as pleomorphism, like the famous biologist Gaston Naessens, have provided evidence over the last three decades of the theory's validity.

The first thing that must be done is to clean out the digestive tract. Most people will present with symptoms of cough, runny nose, headache, chills, fever and aches and pains in the joints. These symptoms are all related to what is known as autointoxication of the body. This means the food that was eaten either did not digest well due to lack of enzymes, poor food quality, poor food combinations, or a variety of these and other factors like stress and poor chewing (as is so common with the typical "rushed" eating habits of many people). Stagnation of the food in the bowel then occurs, irritating the lining of the intestinal tract and colon. When this happens it causes mucus to build up as a protection mechanism in all of the mucus membranes, including the lungs, trachea, sinuses and nose.

The first step in fighting the condition is to begin cleaning out the intestinal tract. For this we can use either enemas (or colonics done professionally) or citrate of magnesia. Drinking half to one whole bottle of citrate of magnesia will clean out the intestines, causing a flushing and diarrhea. Then the patient can be given a coffee or sterile water enema (see Appendix A p. 321-22 for instructions). The enema helps to remove any residual garbage that remains encrusted on the walls of the colon. The second step is to help break up the congestion in the chest. For this we use an inhalation bath. (See p.84 of this section for directions.)

After the inhalation bath, drink plenty of hot water with a wedge of lemon squeezed into it, a tablespoon of whiskey with 1/8–1/4 teaspoon of raw (unheated/unfiltered) honey added. Drink this throughout the day several times. This will help to break up the mucus in the intestinal tract. If the patient has a cough, use zinc lozenges or slippery elm lozenges found in any health food store.

The best expectorant is a homemade remedy using onions (see p.88for instructions on making a natural cough syrup). A reminder, *the goal is not to suppress a cough*! Rather we want only to ease the harsh, painful coughing that may lead to a broken blood vessel in the throat. Coughing is necessary and is the body's attempt at expelling wastes and bacteria. Our goal in doing this is to allow the body to bring out the congested material that has accumulated in the bronchi of the lungs.

Often when medication is given to reduce aches, pains and congestion, the body is being forced to stop its natural mechanisms of healing. Sometimes, the medication only suppresses the symptoms, driving the condition deeper into the body and leaving the patient in an even weaker state. We erroneously equate lack of symptoms with health. This could not be further from the truth.

The following is a list of supplements and other instructions we typically use with much success:

Preventative Care During Cold/Flu Season

1. Echinacea (MediHerb) – take two to three tablets per day
2. Elderberry Extract (trade name Sambucol®) – one teaspoon two to three times per day.
3. Blue Ice™ Fermented Cod Liver Oil – one teaspoon daily.

Do the following at the first signs/symptoms of a cold:

Vitamin Protocol

1. Congaplex® (Standard Process) – two capsules every waking hour for up to 4 days. Then decrease to a dosage of four capsules daily.
2. Immuplex® (Standard Process) – three capsules 3 times daily until cold is resolved. Then take a maintenance dosage of three capsules daily.
3. Thymex® (Standard Process) – five tablets 4 times daily until the cold is resolved.
4. Blue Ice™ Fermented Cod Liver Oil – Take four to five capsules daily until the cold is resolved. Then take three capsules daily as a maintenance dose during the winter months. If the liquid is used, take up to 2 tablespoons per day in divided doses. For children the dose is based on age and the guidelines are provided in the Appendix A p. 320.

5. Pure Radiance Vitamin C (Synergy Company) – powder is best; simply add ½–1 teaspoon to water 2–3 times a day and drink it. It tastes delicious because it is a whole food supplement made from organic berries.

6. Oscillococcinum (Boiron) – one tube twice daily.

Alkalizing Drink

Mix one tablespoon of Bragg's Organic Apple Cider Vinegar or any other organic, unpasteurized apple cider vinegar (to order Omega Nutrition's go to www.healthalertstore.com) in hot water and add 1 teaspoon of raw, unheated, unfiltered honey. Drink this up to three times per day.

Fleet or manual enema: consult a knowledgeable physician's office for direction or see Appendix A p. 321-22 for complete instructions.

Dietary Instructions

Eat *only* fresh green vegetables and/or salad with either fish, chicken, or turkey (broil, bake, boil, steam or sauté). Make soups using homemade stock/broth, recipe from *Nourishing Traditions*, fresh vegetables with either organic, pastured beef, chicken, wild caught fish.

Fresh fruit is permitted as long as it is ripe and in season. It must be eaten separately from any other food.

Drink only water (away from meals), unsweetened herbal teas or fresh squeezed juices.

When the nervous system is freed from mechanical and physiological interference through chiropractic care combined with a healthy, active diet and lifestyle including the use of whole food supplements and phytonutrients, the body will have the tools to stay healthy and fight off anything that comes its way. Medication has its place, especially in emergency care and life-threatening situations. But giving the body drugs laced with other poisons under the guise that this is going to protect you and take the place of living a healthy and active lifestyle free from stress and with adequate rest is nonsense. Expecting to take a pill to fix your ills is foolishness.

SECTION VI
CONDITIONS OF POOR DIGESTION/INTESTINAL TRACT

Indigestion/Gastro-Esophageal Reflux Disease (GERD)

Indigestion is usually caused by a stomach inflamed over a long period of time. Symptoms range from gas, heartburn and acid reflux, to a constant fullness in the upper abdomen or an inability to eat even a moderate amount of food without becoming full. Traditional medical doctors treat this with antacid tablets or protonics (medications designed to shut down the stomach's ability to produce hydrochloric acid). You may even find a patient who, ignoring these symptoms for years just pops Rolaids® or Tums®. Unfortunately, these medications and antacids, while relieving the symptoms never cure anyone because, in the overwhelming number of patients (estimated to be around 95% of cases) with GERD or indigestion, the problem isn't too much acid. It's actually too little stomach acid, a condition known as hypochlorhydria.

An understanding of the stomach's function is important. The stomach's primary task is to produce hydrochloric acid in order to break down the protein portion of our food, producing an enzyme called pepsin to do this. Fat and carbohydrate absorption also rely on stomach acid which causes the release of secretin, thus signalling the pancreas to produce enzymes that digest fats (lipases), protein (proteases) and carbohydrates (amylase). Proper stomach acid production is also needed to absorb certain nutrients like iron. Furthermore, stomach acid destroys most bacteria that gain access to our bodies via our mouths, keeping the body protected from an overgrowth of yeast, bacteria and other disease-causing pathogens. In this way food is transformed into a liquid known as chyme by the time it exits the stomach for the small intestine. Therefore, without hydrochloric acid, we would not only be exposed to far more bacteria from our mouths, we would also not be able to adequately digest our food further down in the intestinal tract.

When in time the stomach cells (known as parietal cells) begin to wear down from the burdens of a poor diet high in processed foods, stress, medications and exposure to bacteria and viruses, the stomach is no longer able to produce hydrochloric acid at its normal, healthy rate. This leads to a rise in the overall pH in the stomach (a measure of acidity or alkalinity, meaning there is a lower acid level in the stomach). An in-depth study of this condition is found in Jonathan Wright, MD's book *Why Stomach Acid Is Good for You*.

When the acid level in the stomach is low, food, especially protein, begins to ferment instead of being digested. As a result, harmful bacteria normally killed by the strong acid produced in the stomach, begin to thrive and multiply consuming these proteins as their own food. One such bacterium is Helicobacter pylori. This bacterium has been linked to anemia as well as implicated in stomach ulcers. It is a bacterium that would not normally survive in a healthy stomach with a low pH.

As the pH in the stomach rises (becomes less acidic) so does the bacterial count. Everything from pathogenic bacteria to yeast begins to grow, fermenting the undigested food in our stomach. Fermentation is the anaerobic conversion of sugars in our food to carbon dioxide and alcohol. Also, fats begin to rancidify. Rancidification is the bacterial breakdown of fats which liberates volatile organic acids like butyrate and propionate. Lastly, bacteria also putrify proteins that sit undigested in the stomach. This breakdown of proteins leads to formation of oxidized organic chemicals that further irritate the stomach lining. It is the result of these byproducts of bacterial metabolism of our undigested food which leads to the acid reflux so commonly felt by sufferers of indigestion. If this situation is allowed to fester in the stomach and even in the beginning section of the intestine (called the duodenum), ulcers and a hiatal hernia may develop. Ulcers, open wounds to the lining of the stomach, can result in bleeding and even infection. A hiatal hernia is when the upper part of the stomach (known as the fundus) rises up through the opening in the diaphragm (the muscle we use to breathe) due to the muscular spasms and gas caused by the inflammation and fermenting food (remember, fermentation produces excess gas and gas wants to rise). The diagram on page 96 illustrates this condition.

With younger patients presenting with this problem, their inflammation most often has its roots in poor eating habits (think of all the modern, processed and vitamin-depleted foods the majority of our young children and young adults eat on a regular basis). Poor food combinations and drinking a lot of fluid while eating also add to the digestive load placed on the stomach. (Refer to the the chart in Section III p. 24 for a detailed explanation of food combining.

The stomach needs acid to function. By drinking a lot of water (or soda, juice, etc.) with meals, one ends up diluting the acid the stomach is trying to produce to digest the food. The first step in healthier eating habits is not to drink a lot of fluid with meals. To learn more on basic rules of healthier eating, see the explanation in Section III of this book.

A second important step toward correcting indigestion and GERD is to take a digestive enzyme. Enzymes are proteins normally found in whole foods. They assist in the breakdown of that specific food. However, overcooking and processing destroy these natural enzymes. Most enzymes are denatured (their structure destroyed) at temperatures above 55-60°C or 140°F. Therefore our digestive tract must pick up the slack, placing a greater burden on our system to produce enough enzymes to completely digest our food. Over time, this leads to a weakening, and ultimately, a failure of digestion bringing the resultant problems of gas, bloating and indigestion. For many people, a digestive enzyme becomes a necessary supplement to ensure the complete breakdown of food.

If a patient's indigestion has progressed to the point of gastric ulcers, it will be necessary to take a digestive enzyme without betaine hydrochloride in it. In cases where the person does not already know whether or not they have ulcers, there is a simple way to test for it. *Always consult with a physician to work with you on this matter.* First, the patient must take either Betaine Hydrochloride by Standard Process (one to two with each meal) or a digestive enzyme containing betaine hydrochloride (often abbreviated betaine HCL on labels). If doing so alleviates the patient's symptoms of indigestion, it is safe to assume they do not have ulcers and can continue using the enzyme with hydrochloric acid. If, however, the symptoms worsen, it is a strong indication that ulcers are present and the patient must temporarily use an enzyme supplement without hydrochloric acid. In this case, I recommend Multizyme® by Standard Process at a starting dosage of one per meal. This can be a simple, cost effective way of identifying whether an ulcer is present without having to do more intensive testing such as gastroscopy/endoscopy.

In dealing with indigestion or GERD, it is recommended that patients blend their food into soups for the first week or two (see the Blended Diet below). Keeping a more liquid diet of rich, homemade bone broths and easy to digest foods will give the stomach the rest it needs to begin healing. The broth is tremendously healing to the gastrointestinal system. I also advise eating smaller meals up to five or six times per day until the stomach is healed and able to handle three larger meals per day. By eating smaller meals and avoiding overeating, the stomach is given less of a burden and can therefore begin to heal. As an adjunct to the healing of the stomach lining, I recommend Gastrex® by Standard Process (two capsules with a full glass of water 15 minutes before meals) and the herb Licorice Root in lozenge form (also abbreviated DGL). It should be chewed or sucked on 10–15 minutes prior to meals. Both products contain compounds effective in healing the stomach and intestinal linings.

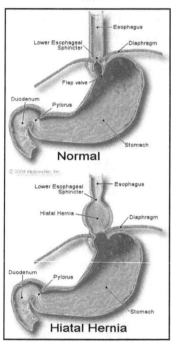

©Kansas Medical Clinic, PA, Copyright image used with permission.

NORMAL STOMACH ANATOMY VS. HIATAL HERNIA COMMON IN GERD

The Blended Diet

Supplements: Only the following supplements should be taken during this diet period for two reasons. The first is to allow the stomach a "rest" from the extra work of breaking down other supplements the patient may be taking. Second, these two supplements are designed specifically to help in the healing of the stomach. This MUST be done first before taking other supplements.

1. DGL (deglycyrhinated licorice root) or GP Soothe (Designs for Health). Chew on two DGL tablets 10-15 minutes prior to each meal OR, if you prefer capsules, take two GP-Soothe capsules in the a.m. before your first meal and two more capsules later

in the day before a meal. You may also use Gastrex® (Standard Process) as described above.

2. Digestive Enzyme with HCL (non-ulcerated stomach) OR Multizyme® (stomach ulcers present). Take one digestive enzyme or Multizyme® capsule per meal with your food.

Breakfast

1. Eggs (soft cooked, scrambled)

2. Fruit (partially cooked) stewed prunes or apricots; baked apple or pear. You should partially bake the pear and apple at first to soften the fruit for ease of digestion. Do not mix the different types of fruits in one meal. You can change types throughout the morning but you must wait 45 minutes before doing so.

Lunch

1. Blended green vegetable soup with homemade bone broth (no potatoes, rice, or beans) using zucchini, escarole, cauliflower, kale, broccoli, asparagus, brussels sprouts, broccoli rabe, etc. Preferably, make your own broth at home according to the directions in *Nourishing Traditons* by Sally Fallon, pages 116-125. However, you may use a quality organic store-bought broth to prepare the soup. If you are not going to make your own broth, I recommend using Pacific Organic Chicken or Vegetable Broth *or* you may use Nature's Promise organic broths from Stop&Shop. Be aware that many other brands contain MSG, salt, and other chemical additives. Also, use herbs like oregano, garlic, and others as long as they are fresh and not spicy or hot. I recommend Celtic sea salt. If you are curious about using other vegetables, please ask the physician first.

2. Dietary/Protein Shake/Fruit Smoothie: Using Whey Cool Protein (Designs for Health, tel. (800) 847-8302) *or* SP Complete® from Standard Process, a shake or fruit smoothie can be made with a blender. Combine six ounces of water, with blueberries, strawberries, pineapple or other fruit to one scoop of Whey Cool powder or SP Complete®. If you are diabetic or do not want to use fruit, substitute a tablespoon of raw almond, cashew, or macadamia nut butter. Add one teaspoon of Tupelo honey and blend.

Caution – This shake is only for patients who are not allergic to milk or dairy as this powder is dairy based. High quality hypoallergenic rice-based protein powders are available through Standard Process and Ortho Molecular. Consult the physician before beginning.

Dinner

1. Green vegetable soup (from above) with chicken, turkey, fish or lamb are the more easily digestible proteins which you must stay with at first. *Make sure to chop the meat up finely into very small pieces.* Organic, pastured animal meats are always best so as to avoid the antibiotics and growth hormones fed to conventional factory farm animals. You may cook the meat by baking, broiling, boiling or grilling. *Absolutely no fried foods.*

In older patients with heartburn or indigestion, we more commonly see a hiatal hernia present. In these cases, we usually see poor circulation occurring in the stomach region with the fundus of the stomach enlarged and dilated (see illustration on p. 96). This dilation, combined with gas from fermenting food causes pressure under the diaphragm muscle. Normally, the stomach contracts with rhythmic movements, breaking the food down into a liquid consistency, and passing it to the lower portion of the stomach to ready it for movement into the intestine. However, in an inflamed and dilated condition, this contraction forces the liquid backward through the cardiac sphincter and up into the esophagus. Eventually, if this condition progresses without resolving, a patient can experience chest pain and pressure in the sternal region (center of the chest) as the stomach pushes up through the diaphragm. The symptoms can simulate those of a heart attack and will often result in a person being rushed to the emergency room. Some who experience this problem even find that they need to sit up in bed to get relief from the heartburn, gas and bloating since in a reclined position, it is much easier for the stomach contents to reflux up into the esophagus as gravity has less effect in this position than it does in the upright position. This condition is becoming more and more common even in middle-aged and younger adults.

In conclusion, if you look at children during the first year of life, they are breastfeeding. Nature planned it this way because their still-developing digestive system is unable to break down solid and more complex foods. After the first year, we give babies blended food and finely shredded or blended meat. Why? Because the specialized cells in the baby's stomach are not fully developed yet (nor are their teeth). Therefore, the stomach cannot handle digesting larger pieces of meat and vegetables. When a patient reaches a certain age in life, food should be made easier for them to digest. Years of poor eating habits combined with aging can damage the stomach causing it to have similar difficulty with certain foods. I always recommend blended/liquified foods made with homemade bone broths for the elderly, especially those with indigestion.

Chiropractic treatment should address the specific subluxation levels relating neurologically to the stomach. We would specifically look to the atlas (C1) vertebra, the 4th through 6th thoracic vertebrae, and of course reflex the abdominal zones as mentioned earlier. Lastly, in cases of hiatal hernia, a specific adjustment to the stomach can be delivered by the chiropractor with the patient supine (on his/her back). The doctor does this by using a reinforced pisiform contact just below and to the left of the Xiphoid bone of the sternum. He then instructs the patient to take a deep breath through his/her nose and release through the mouth. As the breath is releasing, the doctor applies a pressure down and toward the left leg/foot. Then, the patient inhales again while the doctor continues to hold the pressure; this is repeated with each breath for 30-45 seconds with the doctor maintaining a constant, firm pressure. When this is accomplished in combination with the aforementioned diet, you will see an amazing return to normal stomach functioning.

Halitosis (Bad Breath)

I am including my discussion of halitosis in this section on Conditions of the Stomach just after indigestion and GERD for a specific reason. This condition is almost always related to poor digestion in the stomach due to reduced hydrochloric acid production (hypochlorhydria). As a result, foods, especially proteins, sit in the stomach and begin to ferment as previously explained. It can also be related to a wearing down of the liver-kidney-adrenal systems. Therefore, the aforementioned protocol for indigestion must be implemented to resolve the cause of halitosis. No amount of mints, Scope®, or other mouthwash is going to fix this problem. The stomach and digestive system must be treated by a functional and integrative approach.

Here are some suggestions that may help with halitosis:

1. Reduce the amount of meat that is consumed, fish and chicken included, for a period of several weeks up to several months. *Work with a qualified professional well-versed in nutrition and alternative care.*
2. Stay on a bone broth and vegetable-based regimen for a week or two. If you are over 50 years of age you may have to take a digestive enzyme with hydrochloric acid included in it. Consult with your physician for ways to test.
3. Support your adrenal system by taking dessicated adrenal tissue by Standard Process (called Dessicated Adrenal).
4. Perform a Liver and Gallbladder Detoxification. Standard Process has a 21 day Purification Program in the form of a kit, or you can perform the cleanse outlined in this book and printed in Appendix A p. 333-35. Always do so under the guidance of a qualified holistic practitioner.
5. Take liquid chlorophyll or chlorophyll tablets. I prefer to use a product called Kyo-Chlorella at a dosage of six per day. This can be safely increased to support the system during a cleanse. Standard Process also makes a Chlorophyll Complex™ in the form of perles. Dosage is 2–3 perles per meal, or more if needed.
6. The herb Milk Thistle (aka St. Mary's Thistle) – this should be a standardized herb containing approximately 175 mg of silymarin, the active component. Medi-Herb brand herbs are of the highest quality available. LivCo® is an excellent combination product from Medi-Herb. It contains milk thistle as well as extracts of Schisandra and Rosemary leaf. Dosage is one tablet 3–4 times per day.

Flatulence (Gas in the Intestinal Tract)

Gas in the intestinal tract is caused by a few different problems that can be interrelated. They include incomplete digestion of food from poor enzyme production, dysbiosis (a change from the normal, healthy bacteria present in the intestinal tract to more pathogenic strains), and accumulation of yeast in the intestinal tract. Any one of these seemingly different causes can predispose you to the others. For example, in some people, yeast may develop as a result of overuse of antibiotics or overconsumption of carbohydrates; in others the gas could be caused by poor enzyme production in the stomach and intestine. So as yeast build up in the intestinal tract, the enterocytes (cells that line the intestine) that produce the brush border enzymes become damaged. Without these brush border enzymes, our food cannot digest properly. As a result, intestinal motility slows, food begins to ferment and bacterial wastes accumulate. Once the pH of the intestinal tract changes as a result of this waste build-up, the door is open for more and more pathogenic bacteria to thrive. As this happens, enzyme production further diminishes and food begins to ferment, producing gases.

The solution to any of these causes of flatulence starts by changing the diet and eliminating the foods which feed these pathogens. By doing so, we can rid the body of yeast and other gas forming bacteria, improve enzyme function and restore the proper balance to the flora of the intestines. Removal of sweets, flour products, alcohol, refined sugars (candy, soda, ketchup, dressings, etc.), chocolate, vinegar, and juices is essential. These are just a few of the most important foods to eliminate. For a more complete list of foods that must be eliminated, read Natasha Campbell-McBride's masterpiece *The Gut and Psychology Syndrome*. She provides a comprehensive list of allowable foods as well as those which are prohibited.

Once the diet is improved, the next step is to take a high quality probiotic, more commonly referred to as acidophilus. Two high quality supplements are ProSynbiotic by Standard Process and Primal Defense by New Chapter. Start at one per day and increase your way slowly up to 4–8 per day. You have to go slowly because there is often a detoxification reaction known as the Herxheimer response as the body throws off the dead bacteria and toxins. These bacteria, like microscopic warriors, ward off the pathogenic strains and help to keep our intestinal tract healthy. A normal, healthy adult has up to 6 pounds of these bacteria in the intestinal tract!

An even better way to restore the healthy flora to the intestines is to consume naturally lacto-fermented foods. Many people have never heard of lacto-fermented foods, but we have all come across them at some point. They include foods like sauerkraut, kvass, kombucha, yogurt, and kefir. These foods naturally contain the probiotic bacteria needed to stay healthy. People with flatulence who wish to learn more about these foods should consult *Nourishing Traditions* by Sally Fallon. The section on lacto-fermented foods would be helpful. A resource for recipes and a detailed explanation of the importance of fermented foods is *Real Food Fermentation*, by Alex Lewin. An additional help is the Standard Process supplement called Lactic Acid Yeast™ which is designed to help restore the proper pH of the intestinal tract and thereby promote probiotic growth. These wafers can be sucked on before each meal and will help get rid of the pathogenic gas-producing bacteria and yeast.

A final component in the treatment of flatulence is a high quality digestive enzyme to ensure the proper and complete breakdown of food. This is especially important for patients who have a history of intestinal illness and need to repair the damage that has been done to the intestinal enterocytes. Enzymes are effective in helping patients with compromised digestion improve their breakdown of food and assimilation of nutrients. High quality enzymes on the market today include Digestin made by Progressive Labs, Ortho-Digestzyme, by Ortho Molecular and Zypan® or Multizyme® by Standard Process (Appendix D #10 and #23). Start at a dosage of one per meal and increase if necessary to two per meal.

Irritable Bowel Syndrome (IBS)/Inflammatory Bowel Disease

The heading of Irritable Bowel Syndrome includes chronic constipation, cramping, abdominal pain, bloating, gas and diarrhea. Inflammatory bowel disease consists of Crohn's Disease, and ulcerative colitis. These conditions are all related to poor diet, poor food combining, overuse of medications/side effects, lack of proper digestion, and allergic problems. Those suffering with these types of conditions are seldom tested for food allergies, pH imbalances, stress/adrenal fatigue, hypothyroidism and medication side effects (especially from antibiotics), nor is instruction given about what foods to eat and how to combine them more effectively. These sufferers are frequently treated with some form of medication, steroid, or combination of both and left to suffer in this diseased state, never fully overcoming the condition. When the symptoms persist or worsen, a GI series/MRI is often ordered. If the condition worsens, surgical removal of sections of the intestinal tract may be recommended. For sufferers of IBS, their condition can often seem confusing and hopeless.

The most important action to take is to restore the proper gut flora. The flora is a term used for the proper, healthy bacteria (including some good forms of yeast) that are present in our intestinal tract. They are passed on to us from our mothers at birth as we pass through and out of the birth canal, and as we breast feed. They live with us in symbiosis, protecting us from pathogenic strains of bacteria and even helping us to absorb certain nutrients. Without the proper balance of these microorganisms, we cannot have a healthy intestinal lining. The overuse of antibiotics has made this a widespread problem (this is why antibiotics frequently cause digestive symptoms like stomach upset and diarrhea).

When normal flora is disrupted, a condition known as dysbiosis ensues. Dysbiosis is the presence of an imbalance in the natural bacterial flora typically present in a healthy intestinal tract. Some children never develop a healthy flora because they inherit the intestinal problems of the mother from birth or because they are formula fed with conventional soy and milk-based formulas. The more frequent use of cesarean sections is another cause of dysbiosis as the child never passes through the birth canal and is thereby prevented from receiving some of the mother's natural flora. Over time, the intestinal tract becomes encrusted with waste products of incomplete digestion as well as toxins from pathogenic yeast and bacteria. Normally, a healthy intestinal cell (enterocyte) is not encrusted with waste and is protected by the healthy probiotic bacteria. Now, however, the layer of waste that forms on the walls of the intestine prevents the villi and microvilli from doing their job (villi and microvilli are microscopic fingerlike projections of enzyme producing cells that come in contact with the food we eat, thereby helping the food we eat to break down properly). The disease process progresses rapidly until these cells become dysfunctional.

The chiropractic approach to IBS starts with the examination of the spine in the cervical, mid-thoracic and lumbar regions. Through palpation, the physical exam will also reveal which areas of the intestinal tract are sensitive. This is correlated with the correct spinal adjustments. Every organ in the body connects to the spine at a very specific spinal level. Chiropractic adjustments at these specific levels, in a very specific manner correlating to the area of disease, will facilitate the healing process. For example if the vertebra is rotated spinous left, the correction is to adjust it back to the right; if the subluxation is compression, the correction will be traction and so on. Any subluxations found in these regions must be corrected and in some cases, stretches and exercises given to prevent recurrence.

After a complete history and physical exam that includes the abdomen and the spine, testing may need to be ordered to examine different aspects of gut health, uncover any food allergies that may be present, and investigate for the presence of bacterial/parasitic infection. We use Genova Diagnostics Lab's stool testing and IgE and IgG4 Food Allergy testing to accomplish this. These tests enable us to see inside the intestinal tract and glean information that other tests like colonoscopies and ultrasounds do not. For example, we can find out if inflammation is present; we can test for yeast, parasites and pathogenic or opportunistic bacteria as well as probiotic good bacteria. Furthermore, we can assess digestive function through stool testing by evaluating the digestive function of the gallbladder and pancreas. Simply by looking at the contents of the stool, this test can tell us what types of foods are digesting and which are not. If yeast is suspected we will often perform an additional urine test known as D-Arabinitol which is part of the urine organic acids test. We can also use urinary organic acids to further assess intestinal health for dysbiosis. After the proper tests have been identified and ordered, diet must be examined.

Once we have established the specific areas of disease as outlined above, we set up a treatment plan for the patient and start to correct the problem. A proper diet must be appropriate to the specific needs of the patient. In more severe cases, I use my own version of what has become known as the GAPS diet or Specific Carbohydrate Diet (SCD). To learn more about what this entails, I recommend two excellent books on the subject: *The Gut and Psychology Syndrome* by Natasha Campbell-McBride, MD and *Breaking the Vicious Cycle* by Elaine Gottschall. These two books are priceless guides through the often confusing and contradictory world of diets.

There are some golden rules that apply to almost all IBS patients, and others which must be tailored to the specific person involved.

First, IBS patients must first eliminate all conventional, pasteurized dairy and dairy products, including milk, yogurt, cheese, cream. The pasteurization process destroys the nutritive value of these foods. The recommendation to eat pasteurized yogurt because it is healthy for digestion is misleading. For more information on the history and controversy over dairy, read *The Untold Story of Milk, Revised and Updated: The History, Politics and Science of Nature's Perfect Food: Raw Milk from Pasture-Fed Cows* by Ron Schmid. Raw dairy products can often be reintroduced as one progresses.

Second, all refined sugars and carbohydrate foods are to be eliminated. This means no white sugar and products containing high fructose corn syrup. Refined sugars like table, "raw", "natural", turbinado sugar, and Sucanat are not only completely stripped of the vitamins and minerals once found in the whole food form of the cane sugar, they are also unnatural to our system. They act more like a drug than they do a food. Observe how your children behave on a sugar "high." Furthermore, refined sugars are a big part of why diabetes is so prevalent in our country. Young children are now walking around with what was once called adult onset or Type II Diabetes. For an excellent guide to natural sweeteners, see Sally Fallon's book *Nourishing Traditions*, pp. 536–537.

Most grains must be removed from the diet as well, especially bromated, bleached white flour and products made from white flour. Grains as well as nuts, seeds, legumes and beans are very difficult to digest. This is the way that nature intended it. All of these foods have one thing in common in order to release their nutrients for our use. We must first soak them, or allow them to germinate. Seeds, for example, contain the necessary genetic information and nutrition to produce a plant. Nature intended these nutrients to be released only when the conditions were right for growth (temperature, water availability, etc.). These types of foods have their nutrients locked up by compounds called enzyme inhibitors and the organic acids known as lectins and phytic acid. These anti-nutrients prevent our digestive tract from being able to break the foods down properly. In fact, the anti-nutrients like phytic acid found in grains, nuts, seeds and beans can prevent our digestive system from absorbing important minerals like calcium, iron, and magnesium. Properly soaking these foods allows enzymes to break down and neutralize phytic acid and to increase the amounts of many vitamins and minerals found in the food. For example, soaking drastically increases the vitamin C content of grains.

This is one of the main reasons why many of these foods cause gastrointestinal symptoms. Nuts, corn, and seeds are evident culprits. Many people develop allergies and/or constipation when eating nuts. Corn remains undigested. Ask any person with diverticulosis (pockets that form in the intestine that can trap food and become inflamed) and they will tell you they cannot eat seeds for that reason. Properly soaking these foods (see Appendix C p. 344-346 for instructions taken from *Nourishing Traditions*) ensures that they will be more easily digested and their nutrients made available to our system. For a period of time (sometimes weeks, sometimes longer), one may have to *eliminate these foods from the diet* and then *slowly reintroduce them in the properly prepared forms* when the patient's gastrointestinal system can handle them better.

Third and lastly, certain starches must be eliminated from the diet. There are several different theories as to why starches can be such a problem. The most popular is that the long chains of polysachharides (units of multiple single sugars linked in long chains) are too difficult to break down into their component monosachharides (single sugar molecule). Only monosaccharides can be absorbed through the intestinal enterocytes into the bloodstream. As a result, these undigested starches sit in the intestine and serve as food for yeast and pathogenic bacteria creating gas, inflammation, and other symptoms common to IBS. It cannot be stressed enough that every person is unique, so it is often necessary to work with each patient to find exactly what works best for them. A person with a poorly functioning gallbladder will not be able to tolerate certain starches and fats that another person might. For this type of patient, it will first be necessary to cleanse the gallbladder thoroughly in order to augment digestion and ameliorate the irritable bowel. Others may find it necessary to avoid acidic type foods for a while. It all depends on the patient in question.

Several supplements are very helpful in the case of IBS. One, if it can be called a supplement, is actually a food — lacto-fermented vegetables. These naturally fermented foods have been around for thousands of years and were a staple to the health of the traditional cultures documented in the book *Nutrition and Physical Degeneration* by Weston A. Price. Traditional lacto-fermented foods like raw yogurt, kefir, sauerkraut and pickles provide us with many wonderful species of bacteria (also referred to as probiotics) which are tremendously healthy to our digestive tract. Some of these foods are pasteurized, thus destroying their nutritive benefits. The Weston A. Price Foundation's Shopper's Guide (available on their website for $1) suggests proper choices, or learn how to make these foods yourself at home. It is a way for the family to reconnect to the spirituality of food and nature. Introducing these "ancient" and forgotten traditional foods, and many others, is the best way to give the body the probiotics it needs and is crucial in helping the IBS patient recover. Learn more about this in *Nourishing Traditions* by Sally Fallon. I recommend this book to my patients as a great resource for healthy recipes, information and procedures.

A second supplement used is Okra Pepsin E3 by Standard Process. It consists of the vegetable okra, alfalfa extract, Spanish moss (Tillandsia usneoides) and buckwheat leaf. It is designed to support bowel cleansing and function as well as to promote the healing of the mucosal lining of the intestinal tract. Usual dosage is 1–2 capsules after each meal.

A third useful supplement in cases of IBS is Cholacol® II, also by Standard Process. It is made from Bentonite clay (montmorillonite) along with Collinsonia root and bile salts. The clay from the earth carries a chemical charge that allows it to act as a magnet for many of the toxins and wastes which accumulate in the gastrointestinal tract of a person with IBS. Using it frees the enterocytes (cells that line the colon) from all of the encrusted waste that has accumulated in the intestines over time. A dosage is four tablets taken 15 minutes before each meal.

Lastly, a good quality digestive enzyme taken with meals is in order. As in our discussion of GERD we must be careful to consider whether or not the patient has ulcers, this time in the intestine. If so we may have to modify our treatment plan and our choice of enzyme type.

Constipation/Diarrhea

Constipation/diarrhea encompasses two seemingly opposite conditions caused by the very same problem. Constipation and diarrhea persisting over a long period of time can result in a diagnosis of IBS, diverticulosis and even Crohn's disease. A classic misconception about constipation is that the person is not getting enough fiber in the diet. Although in many cases this is true from the standpoint of their SAD diet alone, the real cause of the constipation lies elsewhere.

People with constipation/diarrhea have the beginnings of dysbiosis which is the altering of the natural, healthy flora (or bacteria) of the intestine to that of more pathogenic bacteria and yeast. The result is damage to the mucosal lining of the intestines and poor breakdown and assimilation of nutrients. There can be many different causes of constipation/diarrhea — everything from poor mineral absorption, to lack of whole foods and fiber in the diet, and dysbiosis. With any case of constipation or diarrhea, we must restore the healthy environment of the intestine. This is accomplished with some common sense and a little old-fashioned know-how.

First, it is important to rule out medicine as a cause of the constipation. Good history-taking skills are crucial here because we can learn valuable information about our patient's food choices and dietary habits. Remove processed foods, pasteurized dairy, white flour and any un-soaked nuts from the diet immediately. Try to increase natural, whole foods that are rich in water, fiber and minerals like magnesium. These include homemade bone broths, fresh fruit, green vegetables, eggs (preferably from pastured chickens), lacto-fermented foods, properly soaked brown rice, white and sweet potatoes and soaked beans. Later, once progress is made and the condition is abated, you can introduce raw dairy from organic, grass-fed cows.

Then, administer a coffee or sterile water enema (see Appendix A p. 321-22 for instructions) every night for 3–4 nights in a row. Use a baby fleet enema for children under the age of eight. This will help flush out the waste accumulating in the intestinal tract and make restoring normal bowel function easier. There are many laxative products and stool softeners on the market today, but remember, these are all irritants when used frequently. Furthermore, they are only treating the symptoms and not the true cause of dysbiosis.

One final point: water, our most crucial nutrient, comes from the foods we eat or from drinking it by the glass. People who do not eat a healthy, fruit and vegetable rich whole-food/traditional food diet and do not drink water are at a much greater risk of developing bowel problems like constipation/diarrhea. Avoid drinking water with your meals as this dilutes the stomach acid and prevents proper digestion of food. The more active you are, the hotter climate you live in, the greater your need for water from food or drinking. Today's modern diet contains foods that dehydrate us making the need for water even greater. Coffee, teas, refined and processed foods and medications all dehydrate our system. A good quality water filtration system in your home, preferably reverse osmosis is helpful. Many affordable high-quality units are available. (See Appendix F p. 362 for resources.)

Gallbladder Disease/Gallstones

Gallbladder problems are common today. Roughly 700,000 people have their gallbladders removed each year in the United States, up from 500,000 in the years before laparoscopy was introduced. This is no surprise considering the modern processed diet, SAD, and overuse of medications.

Sadly, very few of these patients are instructed on making dietary changes to compensate for this organ loss. Many are told that they don't need to make any changes at all. They are never warned that they will not be able to digest fats as well, or fat soluble vitamins A, D, E, and K. Author Jeremy Bernal notes, "Vitamins A, D, E, and K need to hitchhike through the intestinal wall on the backs of fat molecules in order for your body to absorb them. If the fats in your digestive tract are not being properly broken down and absorbed, neither are vitamins A, D, E and K."(Bernal J. The gall bladder survival guide. EVEL Media Limited; 2011. p. 62). Many patients are told to "eat a low-fat diet." This is, as Bernal points out, positively backwards. (Ibid p. 14) With your gallbladder removed, you need the good fats more than ever.

The gallbladder's job is multifaceted. On one hand, it is an organ of digestion, secreting bile into the intestinal tract to aid in fat digestion (via emulsification of fats) and to increase intestinal peristalsis (rhythmic movements of the muscles of the intestines to move food along) when food arrives from the stomach. On the other hand, it serves in the removal of old red blood cells that have been broken down by the liver, secreting them into the intestine as part of the bile. Its work in digesting and emulsifying fats with the help of the pancreatic enzyme lipase is what enables us to absorb the incredibly important fat soluble vitamins A, D, E, and K. Without these fat soluble vitamins, we cannot absorb our minerals.

People who have had their gallbladder removed, a procedure known as a cholecystectomy, are told that they do not "need" the gallbladder. There is a difference between "needing" an organ and "you can live without" it. You *can* live without it. However, you definitely "need" something to fulfill its role, if not the organ itself. It is there for a reason. People who have had it removed find themselves in difficulty.

Bile coming from the liver is fundamentally different from that which is found in the gallbladder. As bile is stored in the gallbladder it becomes more concentrated, which increases its potency and intensifies its effects on fats. This concentration of the bile makes it more alkaline as well. Bile from people who have had their gallbladder removed lacks these important characteristics. Their bile is much more acidic in nature, which creates a disruption in fat metabolism and irritation to the intestinal lining. This irritation can even cause bile to back up into the stomach, causing belching, heartburn (GERD) and even ulcers if allowed to persist.

When a patient presents with excessive belching and constipation, it is sure that he or she has developed some level of gallbladder dysfunction, though it may be subclinical with very few if any other symptoms. Occasionally a patient will present with more severe symptoms known as Habba Syndrome. "Habba Syndrome, named for Dr. Saad Habba, its discoverer, is often misdiagnosed as IBS. Most often it results in chronic and urgent watery diarrhea, especially after meals as a result of malabsorption of bile salts in the small intestine." (Bernal J. The gall bladder p. 82) Sometimes it is because the bile is not concentrated enough, rendering it ineffective in the intestinal tract. At other times the bile is too thick, like sludge or sand, and does not release into the small intestine from the gallbladder in sufficient amounts. Lastly, the bile may not be alkaline enough (as in those patients who have had a cholecystectomy). This is related to poor diet and improper body pH. If the body's fluids are not alkaline then the bile is affected and this causes the ensuing constipation. Gallbladder dysfunction in this manner has been linked to all types of health problems from constipation to skin conditions, IBS and more.

Another problem very common with today's processed diet is the formation of gallstones. Although the specific cause of gallstones is still unknown, it is theorized that, as the gallbladder removes water from the bile and concentrates it, certain elements in the solution which are not chemically balanced begin to crystallize into grains and sediment, which eventually build up to form stones. (Ibid p. 31) A gallstone is a crystalline concretion formed within the gallbladder. As they build up, these stones not only disrupt the normal flow of bile into the intestine, they can also pass distally into the biliary tract blocking the cystic duct, common bile duct, pancreatic duct, or the ampulla of Vater (see diagram on p. 113). Gallstones may lead to inflammation of the gallbladder (cholecystitis) and often infection. Even worse, life-threatening conditions like pancreatitis or cholangitis can arise as well, and are medical emergencies. In the majority of cases, however, these surgeries can be avoided by using some simple preventative measures and good old-fashioned common sense.

In the diagram it is clear to see how stones can easily obstruct the flow of bile along the pathway to the intestine, even obstructing the pancreas. Gallstones can be removed/flushed out of the gallbladder and surgery avoided using a very simple at-home procedure. The Seven Day Liver and Gallbladder flush is explained in detail in *The Liver and Gallbladder Miracle Cleanse* by Andreas Moritz, as well as more specifics on the benefits of the procedure.

The diet of the average American is too high in refined carbohydrates, sugar, and processed, rancid vegetable oils and trans fats. These are the main culprits in gallbladder disease. Perhaps the major dietary player in gallbladder disease, however, is gluten. In his personal journey through gallbladder disease, removal and recovery, author Jeremy Bernal notes in *The Gall Bladder Survival Guide* that "The thing that had the biggest effect, believe it or not, was going on a low-gluten diet." (Ibid p. 125) Either way, these foods, especially gluten, all strain the gallbladder, clogging it up over time. This renders the quantity of bile secreted insufficient and ineffective.

I have treated my gallbladder patients using a specific gallbladder diet and specific supplements until they were back on track. For those who are interested, this diet can be found in Appendix C p. 351. Supplementation to aid in the recovery of gallbladder symptoms is straightforward. We want to stimulate better movement and flow of the bile from the gallbladder into the intestinal tract while using the aforementioned flush to remove any accumulated stones. The first step in doing this is using Standard Process A-F Betafood® and Cholacol®. In most cases each is to be taken at a dose of 2 per meal. Both of these products help to support gallbladder function by aiding in fat metabolism, bile flow, and healthy bowel elimination. They do so by using a mixture of bile salts, the herb collinsonia, glandular extracts and many other nutrients.

To facilitate better digestion and alleviate some of the symptoms for the patient, I recommend using the bitter herbs to stimulate what is known as the Bitter Reflex.

"When a Bitter substance is recognized by bitter receptors on the tongue, a chain of neural and endocrine events begins, labeled as the "bitter reflex." Mediated by the release of the gastric hormone gastrin, this reflex results in an overall stimulation of digestive function, which over time strengthens the structure and function of all digestive organs (liver, stomach, gallbladder, pancreas, etc.)." (Charles-Davis D. Bitters: the revival of a forgotten flavor. Wise Traditions. WAPF. 11(4):35.)

Successful products used to stimulate this reflex are Swedish Bitters (www. Florahealth.com) and Urban Moonshine (www. urbanmoonshine.com). Bitters have a tremendous effect on the digestive tract, specifically the gallbladder and have been used safely for centuries to treat reflux and to increase the liver's production of bile as well as the gallbladder's excretion of bile. To learn more, I highly recommend reading Danielle Charles-Davies' article in *Wise Traditions*, men-tioned above.

Patients with gallbladder problems are encouraged to incorporate bitter vegetables and greens into their diet more often. This includes chicory, dandelion, arugula, radicchio, endive, broccoli, rape, and burdock. One last thought here is the little-known fact that lemons are very good for the liver and gallbladder. They can even be eaten in their entirety, skin and all, or included in a juicing regimen. Remember to always buy organic so as to avoid toxic pesticide sprays and take advantage of the greater nutrition.

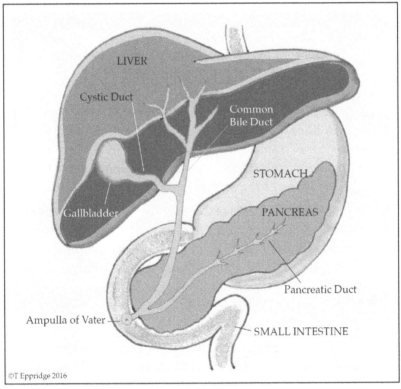

ANATOMY OF THE BILIARY TREE INCLUDING THE LIVER, GALLBLADDER, AND PANCREAS

SECTION VII
COMMON CONDITIONS OF THE JOINTS AND CONNECTIVE TISSUE

Carpal Tunnel Syndrome (CTS)

Carpal Tunnel Syndrome (CTS) is a condition that causes a great deal of discomfort in the hand, and occasionally both hands. According to the Mayo Clinic, CTS is a progressively painful hand and arm condition caused by a pinched nerve in the wrist. A number of factors can contribute to CTS, including the anatomy of the wrist, certain underlying health problems and possibly patterns of hand use. Bound by bones and ligaments, the carpal tunnel is a narrow passageway, about as big around as the thumb, located on the palm side of your wrist. This tunnel protects a main nerve to the hand and nine tendons that bend the fingers. Compression of the nerve produces the numbness, pain, and, eventually, hand weakness that characterize CTS. The medical profession will usually first treat the condition with splinting of the wrist, nonsteroidal anti-inflammatory medications (NSAIDs) and even corticosteroids. If these do not work, and in most cases they do not offer a long-term cure, surgery and/or physical therapy will be recommended.

In the chiropractic office we see this syndrome as most often caused by a weakness of the wrist joint and the associated tendons of the forearm musculature. There is often a concomitant nutritional deficiency of some of the B vitamins as well as a repetitive movement component involved in the syndrome. For example, CTS is common in people who have to work with their hands doing manual labor, typing, or other occupations that require intensive hand use.

Some patients will require manipulation of the area of the wrist joint. This will vary based on the individual's structural problems and may require manipulation of the carpal-metacarpal, radio-carpal, ulno-carpal, or radio-ulnar joints respectively as well as respective spinal regions in the neck. Some patients presenting with CTS have musculo-tendonous spasm and inflammation at the elbow. They will require soft tissue work to the elbow and forearm as well as chiropractic adjustment. This treatment often yields good results in a very short period of time. Obviously if there is a repetitive action that is causing this inflammation, then rest must be the primary treatment in order to remove the causative action. Without removing the noxious stimulus, all adjusting and soft tissue treatment will not yield good results. In some cases, it may be impractical for the patient to completely stop using the hands because of their work. In these cases, helping the patient to develop better posture, to stretch, and even bracing may be most important.

Furthermore, some studies have shown a relationship between a deficiency in vitamins B2 and B6 and CTS. ("Successful Therapy with Vitamin B6 and Vitamin B2 of the Carpal Syndrome and Need for Determination of the RDAs for Vitamin B6 and Vitamin B2 for Disease States," Folkers, K. Ellis, J. Annals of the New York Academy of Sciences, 1990. pp. 295–301) Therefore it is important to address the nutritional component as well. Organic acid testing is an affordable and accurate way to assess the need for the B vitamins. Another nutritional component used to treat the inflammatory component of CTS is a natural anti-inflammatory such as Inflammatone by Designs for Health or Zyflamend by New Chapter. These products contain proteolytic enzymes and anti-inflammatory herbs like boswelia that help control inflammation and encourage wound healing without the gastro-intestinal side effects of NSAIDS.

Lastly, cold laser treatment may be used to reduce the inflammation of the affected area and provide relief for the patient. This works hand-in-hand with the soft tissue and the chiropractic manipulation of the involved joints to remove inflammation and encourage healing.

Sprains and Strains of the Knee

If a person is running or makes a sudden turn and sprains one of the collateral ligaments on the side of the knee or even one of the cruciate ligaments, he or she should be treated by a chiropractor immediately because if the ligaments are stretched and the cartilage shifts out of position, it is best not to walk on it. This will only create further inflammation and damage as well as compensatory problems with gait and low back pain. The first thing that should be done is to have the knee adjusted in order to bring the tibia and femur back into proper alignment with the two menisci, medially and laterally. This is done simply by using common sense and having faith in the innate intelligence of the body to heal.

Treatment protocol

First, soft tissue massaging to the medial and lateral aspects of the knee should be performed to gently release some of the spasm that occurs in the soft tissue. This is especially important along the joint line medially as most injuries of this nature overstretch this area. Then, the hamstrings and quadriceps muscles should be gently stretched as well. Physical therapy modalities like cold laser, electric stimulation, and ultrasound are great during the acute phase for reducing inflammation, swelling, and reducing pain. Once this is accomplished, the knee will be much easier to adjust and reposition. Finally, ice should be used on the knee joint at 10 minute intervals (10 minutes on the joint and then 10 minutes off) for the first 24 hours.

Rest is very critical here, too. Keep off the leg for 24–48 hours in order to allow the knee to rest and properly heal. Doing so allows the synovial fluid to flow into the joint space properly and to heal the tissue damage. The use of natural anti-inflammatories is helpful in aiding the healing process. Zyflamend by New Chapter is a well-researched and natural combination of herbs designed specifically to alleviate joint inflammation by acting on the cyclooxygenase pathways of inflammation. Generally, a dosage of 3–4 for the first few days is necessary until the joint heals. In more severe cases a ligament or cartilage may be torn or ruptured and will therefore require surgery. However, in most cases surgery can be avoided with prompt, conservative treatment.

Knee Pain and Other Knee Injuries

Structural Injury

Most people experience knee pain of some kind at one time or another. Sometimes it is caused by arthritis, at other times by a specific injury, while some knee pain seems unexplained. Let me start with the unexplained incidences. Here the patient presents with knee pain without any history of trauma, arthritis, or known cause. Upon examination we will almost always find that there is a concomitant dysfunction in one or both arches of the feet. When this movement of the arch of the foot occurs, it brings with it the tibia and fibula and therefore the femur and everything above it. As a result, there is a malposition of the knee joint, most commonly with a valgus strain. This compresses the lateral knee joint, while overstretching the medial knee joint, and creates an internal rotation of the knee joint. Uncorrected, it can result in degeneration of the ligaments and menisci and cause pain.

Treatment of this type of knee problem starts by scanning the foot with the Foot Levelers 3D scanner (see Appendix D p. 358 #29) and assessing the specific problems. Then custom orthotics are made by Foot Levelers directly from the scan. Having the patient wear the orthotics will ensure that the joints of the feet and therefore the knee and hip above will remain in the proper structural position during weightbearing. Next, based on our physical exam findings as well as the scan, we correct the specific malpositions of the arches of the feet as well as the knee joint. This is done by using soft tissue to stretch the muscles and tendons and by using chiropractic adjustment.

As a palliative treatment, we may also use electrical stimulation and cold laser to assuage the pain and swelling and to facilitate the chiropractic adjustment. We use nutritional anti-inflammatory compounds like Zyflamend by New Chapter to reduce pain and swelling and thereby encourage healing.

Arthritic Type

The most important aspect of an arthritic knee is to determine the nature of the arthritis. Is it caused by a generalized, systemic physiological and nutritional breakdown or is it caused by a repetitive, chronic structural irritation? Possibly it may be both. If it is the latter, then we first refer to the protocol mentioned above for structural knee treatment. However, if it is the former or both at the same time, then we first do a complete nutritional assessment of the patient from top to bottom. Otherwise, the structural treatment we employ will be only temporary. We typically begin with Genova Diagnostics Lab's nutritional and metabolic testing as well as assessing digestive function and body pH. Refer to the section on arthritis for dietary and supplement protocols.

Injury to the Knee

In treating a knee injury, it is of paramount importance to take a thorough history of the nature of the injury. Essentially we want to reverse engineer exactly what happened when the injury occurred. This enables us to make an assessment as to what tissues were injured, overstretched, compressed, etc. Once this information is gathered, we can determine the type of treatment necessary to correct the injury.

Most knee injuries involve damage to the soft tissue in three specific areas, referred to as the terrible triad — the medial meniscus, medial collateral ligament and the anterior cruciate ligament. Sometimes the medial cartilage, or medial meniscus as it is called, is moved out of position and has to be adjusted back into proper position. At other times, the medial collateral ligament is overstretched and, as a result, the muscles surrounding the medial knee joint are in spasm. In each case we must evaluate the tissue and use stretching, ice, physical therapy and adjustment to reverse the damage.

Some very specific things may be used to treat almost all knee injuries regardless of the mechanics of the injury. First, ice helps remove any swelling/fluid in the joint. Since fluid is non-compressible, it is very difficult to move and stretch the knee without first reducing the swelling. Therefore it is best to start the patient icing the knee immediately. Second, cold laser and other physical therapy modalities are used to further reduce swelling and inflammation. This will make our soft tissue work and manipulation that much more effective. Third, expeller-pressed unrefined peanut oil is used to restore the elasticity to the ligaments. Peanut oil should be applied liberally to the entire joint each night until complete recovery is established. Fourth and finally, we begin to mobilize the joint more and more using soft tissue and stretching followed by chiropractic manipulation. It is important to note that natural anti-inflammatory supplements are a crucial part of reducing the swelling and inflammation throughout this protocol.

As mentioned previously, it may also be necessary to address any pedial foundation problems in a patient with a knee injury. Even if the trauma occurred only to the knee, malposition of the foot may have served to predispose the knee to injury, and may even prolong or prevent a full recovery. Therefore, we always scan the patient's feet to rule this factor out.

Sprained Ankle Treatment

A sprained ankle can be treated in much the same manner as the knee. Ankle injuries are most often inversion sprains in which the ankle is "rolled" over on or bent inward. This commonly occurs with a misstep off a curb or while walking or jogging. Many doctors recommend bathing the ankle in warm water and Epsom salts and staying off of the foot. However, in chiropractic we are trained to bring the ankle back into the normal position with soft tissue stretching followed by a simple adjustment. Then, the arch of the foot is strapped with sports tape to stabilize the ankle joint. In cases where there is swelling, we bathe the foot in a mixture of 4 tablespoons of kosher salt and 4 ounces of apple cider vinegar in a basin of cold water. This is done for 30 minutes, three times a day for the first 48 hours. Then reduce to two times per day on the third day and once a day thereafter until the swelling and pain are gone. Soaking the ankle like this will facilitate the osmotic movement of fluid in the tissue and aid in healing.

To aid the healing of the ligaments and tendons and restore their elasticity, use peanut oil rubbed into the affected area once or twice a day. Also soak the ankle in one cup of Burow's solution, (an over-the-counter drug for topical administration) added to a basin of water.

Plantar Fasciitis

Plantar fasciitis is inflammation of the plantar fascia, the thick tissue on the bottom of the foot. It connects the heel bone to the toes and creates the arch of the foot. Plantar fasciitis occurs when the thick band of tissue on the bottom of the foot is overstretched or overused. This can be painful and make walking more difficult. You are more likely to get plantar fasciitis from the following: foot arch dysfunction (either flat feet or high arches), long distance running especially running downhill or on uneven surfaces, sudden weight gain/obesity, standing on your feet all day especially in shoes with poor arch support, tightness in your achilles tendon of the calf muscle. Plantar fasciitis is seen in both men and women. However, it most often affects active men ages 40 – 70. It is one of the most common orthopedic complaints relating to the foot. Plantar fasciitis is commonly thought to be caused by a heel spur, but research has found that this is not the case. On x-ray, heel spurs are seen in people with and without plantar fasciitis.

The treatment of plantar fasciitis is multifaceted. First, it is best to treat the inflammation of the foot using the cold laser, which uses light with a wavelength above that of the infrared spectrum and is therefore non-visible. This light has the ability to penetrate the deep tissue, reduce inflammation and restore circulation. It also encourages faster wound healing and reduces pain. Second, the physician must gently stretch the soft tissue on the bottom of the foot. This can be done with the patient lying prone and using a muscle liniment like Arnica or Kool'N Fit®/CryoDerm®.

Chiropractic Treatment

The third aspect of treatment protocol is to adjust the foot using chiropractic techniques to correct the malposition of the bones of the foot. The bones most commonly involved are the calcaneus, navicular, cuboid and even the metatarsal heads. Plantar fasciitis is typically caused by one of the most common conditions of the body, excessive foot pronation. We find that the patient presents with the following malposition of the arches and bones of the foot:

- Posterior/lateral heel wear
- Foot flare/external foot rotation
- Patella/knee joint rotation/flaring
- Valgus position of the Achilles tendon
- Dropped medial/longitudinal arch with accompanying dropped navicular bone
- Callous formation at the 2nd–4th metatarsal heads

Typically we will adjust the navicular bone first, with the patient lying in a prone position and the leg bent at the knee to 90 degrees. We then adjust the navicular by stabilizing the lateral ankle with our outside hand and using our medial hand to make an index contact on the navicular bone. The foot is brought into inversion and the thrust is made plantar to dorsal and medial to lateral. This adjustment may also be done with the thenar pad of the inside hand. Secondly, we will commonly see an inferior-lateral subluxation of the cuboid bone. To correct this, the doctor, with the patient again prone and with knee bent to 90 degrees, takes the inside hand and stabilizes the ankle. The doctor then uses his outside hand to make a contact just posterior to the base of the 5th metatarsal (which can be easily located by palpating the styloid of the 5th metatarsal and moving posterior just slightly) on the cuboid bone with his/her thenar pad. The thrust is made in a superior to medial direction.

Often it will also be necessary to adjust the cuneiform bones as they will typically collapse inferiorly (toward the ground) in these cases as well. This can be accomplished in many ways, but I prefer to stand facing the involved leg on the same side; the patient is prone and knee bent to 90°. Keeping the forearm of the superior arm parallel with the tibia, a contact is made "cupping" the heel with the fingers contacting the medial calcaneus. The inferior hand then contacts the plantar surface of the foot directly under the three cuneiforms. Keeping this forearm parallel to the tibia as well, the doctor tractions the calcaneus inferiorly (which will actually be toward the ceiling with the patient prone and knee bent) with the superior hand while thrusting superiorly with the inferior hand (which will be toward the floor in this position).

Since each person is unique, one should be examined by a qualified chiropractic physician with experience in extremity adjusting in order to have these and any other subluxation patterns evaluated. After treatment with the laser and the adjustment, I advise my patients to soak the foot in warm water (a bucket will suffice) with 4 tablespoons of Epsom salts. The foot should be bathed for 30 minutes three times per day, including just before bed, until directed otherwise. I find this soaking to be an excellent way to relax the fascia underneath the foot and promote healing.

Supplementation for this condition is primarily focused on using a natural anti-inflammatory approach. For this we use Inflammatone from Designs for Health at a dose of two in the morning on an empty stomach and two again at bed time. Another excellent product made by New Chapter is Zyflamend™. You can take up to four a day on an empty stomach. Be aware that it may irritate the stomach in sensitive people due to the volatile oils found in the herbs used in the product. The symptoms generally resolve quickly and are not serious but this may not be a good option for some patients.

It is wise to advise the patient to stay off their feet as much as possible for at least a few days. Unfortunately most working people do not have this option. Therefore we recommend they wear a special boot at night which holds the foot in a more relaxed position to take the strain off of the fascia. There are many different versions of this boot, so work with your doctor to find an appropriate one.

Lastly, and perhaps most important, the patient should be evaluated for orthotics. My patients have used Foot Levelers brand (see Appendix D) custom orthotics with great success. A 3D laser scanner enables both the physician and the patient to see the foot three-dimensionally. This not only helps the doctor to see the structural dysfunction of the foot, it also enables the patient to better understand the cause and nature of the fasciitis. Foot Levelers custom make a pair of orthotics that fit the patient's unique specifications. Once the orthotics are made, the patient must wear them as much as possible, especially in the morning when first stepping out of bed. The orthotic supports the arch properly, taking the strain off the ligaments and tendons and hastening recovery.

Bursitis

According to WebMD's medical reference, bursitis is defined as inflammation of the fluid-filled sac (bursa) that lies between a tendon and skin or between a tendon and bone. The purpose of the bursa is to decrease rubbing, friction and irritation during normal movements of the joints. However, when there is trauma, overuse, or other damage to the bursa, it can become inflamed and swell. Aging and poor nutrition can also play a role. Andreas Moritz, writes on p. 181 of his book, *The Liver and Gallbladder Miracle Cleanse*, that bursitis can also be related to stagnant bile and gallbladder dysfunction. This can make movement of the joint very painful and therefore limited. Bursitis is most often the result of an impact injury to the joint or improper repetitive movements such as are commonly experienced with shoveling, exercising, etc. The most common areas for bursitis are the shoulder, elbow, knee, and hip.

Many cases of bursitis, especially shoulder bursitis, are *not related to an injury, fall, or repetitive movements*. Bursitis can be triggered by a physiologic problem just as easily as it can be caused by repetitive movements or injury. If a person has a diet that is overly acidic as a result of eating too much processed and refined foods, then calcium will begin to deposit in the joint. This can lead to tendonosis (which often includes calcification of the tendon) and eventually inflammation of the bursa sac.

Either way, this condition must be treated with several different techniques. In cases where there is a physiologic cause, we must alkalize the patient's diet first. This can be done as discussed in the section on arthritis. Refer to the alkaline foods list in Appendix G p. 368. This will help move calcium out of the joint and soft tissues and back where it belongs, in our teeth and bones.

Patients with bursitis (and even frozen shoulder), as mentioned above, are also likely to have gallbladder congestion and gallstones. This should be examined by a qualified holistic practitioner, and necessary testing performed. If there is congestion of the gallbladder, a flushing protocol must be followed to get to the real root of the problem. I recommend the 7-day gallbladder and liver flush as outlined in the book *The Liver and Gallbladder Miracle Cleanse* by Andreas Moritz. A diet specifically designed to relieve gallbladder problems can be found in Appendix C p. 351-53.

Next, bursitis must be treated with soft tissue work and mobilization. A combination of chiropractic adjustment, physical therapy including cold laser treatment, and soft tissue stretching on the glenohumeral joint (shoulder) and the scapular muscles can be used. One of the main focal points of this treatment is to work with the patient's arm behind their back while they are lying prone (face down). In this position I work to get under the shoulder blade, stretching the scapula laterally and superiorly. This is very painful for most patients, so it has to be done slowly and gently, with the patient exhaling as the stretch is performed. The procedure should be explained to the patient and they should be made aware that it will be painful. Take your time with the stretching and be firm but never, ever force.

Next, the patient must also be given home exercises to do. I use a combination of wall crawl exercises and simple circumduction movements in both clockwise and counterclockwise directions. Thera-Band® brand exercise equipment including the pulley system is extremely helpful for the patient and doctor in rehabilitating the shoulder. Thera-Band® even has a website at www.thera-bandacademy.com which offers patients and doctors different exercises complete with pictures and explanations. Patients and doctors may also purchase equipment online. I advise the patient not to be afraid to work through the pain to the best of their ability.

After each treatment and after doing the exercises, the patient is always advised to ice down ten minutes on, ten minutes off, especially during the first 24–48 hours of onset. Then, alternating ice and heat can be used to serve as a type of pumping for the circulation. This will aid in getting the swelling down. Prolonged ice or heat will aggravate the condition.

Anti-inflammatory supplements can be very helpful in quelling the inflammation as the shoulder is worked on. One of the best is Zyflamend by New Chapter. It can be taken up to four per day in the short term until the inflammation is controlled. It should NOT be taken if you are on blood thinning medication. If you cannot find this supplement, I recommend using bromelain and/or turmeric at a dosage of 1,500 milligrams per day. I use Medi Herb products which are of the highest quality and always standardized. Inflammatone, made by Designs for Health, is also a wonderful product for aiding in naturally reducing inflammation.

One final yet very important consideration regarding bursitis is a deficiency in vitamins D, F, and K. Without adequate vitamin D and vitamin F status, the body cannot absorb and use calcium properly. These deficiencies are prevalent. Rarely do I see a bloodwork with adequate vitamin D levels. I consider a range of 50 ng/mL–80 ng/mL to be optimal. Many doctors will say that 30 ng/mL is adequate, but I find this not to be the case for most people. Since no clear gold standard exists for bloodwork levels of vitamin D, it is important to take a food diary on the patient to see if he or she is obtaining adequate dietary vitamin D. Those living in a cooler climate will not be exposed to as much sunlight and will therefore make less vitamin D throughout the year. Lack of regular exposure to sunlight, lack of natural vitamin D in our food supply (see Section III page 29 on General Dietary Guidelines), living in northern climates, and the overuse of sunscreens from what I like to call "sunshinephobia" are all culprits in this problem.

To check vitamin F (unsaturated fatty acids) status on my patients I use the Genova Diagnostics Lab based in Georgia. They have a blood test for this that gives a patient's omega 3 and omega 6 ratios as well as omega 9. Many researchers believe that traditional cultures once maintained a nearly 1:1 ratio of omega 3 to omega 6 fatty acids. Unfortunately, the Standard American Diet (SAD) puts most people somewhere between 15–30:1 omega 6 to omega 3. This imbalance, researchers believe, points to the overwhelming occurrence of inflammatory conditions so prevalent in our society. Vitamins F, D, and K are critical for ensuring that calcium is taken from the intestines, into the bloodstream and from the bloodstream into the bone and teeth where it belongs. Without these critical osteofactors, calcium can precipitate out of the blood and into the tissues and joints where it does not belong. To find a doctor in your area who can assist you in getting tested, go to the Genova Diagnostics Institute website www.gdx.net.

Good food sources of vitamin K include lacto-fermented vegetables, natto, meat and organ meats of pastured animals, eggs and raw dairy from cattle grazing on fast growing grass in spring and fall.

Lyme Disease

Over the last 20–30 years, Lyme disease, sometimes referred to as Borreliosis, has become a more prevalent and serious health problem, especially in the Northeastern United States. It is difficult to diagnose even with current sophisticated testing, and often has debilitating health consequences. It is caused by transmission of Borrelia burgdorferi, a spirochete (a unique spiral-shaped bacterium) via a tick (called the vector of the disease) belonging to the genus Ixodes. This disease is initially characterized by a bull's-eye rash, more properly termed erythema migrans, which appears in the majority of cases (70%–80%). There are many other symptoms which can vary widely from person to person. The most common symptoms aside from the erythema migrans are muscle and joint pain, fever, chills, flu-like symptoms and frequent headaches.

Untreated Lyme disease can have more serious health sequelae including neurological, cardio-vascular, memory and cognitive impairment, and even damage to the eyes. As Stephen Harrod Buhner notes in his book *Healing Lyme*, "results show that for many, antibiotic treatment alone is insufficient. . . . and studies indicate that additional supportive protocols are necessary to help correct brain impacts from the infection." (p. 49) He continues, "while pharmaceuticals are inept for this purpose, plants are not, and in many instances have been found specific for the problems that occur in post-Lyme-disease syndrome."

Unfortunately, testing for Lyme borreliosis can be confounding and unreliable due to the ability of the spirochete to mask itself and evade the immune system. Regarding this ability, Buhner comments, "Lyme spirochetes. . . . can change their outer membrane structure quickly and often. . . . and can take on or create completely different spirochetal forms." Therefore, diagnosis of Lyme borreliosis must be based upon a thorough history, proper testing which often must be repeated, and symptomatology.

A more thorough discussion of Lyme borreliosis is beyond the scope of this book. However, I have summarized the important information regarding prevention and treatment of the disease. Much of this information combined with the insightful knowledge of Stephen Buhner is a protocol I have used successfully for treating many cases of Lyme. Many of these protocols are from *Healing Lyme* which is a must-read for anyone with Lyme.

Lyme Disease Information/Protocol

What You Must Know About Lyme Disease

Consult *Healing Lyme* by Stephen Buhner. Also visit the online support group at www.planetthrive.com (click on *connect with others* in the masthead) for questions and answers about this protocol and people's experience with it.

Lyme disease is typically transmitted (vector) by ticks, but may also be transferred by fleas, mites, etc. Standard treatment for Lyme in the United States is antibiotics (typically amoxicillin, doxycycline, clarithromycin, etc.) for 10–28 days. Studies show up to a 35% relapse rate for those taking antibiotics to treat Lyme. They are not as effective as purported to be.

Up to two-thirds of those infected with Borrelia have no rash at all and many never see the ticks. Since testing for Lyme disease is unreliable, it is important to know the following information: In the first 2–4 weeks of infection, only about half of infected people produce measurable antibodies to Lyme spirochetes. Borrelia may encyst, making it even harder for them to be detected.

The most common tests include:

Elisa – exceptionally unreliable and not to be relied upon solely for a diagnosis.

Western Blot (aka Immunoblot) – may be oriented around IgG or IgM antibodies. This test should always be reported by showing which bands are reactive, *not* simply as positive or negative. The 18kd, 37kd, 39kd, 83kd, 93kd, 23–25kd, 31kd, and 34kd bands are the most specific for Lyme infection. In order for a Lyme test to be considered positive, the 41kd band and at least one of the others have to appear at testing.

Polymerase Chain Reaction (PCR) – not a very sensitive test (and therefore unreliable).

Other Tests Showing Promise:

Reverse Western Blot (RWB) – tests for antigen presence in urine.

Lyme Dot Blot Assay (LDA) – tests for Lyme antigen presence in urine. Available through IgeneX in Palo Alto, California (www.igenex.com).

Phillips/Mattman – perhaps best of the newer tests and reported to have 100% accuracy. A similar test, Rapid Identification of Borrelia burgdorferi or Q-Ribb test, available through Bowen Laboratories, gives results within 24–48 hours (www.Bowen.org).

Prevention of Lyme Disease

1. Astragalus (Astragalus membranaceous) – dosage is 1,000 mg 3 times daily working slowly up to a maximum of 4,000 mg 4 times daily for at least 60 days, then decrease to a lower dose. Take for 8–12 months. Highly indicated in pre to early and early disseminated Lyme infection. However, it is *contraindicated* in later stage Lyme infection.

2. Thymex® by Standard Process – begin dosage at one tablet 3 times daily and increase slowly up to three tablets 4 times daily. Begin dosing one week prior to visiting endemic area and continue to take one week after leaving. Contraindicated in later stages of Lyme.

Acute Onset of Lyme Disease

1. Eleuthero (aka Siberian Ginseng) – I recommend MediHerb's Eleuthero — 450 mg capsules (200 mg of whole herb and 250 mg of standardized extract) at a dosage of 2 capsules 4 times daily for 8–12 months. It should be standardized to 0.8% eleutherosides B and E.

2. Thymex® (see above)

These 2 products should be taken immediately at the onset of the infection and continued throughout the early stages of the disease.

The Basic Core Protocol for Lyme Disease

The Core Protocol can be used along with antibiotic therapy and will increase considerably the positive outcomes from antibiotics.

1. Andrographis paniculata – must be standardized to 10% andrographolides. Take 400 mg, one to four capsules or tablets 3–4 times daily for 8–12 months. It is best to begin gradually, starting with the lower dose and increasing the dosage by one capsule/tablet every 7 days. Gradually increase dosage to a maximum of four capsules/tablets 4 times daily. Maintain this dosage for at least 60 days and then gradually decrease to the minimum dosage of one capsule/tablet 3 times daily.

2. Japanese Knotweed (Resveratrol) – one to four tablets 3–4 times daily for 8–12 months. Increase the dosage slowly, increasing by one tablet each week and working up to the maximum dosage of four tablets 4 times daily and remain at this dosage for 60 days. As symptoms decrease, slowly decrease the dosage down to a maintenance dose of one tablet 3 times daily. I recommend Source Naturals brand. The standardized tablets contain 500 mg of standardized polygonum cuspidatum whole herb.

Warning: *Do not use this herb along with blood-thinning medications. Discontinue use of the herb 10 days prior to any scheduled surgery.*

SYMPTOMS OF LYME BORRELIOSIS

Erythema migrans (EM) or bull's eye rash (only in 1/3 of those infected)
Multiple EM lesions (in about 1/5 of those infected)
Acrodermatitis chronic atrophicans (later stages)
Borrelial lymphocytoma
Continual low-grade fever
High fever, chills, or sweating (generally indicates bacterial coinfections)
General flu-like symptoms
Frequent headaches, neck stiffness
Regular mild-to-moderate muscle and joint pain
Severe unremitting headache (generally indicates bacterial coinfections)
Bell's Palsy (partial face paralysis)
Mental confusion or difficulty thinking
Disorientation, getting lost, going to wrong places
Lightheadedness, wooziness
Mood swings, irritability, depression
Disturbed sleep
Fatigue, tiredness, poor stamina
Blurry vision with floaters and/or light sensitivity
Feeling pressure in eyes
Stiffness in joints or back
Twitching of face or other muscles
Neck creaks, cracks, stiffness, pain
Tingling, numbness, burning or stabbing sensations, shooting pains
Chest pain, heart palpitations
Shortness of breath, cough
Buzzing or ringing in ears, sound sensitivity
Motion sickness, vertigo, poor balance
Sudden hearing loss
Tremors
Weight gain or loss
Swollen glands (can also be from coinfection)
Menstrual irregularity
Irritable bladder or bladder dysfunction
Upset stomach and/or abdominal pain
Galactorrhea

3. Cat's Claw (Uncaria tomentosa) – 500 mg, one to four capsules 3–4 times daily for 8–12 months. Begin at the lowest dose and increase incrementally every seven days. Maintain the maximum dosage for 60 days and then slowly decrease in the same manner to a maintenance dose of one capsule 3 times daily. I recommend Raintree Cat's Claw only (purchase at www.

raintree.com). ***Do not use*** if you have had an organ transplant or are using immunosuppressive drugs. ***Do not use*** if you are trying to become pregnant, if you are on acid-blocking medication or if you are using blood-thinning medication.

4. Congaplex® by Standard Process – an excellent multivitamin for the immune system. It consists of calcium, vitamin A, and many other nutrients specifically designed to support the immune system. Dosage should be two capsules every waking hour for the first week then decreased to a maintenance dose of six per day. This is to be taken indefinitely at the maintenance level.

5. Argentyn 23 Silver Hydrosol – a potent antibiotic/antiviral which can be taken safely without damaging the natural gut flora. Dosage is given according to body weight (ask for specific dosage instructions from the physician).

Collagen Support Protocol

Lyme spirochetes cause a destruction to collagenous tissues throughout the body. The core protocol outlined above will help with this, but if you are suffering severe side effects of the disease or suspect that its course might be severe, you should consider initiating a regimen as outlined below to support the collagenous structures of the body:

Homemade Bone Broth: Drink/consume 2–3 cups per day; made according to the *Nourishing Traditions*/Nourishing Broth recipes. It may be used as a drink with added parsley and Celtic or Himalayan sea salt *or* you may consume it as the broth of vegetable/chicken/beef soups. Ask the doctor for the proper recipes or you may purchase bone broth at US Wellness by visiting our website at www.dramoruso.com and clicking on the round US Wellness link in the upper left hand corner.

Pure Radiance vitamin C – can be taken as a powder at a dosage of two teaspoons mixed in water daily *or* eight capsules.

Zinc Picolinate with Copper – 20–30 mg daily. Zinc and copper are essential for repairing the damage caused to the cartilage and connective tissue as a result of Lyme disease.

Glucosamine Synergy® – recommended dosage is 500 mg. 3 times daily. Use Standard Process brand only.

Silicon – 6–20 drops added to ¼ cup water daily. Use only the orthosilicic acid version of this supplement.

Dietary Recommendations Regarding Lyme Disease

Since the etiology of Lyme Disease is immunosuppressive, it is important that the dietary approach be anti-inflammatory in nature and course.

Seeing that refined sugar is immunosuppressive, the diet should be low in overall sugar, with careful attention given to removing any and all refined sources of sugar. Consult with the doctor for more specifics.

The diet should be centered upon traditional foods which nourish the immune system and with special attention to supporting the connective tissues. Homemade bone and fish stocks should be incorporated into the diet on a daily basis. Consult with the physician for specifics and recipes, or see the book *Nourishing Traditions* by Sally Fallon Morell.

Avoid all industrialized fats including but not limited to: hydrogenated or partially hydrogenated oils, soybean oil, corn oil, canola oil, safflower and cottonseed oils, margarines and other man-made spreads, and vegetable oils (mixes). These oils are all immunosuppressive and related to all types of degenerative illness. Instead, increase your intake of organic, pastured animal fats, extra virgin coconut oil, flaxseed oil, and raw, pastured butter. For more information on the specifics, visit the Weston A. Price Foundation's website at www.westonaprice.org.

Lyme Prevention Protocol

Much of this is from Stephen Buhner's book *Healing Lyme*.

For prevention of Lyme if you live in a Lyme-endemic area or will be visiting such an area:

1. Astragalus – 1,000 mg taken twice daily all year-round if living in a Lyme endemic area; take temporarily for several weeks before and after visiting such an area. Use MediHerb or Planetary Herbs formula or equivalent.
2. Andrographis (400 mg) – one capsule 3 times daily taken throughout the season.

3. Cat's Claw (500 mg) – two capsules 3 times daily taken throughout the season. I recommend using Raintree Cat's Claw only (purchase at www.raintree.com). *Do not use* if you have had an organ transplant or are using immunosuppressive drugs. *Do not use* if you are trying to become pregnant, are on acid-blocking medication or are using blood thinning medication.

My Protocol – Blue Ice™ Fermented Cod Liver Oil made by Green Pasture™, the highest quality product on the market. Take one teaspoon per day with meals for prevention and immune support.

My Protocol – Congaplex® (Standard Process): two capsules every waking hour for up to one week, then decrease to a maintenance dose of six a day for the remainder.

At the First Sign of a Bull's Eye Rash (EM) or Embedded Tick

For Rash, Homeopathic Apis – 30C 3 times daily for three days.

For Tick Bite, Homeopathic ledum: 1M – 3 times daily for three days. (M= dilution rate of 1/1000.)

Begin Core Protocol for Lyme Disease

Eleuthero (aka Siberian Ginseng) – 450 mg capsule of a formulation standardized to 0.8% eleutherosides B and E. MediHerb and Nature's Way are better quality brands. Take two capsules 4 times daily for 30–60 days.

My Protocol – Blue Ice™ Fermented Cod Liver Oil: made by Green Pasture™. This is the highest quality product on the market. Take one teaspoon 3 times daily with meals for up to 2 weeks then slowly wean down to one teaspoon a day.

Joint Pain in Young Children
(under the age of 12)

In children, joint pain is often related to a high acid condition of the body. Why this happens is a matter of basic chemistry. When the body becomes overly acidic from poor diet, lack of proper rest, stress, etc. it will draw alkaline minerals like calcium and magnesium out of the tissue (bones, muscle, etc.) in order to buffer the blood's pH. (Our blood's pH must be strictly controlled or death can result). This loss of calcium from the tissue is often compounded in today's children by deficiencies of vitamins D, F, and K (unsaturated fatty acids). These deficiencies make it difficult for the body to absorb calcium present in the diet. As a result, the acidic pH along with vitamin D, F, and K deficiencies work together to compound the problem. Every family should have litmus paper (pH paper) to test first morning urine as well as oral pH (this tape can be purchased in any health food store). It is important that every child on the SAD should be checked for vitamin D, F, and K deficiencies. To have your child tested, visit the Genova Diagnostic's website at www.gdx.net to find a doctor in your area familiar with fatty acid testing. Once you have established the child's pH and vitamin D, F, and K status, you can adjust the diet accordingly. Without the proper fats in the diet, including saturated fats, minerals cannot be absorbed. The general dietary guidelines in Section III indicate which fats are good and which to avoid.

Joint pain in children can be a simple condition caused by poor diet and/or lack of calcium absorption. Children will most commonly complain about pain in the knees. They will say that the knees are painful in the mornings and especially after exercising. Occasionally there can be pain and discomfort doing nothing at all. Some doctors tell the parents that the children are merely having "growing pains." Nothing could be farther from the truth. Very few doctors, whether MDs or chiropractors, are properly schooled in nutrition. Furthermore, most allopathic doctors know very little about chiropractic and how it works to help the body heal itself.

Many children eat too many simple carbohydrates, especially in the form of refined white sugar and white flour. Compounding this problem, they also eat the wrong types of fats. Typically their diet is too high in trans fats found in rancid vegetable oils and processed/packaged foods, and too low in pastured animal fats, fats found in wild caught fish, palm oil, and coconut oil. The main culprit however, is refined sugar. The high-sugar American diet is the driving force behind calcium-phosphorus imbalance and therefore a leading factor in bone loss and tooth decay. The high sugar diet causes the body to excrete calcium and magnesium, resulting in an improper calcium-phosphorus ratio. (Albritton J. Zapping sugar cravings. Wise Traditions. WAPF. 2010 Winter;11(4):54.)

Children are particularly at risk. Obesity, lethargy, lack of interest, diabetes, learning disabilities, ADHD, and autism are all caused or influenced by excessive sugar consumption. Refined carbohydrates in the grain family and in white sugar rob children's bodies of important minerals, especially calcium and magnesium. The culprits include cereals, pasta, cakes and cookies. *Nourishing Traditions* by Fallon Morell is a reference to help you read labels and learn the facts. She gives an excellent guide to natural sweeteners on pages 536–537. Become familiar with Vani Hari, aka the Food Babe and her book *The Food Babe Way*, an excellent guide for parents. Introduce whole foods like fresh fruits and vegetables into your children's diets as well as nutritious fats from pastured animals, one at a time if you have to. Cook with your own homemade bone stocks. Be diligent and your children's health will be greatly benefitted.

There are a few main supplements children need to help their joints and their health. First give them Catalyn® Chewable by Standard Process at a starting dosage of three per day. This is an excellent whole-food multivitamin. Secondly, they should take a cod liver oil/butter oil mixture at a dose ½ to 1 teaspoon per day. Butter oil supplies many nutrients, most importantly Activator X (now known to be vitamin K2). This nutrient is found only in dairy and beef from grass-fed cows feeding on rapidly growing grasses in the spring and fall. It also provides vitamin D so desperately needed to feed growing bones and to help absorb calcium in the diet. Lastly, give a good form of calcium like Calcium Lactate by Standard Process. It's gentle on the digestive tract and easy to assimilate. A typical dose is 6/day or more if the child is very active.

Joint Pain in Older Children
(over the age of 12)

Older children may experience joint pains for reasons such as food allergies, improper diet, and/or a lack of vitamins and minerals. Early teens diagnosed with juvenile arthritis by a family physician because of a positive blood test may be given cortisone to treat the symptoms. The real cause of the problem — the body's metabolic and physiologic breakdown — is left untreated. Medications like cortisone can permanently damage the adrenal glands, encourage yeast overgrowth and even predispose to diabetes.

Dr. Angelo Rose; Dr. Christopher Amoruso

In my practice, we utilize food diaries and allergy tests to isolate what offensive foods are being eaten, and those that the child may be allergic to. We look at their food diaries to determine what foods the child isn't eating. This is valuable information in ascertaining what nutrients the child may not be getting from his/her diet. We also look at the pH of their saliva and urine to determine whether or not they are too acidic or too alkaline. This allows us to adjust their diet accordingly. Refer to the section on pH balance in the diet in Section III of this book.

After the diet is analyzed, we examine the spine for subluxations and postural abnormalities. Next, we look at the digestive system to find out what zones on the abdominal wall are showing irritation. This gives valuable information as to which areas of the digestive system are not functioning. Once this is done, a chiropractic adjustment is given to specifically address the areas of malfunction.

Supplementally, calcium and magnesium are probably the two most important minerals for young people to receive. Children may not get calcium from conventional pasteurized dairy because the absorption-necessary enzyme, phosphatase, is destroyed during pasteurization. The heat of this process destroys the enzymes naturally found in milk along with many vitamins and minerals. Increasing the child's intake of dark, leafy green vegetables as well as raw dairy will supply dietary calcium from food. Magnesium-rich foods like organic broccoli, black and navy beans, lentils and seafood like halibut, salmon and shrimp should be included in the diet. Remember, beans and lentils must be soaked. See Appendix C p. 344-346 for proper soaking procedures.

Another important consideration in these cases is to have the thyroid and adrenal glands checked by an alternative physician. These two glands play an important role in our ability to digest and assimilate calcium and other nutrients. Simple home testing of the thyroid gland using the Axillary Temperature Test and Survey (see Appendix B p. 338 for instructions) can be performed to identify poor thyroid function. For the adrenal glands, salivary hormone testing and Ragland's blood pressure test can be used to identify poor adrenal function. We also make use of an Adrenal Survey/Questionnaire to gauge the likelihood of adrenal insufficiency (see

Appendix B p. 338). Once a problem with either of these glands is identified, supplementation can be initiated to resolve it. Glandulars made by Standard Process are helpful in enabling these glands to regain their function. Thytrophin® is used to support the thyroid and Drenatrophin® for the adrenals. Further supplementation may be needed based on the results of testing and examination. These basic principles will get the child on the way back to health. Consult with your chiropractor or alternative physician as further supplementation and guidance may be necessary.

Arthritis in the Adult

There are many different types of arthritis including but not limited to osteoarthritis, rheumatoid, gout, and ankylosing spondylitis. Many of these conditions are under the umbrella of autoimmune disorders where the body's immune system begins to have trouble identifying self from non-self. As a result the immune system begins to attack the body — in this case, the joints. In my experience, poor nutrition is at the heart of many of these conditions. Furthermore, in many cases there is an involvement of food allergies, a build-up of yeast/fungi, bacteria and parasites.

All types of arthritis involve a degeneration or breakdown of the joint. In some cases we see erosions of the joint and in others we see immune/antibody complexes involved. Positive results occur in most arthritic patients when they change their diet. For osteoarthritis, a basic dietary platform exists which will improve the patient's condition. We start by removing refined white flour, conventional pasteurized dairy, and refined white sugars. This means an abstention from bagels, conventional store-bought breads, pasta, cookies, and other processed wheat products. The vitamins and minerals in these foods have been depleted by over-processing. They are highly acidic (as are all industrially processed and refined foods) and will draw alkaline minerals away from the joints and bones. The same is true for white sugars indiscriminately added to many commercially prepared foods. Lastly, we must remove all of the nightshade vegetables. These include tomatoes, white potatos, eggplants, and peppers. The reason for this is believed to be that nightshade vegetables contain a glycoalkaloid called solanine which irritates the joints.

Dr. Angelo Rose; Dr. Christopher Amoruso

The topic of grains must be discussed regarding arthritis. A very important aspect of grains that is overlooked by many of today's nutritionists and physicians is the subject of phytate. Phytate, or phytic acid, is the principal storage form of phosphorus in many plants, and is especially high in the hulls of seeds, nuts, beans, and grains. The chemical properties of phytate make this important regarding arthritis. Due to its chemical properties, it is a powerful chelator of positively charged minerals like zinc, iron, calcium and magnesium. Chelation is the process by which multiple bonds are formed between the chelator and a single central atom. Once these important minerals are chelated to phytate, they are carried out of the digestive tract without being absorbed. In layman's terms, regarding arthritis, the more grains consumed (nuts and seeds as well), the more unable we are to absorb the aforementioned minerals due to their chelation by phytate in the intestinal tract.

Fortunately, traditional wisdom instructs us how to properly prepare these foods and reduce their phytate content. Through the processes of acid soaking, lactic acid fermentation, and sprouting, we can reduce the amount of phytate present in grains, seeds, nuts, beans and legumes (Fallon S. Nourishing Traditions. Washington DC: New Trends Publishing; 2001. p. 452-54). Furthermore, the lactobacilli genus of bacteria, as well as many others found in a healthy intestinal tract, naturally produce the enzyme phytase. Phytase catalyses the release of phosphate from phytate and hydrolyses the complexes formed with calcium and the other positively charged minerals. Therefore, the healthier we keep the flora of our intestine, the less likely we are to lose the important minerals like calcium from our diet.

There is one major caveat here. The overzealous use of antibiotics as well as other medications like BCPs and Prednisone has led to poor gastrointestinal health of epidemic proportions. As a result, the average American does not have a healthy intestinal flora. This when combined with a diet high in processed, unsoaked/unsprouted grains, nuts, seeds and beans, is a recipe for osteoporosis and joint degeneration. This is where the problem originates. The American diet is overloaded with cheap, processed grain products and refined sugars. Furthermore, the average person has never heard of soaking or fermenting grains and nuts in order to prepare them for better digestion. Add to this an overuse of antibiotics and we have a recipe for mineral depletion and poor joint function.

Once the majority of the offending foods have been removed, we focus on alkalizing the body with nutritionally dense whole foods and supplying supplements that help normalize and improve joint function. The diet must be roughly 80% alkaline foods and 20% acidic. Examine the acid/alkaline list on the website found in Appendix D p. 358 #28. Suggested reading on this topic is *Alkalize or Die* by James Baroody. We must increase the patient's intake of green vegetables and salads as well as alkaline fruits, and organic meats, including chicken and fish which must be eaten, though not in large amounts. Important to patients with any type of arthritis is mineral absorption. We stress that minerals, especially alkaline ash minerals like magnesium, cannot be absorbed without proper fats in the diet. Healthy fats taken in the form of fresh, raw, organic dairy from grass-fed animals, organic pastured organ meats and pastured animal fat are important sources of needed saturated fats and fat soluble vitamins, particularly vitamins D and K. Brown and wild whole grain rices, lentils, beans and nuts are all included, but must be soaked. Raw organic dairy from cows fed on rapidly growing grasses is also important because it supplies an important joint nutrient which Weston A. Price identified as Activator X (later discovered to be a form of vitamin K2). This nutrient is also known as the anti-stiffness factor. It has been found by research to support proper growth and development in children, to support endocrine function, and to reduce chronic inflammation due to heart disease. This means we must use raw butter and dairy products from organic, grass-fed cows. Visit www.westonaprice.org and www.realmilk.org for more information and for local sources of these products. Perhaps most important is the daily use of bone broths to supply necessary nutrients to support cartilage and bone health.

DR. ANGELO ROSE; DR. CHRISTOPHER AMORUSO

Diet for Arthritis Patients

DOs
- All seafood (see clean list)
- Raw organic pastured dairy
- Nuts and seeds (must be soaked).
- Whole grain/wild rice (soaked).
- Unrefined safflower seed oil
- Egg whites
- Coffee (kava).
- Parsley, onions, garlic
- Bay leaf
- Unbleached/unbromated 100% whole grain flour, pre-sprouted, soaked
- Homemade/organic chicken broth
- Raw honey (local is best)
- Sourdough/sprouted bread (See WPF Shopper's Guide)
- Chicken (pastured organic)
- Vegetables – raw or half-cooked

DON'Ts
- Citrus fruits
- Conventional pasteurized/homogenized dairy
- Eggs (yolk)
- Non-organic red meats
- Tomatoes
- Vinegar
- Peppers
- Dry roasted nuts
- Soft drinks
- Chocolate
- Processed salts
- Black pepper
- Alcohol (all kinds)
- All chemical/processed foods

Breakfast

Cereal – hot only, presoaked overnight in acidic medium. You may use cinnamon for flavor and Celtic sea salt.

Choices include – steel cut oatmeal, rice, corn (organic only), whole grain, barley, rye, millet, wheat

Fresh Fruit – eat as much fruit during the morning hours as you want. Do not mix fruit varieties, and remember, no citrus.

Take the following drink either before lunch or before dinner:
- 1 heaping tablespoon of Great Lakes Gelatin
- 3 ounces of Welch's Unsweetened Grape Juice
- 3 ounces water

Note: Try to chew the drink and not just swallow it.

Lunch

Use bone broth – to make soup, sauces, or just to drink

Small Salad – onions, parsley, lettuce, spinach, celery, radish. You may use extra virgin olive oil only as dressing

Meat choice – have a different meat or fish every day: choose from fresh wild caught fish (see list), Cornish hen, lamb (rare), wild game and organic calf's liver

Vegetables choice – should be eaten in abundance: squash, Swiss chard, watercress, mustard greens, beets, beet tops, all types of lettuce, celery, carrots, stringbeans

Dinner
Use bone broth – to make soup, sauces, or just to drink
Small Salad – onions, parsley, lettuce, spinach, celery, radish, (no dressing; extra virgin olive oil only)
Meat choice – fresh wild caught fish (see list), Cornish hen, lamb (rare), wild game and organic calf's liver
Vegetables choice – squash, Swiss chard, watercress, beets, beet tops, mustard greens, celery, carrots, stringbeans, all types of lettuce

Snacks
Nuts must be raw and presoaked overnight (Appendix C p. 344) sunflower, filbert, almond, cashew

Beverages
Vegetable juice: freshly-juiced and no more than 4 ounces
Herbal Tea: organic, non-GMO certified
Choose from these brands – Numi, traditional medicinals, Rishi tea
Cinnamon tea – six drops of cinnamon oil in a cup of hot water
Fresh squeezed fruit juice (no citrus)

Juvenile Arthritis

This condition can be multifaceted in nature. Factors such as poor diet, leaky gut syndrome, a weak immune system and mineral imbalances can all be involved in causing juvenile arthritis. Typically these young patients have a very restricted diet. The children are often picky eaters and have often "trained" their parents to give them the foods they like (often sweets, processed foods and junk foods) whether through crying, throwing tantrums or just refusing to eat the food placed in front of them. For success with these children, parents must be willing to stick to a plan to "retrain" their children and get back the balance of power they lost along the way.

To do this, I recommend parents read *The Gut and Psychology Syndrome* by Natasha Campbell-McBride, MD. The author explains the connection between the intestinal tract, digestion and health. Although the focus of the book is on disorders of the brain like ADHD and Autism, it provides incredible insight into how deterioration of the intestinal lining/environment can lead to all types of illnesses. She also discusses a behavioral modification technique that can be used with fussy eaters known as Applied Behavioral Analysis (ABA). Use the following link to read more about ABA and how it can help you help your child — http://www.gaps.me/preview/.

When parents start feeding a baby a variety of fruits and vegetables in its first year, that child is more likely to grow up eating a varied and healthy diet. Parents who fed their children a restricted/convenience diet at a young age, encourage them to grow up as fussy, picky eaters more likely to become ill. Diet is the first issue to be addressed if the patient is to overcome juvenile arthritis.

Some important warning signs to look for in children are constipation, bad breath, tartar on the teeth, and allergies. A thorough examination of the child's digestion should be performed by the physician including stool and allergy testing to rule out Leaky Gut Syndrome (LGS). Leaky Gut Syndrome can lead to the formation of antigen-antibody complexes that can deposit in joints and create inflammation. See Section III on Intestinal Health for more on this.

The thyroid gland must be examined in juveniles to rule out dysfunction. The thyroid is crucial in calcium utilization and movement throughout the body and has been linked to arthritis. Performing the axillary temperature test and thorough blood tests is crucial in ruling out thyroid dysfunction. (See the recommended panel in Appendix B p. 338 under Axillary Temperature.)

It is also important to examine copper/zinc ratios using a simple hair analysis test. If, in the teen years, a copper/zinc problem exists, it can interfere with hormone balance and cause the sexual organs to malfunction. This can create problems with the joints, growth, and development. It can also create adrenal gland malfunction and loss of control of the body's inflammatory processes.

Menopausal Arthritis

Menopausal arthritis afflicts women in great numbers in this country. I believe there is a causal link between this type of arthritis and the overuse of birth control therapies, hormone therapy, and hysterectomies. In almost all other developed countries, this type of arthritis is less prevalent. In the United States, osteoporosis and menopausal arthritis are an epidemic. Women are often told that as they pass through menopause, their estrogen level drops off and they need to address this. They are told that they can prevent osteoporosis/arthritis by going on a synthetic hormone to supplement this estrogen loss. In a majority of cases, this is incorrect.

What is the connection between these factors and arthritis? Take, for example, a woman who has a hysterectomy. It may have been due to fibroids, or conditions like endometriosis. Having had the uterus removed (and oftentimes the ovaries as well) this woman's system will no longer produce the proper hormonal balance. This can result in hot flashes, night sweats, and even emotional changes. And so, her medical doctor prescribes a hormone replacement such as Premarin adding that it will protect her from both heart disease and osteoporosis. Researchers have frequently found that these powerful hormones increase the odds of developing cancer, stroke, and many other problems.

Let us look at the natural approach. The thyroid and pituitary gland in the brain are crucial in helping regulate female hormone levels. Furthermore, these two glands work to regulate blood calcium and its effects on the body. Therefore, it isn't hard to see why proper pituitary/thyroid function is so vital to menopausal arthritis.

To support these glands we use glandular supplements from Standard Process. They are Thytrophin PMG® and Pituitrophin® PMG. Each contains the protomorphogen nuclear extracts that will feed the glands the nutrients they need to repair themselves. Protomorphogens are extracts from specific organs and glands that contain cell determinants that function in cell regulation and maintenance. As such, they will help these crucial glands heal and function more efficiently on their own.

One of the most helpful supplements is calcium. Calcium aids by asserting its effects in conjunction with the thyroid gland. For calcium absorption by the bone to occur properly, good thyroid function is necessary (the thyroid produces the hormone calcitonin which helps to move calcium into the bone). Proper dietary calcium absorption in the intestine, as noted earlier, relies on adequate vitamins D, K, and F. Due to the overuse of sunscreens and a processed diet, vitamins D and K deficiency has become an epidemic. The solution to this is to take a high vitamin, naturally fermented cod liver oil/butter oil mixture along with a good form of calcium like calcium lactate. For vitamin F we can use a high quality, unrefined flax seed oil at a dosage of 2 tablespoons per day on average (see Appendix D #24). If you do not wish to use a liquid oil, it comes in capsules or you can use Cataplex® F (vitamin F) tablets by Standard Process. Wisely, Standard Process has included iodine and liver extract in their Cataplex® F to assist the thyroid with calcium balance.

In cases of menopausal arthritis, one last consideration is hormone balance. It is best to send the patient for a salivary menopausal hormone panel using the recommended labs listed in Appendix D. In this way, any imbalances among estrogen, progesterone, testosterone, FSH and LH can be identified. This will ultimately help determine how the pituitary-thyroid-ovaries/uterus are functioning. Frequently the problem is one of low progesterone relative to estrogen. This may have something to do with the predominance of estrogen-mimicking pollutants in our environment. Everything from the plastics used in bottling and packaging to birth control therapies and food additives can cause estrogenic effects on the body. This displaces the delicate balance between estrogen and progesterone. A majority of woman on estrogen replacement or any combination of these hormones including the birth control pill, begin to put weight on around the midsection of the body, especially the hips and thighs. This is an indication of just such a hormonal imbalance. It is not genetics in the pure sense, although genetics are involved. Hormone receptors throughout the body largely determine where fat will be stored.

Other herbal supplements useful as adjuncts to correct hormonal imbalances that contribute to joint pains are dong quai (angelica root), black cohosh, wild yam, and gotu kola. I have used with good success a wild yam product called Progest E to help balance the progesterone/estrogen levels. Seek the counsel of a qualified nutritionist/herbalist for guidance using these herbs. Two more supplements helpful in balancing the hormonal system naturally are Ovex® and Symplex® F made by Standard Process. The average dosage is three Ovex® per day (it is best to chew and taste the supplement) and six Symplex® F per day (two with each meal).

It is very important to remember the concepts discussed earlier regarding diet and arthritis. For more details on the proper dietary approach see the earlier section in this book. Remember that alcohol, conventional dairy, refined sugars and caffeine will aggravate menopausal symptoms.

SECTION VIII
BACK PAIN AND NECK PAIN
DEGENERATIVE DISC DISEASE AND OSTEOPOROSIS

Cervical Disc Syndrome

Many people who suffer with pins and needles in the fingers, pain in the shoulder blade region on one side or even pain into the arm are often suffering with a compressed disc in the cervical spine. The disc compresses and can bulge or herniate into either intervertebral foramina (IVF), irritating the nerve exiting the spinal cord at that level. The sensation can come and go on a daily basis, and can be prevalent when getting up in the morning and last all day. Some patients note that the pain is worse at night while lying down. When there is pressure on a nerve root, there can be tingling along the path of that particular nerve exiting the spine (see diagram p. 147). If the nerve root itself becomes inflamed enough, neck pain and pain into the shoulder blade region can be severe, and no amount of positioning of the head or neck will relieve it.

Many patients go from doctor to doctor without relief. Some may need surgery. However, proper chiropractic treatment combined with nutritional guidance and specific neck exercises, can be effective in over 95% of these cases. In some cases where the patient has been unsuccessfully treated over a long period, atrophy in the muscles of the arm with a concomitant weakness of the affected area can develop. Although it is usually one-sided, I have seen in more severe, degenerative cases both arms affected. One side is typically affected because this type of condition is usually associated with a specific injury or with how a person uses their body. Repetitive movements, like those performed by dentists, hair stylists, and people who work at a computer all day typically favor one side. These repetitive movements can weaken the soft tissue and create inflammation and irritation predominantly on one side of the neck. Eventually, arthritic changes occur and with poor nutrition, poor posture and other factors, a severe problem soon develops.

The inflammation, degeneration and damage that occur to the discs, vertebrae and muscles results in a decrease in the site of the IVF, creating a compression and irritation of the spinal nerve root exiting from the spinal cord at that level. Depending on what level of the cervical spine is injured, the pattern of tingling and pain will follow the path of the specific nerve that is affected. It is somewhat akin to damming a river — whatever lies downstream from that river will be affected or cut off. The same is true for a cervical disc syndrome. In many cases, an astute physician will be able to identify the exact level of involvement in the neck (which nerve root is irritated) simply by the pattern described by the patient. Of course, people do not present exactly as the textbook says they will, but generally the symptoms will identify the spinal level that is involved. In many cases the physician may need to employ the use of x-ray or MRI to assess the specific spinal level(s) involved.

A caution regarding this treatment: when significant arthritis is present with spurring/osteophyte formation, care must be taken with chiropractic manipulation to avoid aggravating the condition. Work with a practitioner familiar with alternative adjusting techniques like the Activator and Non-Force Technique to evaluate this possibility and determine the appropriate course of action.

Typical allopathic treatment of this type of injury involves treatment of the inflammation with muscle relaxants, anti-inflammatory injections of cortisone, and other medications along with physical therapy. If this does not work, surgery is often recommended. However, in my opinion this treatment will never work to help solve the real cause of the problem. The cause of the problem isn't the inflammation itself, but rather what *caused* the inflammation.

We must treat what caused the compression in the first place. In most cases, there are several factors.

Cervical Compression Diagnosis/Chiropractic Adjustment

First we should address cervical compression injuries where the head is compressed from the top of the head axially down the spine via some type of blunt trauma, whether it be a fall, sport injury, etc. This injury occurs in football, soccer and other contact sports where an impact to the head down the spine from top to bottom is common. It can also happen in car accidents, falls and with other trauma where a blow is delivered to the top of the head axially, in a downward direction. The first step in resolving this type of problem is to reverse the compression using traction. In my practice I begin by doing gentle soft tissue work to the paraspinal muscles of the cervical spine including the sternocleidomastoid (SCM), trapezius, and the suboccipital muscles. This often includes resistive stretches and even physical therapy modalities to pre-stretch and loosen the tight cervical musculature. This will vary depending on the physician and his or her area of comfort, but generally combo therapy works well for trigger points in the neck and upper back.

After this is accomplished, a chiropractic traction adjustment should be given. A prone maneuver using two positions: one with the patient's head turned to the right and the other with the patient's head turned to the left, is effective. A traction is applied axially in each position followed by a gentle but quick high velocity low amplitude thrust (HVLAT). Audible releases will invariably be heard as the carbon dioxide gas is released from the tense neck muscles. A point of importance - the patient's neck and chin may need to be brought into a slight extension prior to the traction adjustment if they have an anterior posture and straightened cervical spine. This is to position the cervical pillars (joints that form between each vertebra and the one above and below) into their natural position and restore the normal cervical lordosis. Of course care must be taken in cases of the elderly and those with severe degenerative arthritis and/or spurring. Accompanying x-rays and/or and MRI may be necessary to determine the appropriateness of the adjustment. Speak with a qualified and well-trained chiropractor experienced in these types of injuries and conditions.

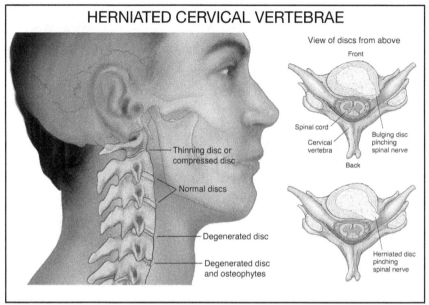

CervicalVertebrae ©Dave Carlson

A second adjustment involves the patient in a prone position, but this time focuses on releasing the tension of the trapezeii muscles and lateral compressive subluxations. Almost without exception the patient will have one "higher" shoulder than the other indicating a weakened and spastic trapezius muscle. To release this type of subluxation, I use a cross-hand technique contacting the mastoid process of the occipital bone (for example the left mastoid is contacted with my left hand's hypothenar compartment [area just proximal to the pinky finger] while the right hand hypothenar compartment contacts the belly of the patient's left trapezius). The head is tractioned gently with a slight ipsilateral rotation while tension is held on the trapezius with doctor's right hand. A high velocity low amplitude thrust (HVLAT) is applied to the trapezius muscle with the right hand in this example. Loud audible releases are heard almost without exception. Several different angles and positions on the trapezius can be adjusted in this manner correlating to the lower cervical spine. Typically these types of conditions resolve with this protocol in 5–7 weeks with one adjustment per week.

Perhaps the most important aspect of the treatment plan for cervical disc problems occurs when the patient leaves the office. We will normally recommend that a soft cervical collar be worn at all times (except while driving), even to bed. This is to prevent the head from approaching a position of further compression: either ear to shoulder, chin to chest, extension of the head or a combination of these compressive movements. The longer we can remove pressure from the nerve root, the faster the healing will occur. The soft cervical collar is often most important in cases where a patient states that they wake up with a stiff neck or find that sleeping at night is uncomfortable for them.

Also, we advise our patients to perform over-the-door-traction at home and/or make use of some of the manual traction devices available on the market. A great product for this is Meditrac's Cervico 2000 traction collar. It is portable and easy to use and allows the patient to be mobile while performing traction. For more information visit Meditrac's website at www.meditrac.co.il or ask your physician to look at it with you if he or she is not familiar with it. It is also covered by many insurance plans. *Please refer to our outline below for the protocol instructions.*

After some progress is made via the soft tissue work, physical therapy, and chiropractic adjustments, we will recommend neck exercises and stretches. These exercises never place a compressive force on the neck in any position. Rather they seek to stretch the neck with traction and some rotation.

A very specific chiropractic adjustment is given with the patient prone (face down) to release the axial or long muscles of the back of the neck. The adjustment is not painful and often provides immediate, notable relief to the patient. It is called a *prone, bilateral cervical traction adjustment.* Consult with a qualified chiropractor familiar with this adjustment technique. Also, work with a knowledgeable chiropractor or physical therapist to discuss appropriate exercises.

As an aside, if arthritis is involved, nutrition must be looked at as a primary cause. I have seen this most commonly in smokers and in those who eat a highly refined diet heavy in commercial wheat and wheat products. Refer to our guidelines on osteoporosis and arthritis in Section VIII of this book for further details. As you will see below, we also make use of some anti-inflammatory compounds to ameliorate the swelling and pain involved in these cases.

Cervical Disc Procedure Outline

Equipment Required: soft cervical collar; over-the-door traction unit; ice; Knox gelatin; Welch's unsweetened grape juice (no sugar added). *Note: Diabetics must use grapefruit juice.*

Procedure:

1. Over-the-Door Traction – optional/preferred – Meditrac's Cervico 2000 neck traction unit. *Work with your individual practitioner for instructions.*

Step 1. Using the setup described, begin with 4 pounds of water in the unit for the first week.

Step 2. Set up the unit and begin by facing away from the door. Stay in the unit for 10 minutes, twice each day.

Step 3. Add one pound of water each week up to a maximum of 14 lbs. Continue using the device for 10 minutes twice each day.

Step 4. If unable to get into a comfortable position in the unit, you may face toward the door.

Step 5. After finishing each session of traction, an ice pack should be used for 1 hour, placing the ice between the neck and top of shoulders. You should ice one side at a time, 10 minutes on one side, and 10 minutes on the other.

2. Knox Gelatin – you need Knox unflavored gelatin and Welch's unsweetened grape juice (The purple type with no sugar added)

Step 1. Add one packet of Knox/or Great Lakes gelatin to 4 ounces of Welch's unsweetened grape juice. *Note – If you are a diabetic or have a history of problems controlling your blood sugar, you MUST substitute 3 ounces of grapefruit juice for the grape juice.*

Step 2. Drink down immediately.

Step 3. Do this once every day for the first week. Then, only once every other day indefinitely.

3. Bone Broth/Soup Stock – make according to directions in *Nourishing Traditions* by Fallon. Try to consume the broth on a daily basis in soups, using it to sauté vegetables, and drinking as a healing tea.

(See recipes in the "Nourishing Traditions" pp. 116-125.) If you do not wish to make the broth, two organic brands on supermarket shelves are Pacific Organic and Nature's Promise, but be aware that they are inferior products.

4. Soft Cervical Collar – you will need to purchase a soft cervical collar. How to wear the collar will be explained to you by the doctor. This collar should be worn to bed and as much as possible during the day. *You should not wear the collar while driving.*

5. Synflex – you can order this online at amazon.com or through another search engine. Synflex is a mixture of a special glucosamine supplement along with anti-inflammatories that aid in the healing of the disc and neck joints.

6. Zyflamend – this product is a very effective natural anti-inflammatory utilizing mixed herbs. It can be purchased at Vitamin Shoppe and most reputable health food stores. Take in a dosage of up to 4–6 per day or as little as two per day depending on the situation. Check with physician before proceeding. *Do not take if you are taking blood-thinning medication such as warfarin or Coumadin.*

7. Neck Exercises – demonstrated by the physician. If you have any questions pertaining to the exercises and how to perform them, please ask your physician.

Degenerative Disc Disease, Back Pain/Sciatica

There is no better first option for treating degenerative disc disease (DDD) and back pain than a chiropractor, especially a chiropractor well-versed in nutrition. There are many reasons why people suffer with DDD and back pain, but the most common cause is poor nutrition combined with weak muscles of the abdominal wall. There is certainly an association with sedentary jobs such as those requiring a person to sit at a desk/computer for eight or more hours a day. Sedentary jobs put prolonged stress on the discs in the back. They also cause a slow-down of the circulation and movement of fluids. Furthermore, the sitting/flexed position for long periods of time weakens the abdominal musculature. Since the discs themselves do not have a blood supply, they require movement (alternating compression and relaxation and known as imbibition) to pump nutrients in and waste out. Therefore exercise is necessary for the good health of the discs.

Let us consider some simple disc nutrition and evaluate where the shortcomings are in the Standard American Diet. Our discs are made up of a special mucopolysaccharide structure called glycosaminoglycans (GAGs), that is especially adept at holding water. GAGs form an important component of connective tissues. GAG chains may be covalently linked to a protein to form proteoglycans. Water sticks to GAGs, and since water is resistant to compression, GAGS are able to absorb a lot of pressure without deforming. They use this pressure resistance to protect our spine and maintain the proper spacing of the nerve roots exiting between the vertebra (see Annulus Fibrosus and Nucleus Pulposus illustration below).

Intervertebral discs are composed of an outer annulus fibrosus and a central nucleus pulposus. The annulus fibrosus is a strong radial tire-like structure made up of lamellae. Lamellae are concentric sheets of collagen fibers connected to the vertebral end plates. The collagen protein is made from amino acids (especially lysine and proline) that are cross-linked through complex hydroxylation reactions which require vitamin C. The sheets are orientated at various angles to give added strength to the annulus. The annulus fibrosus encloses the nucleus pulposus. Although both the annulus fibrosus and nucleus pulposus are composed of water, collagen, and proteoglycans (PGs), the amount of fluid (water and PGs) is greatest in the nucleus pulposus. PG molecules are important because they attract and retain water. The nucleus pulposus contains a hydrated gel-like matter that resists compression. The amount of water in the nucleus varies throughout the day depending on activity.

Vitamin C, water, amino acids from protein, and carbohydrates are all crucial to providing the structural

VERTEBRAL DISC ANATOMY

Annulus Fibrosus
and Nucleus Pulposus
Axial (Overhead) View
of Intervertebral Disc

Annulus Fibrosus   Nucleus Pulposus

©T. Eppridge 2016

components needed for strong disc structure. Smoking significantly depletes both water and vitamin C, so it is no surprise to find Degenerative Disc Disorder (DDD) and arthritis in patients who smoke. In my opinion vitamin C deficiency is becoming more and more common as a result of the SAD. Vitamin C is readily destroyed by most food processing procedures including canning. Also, a large percentage of Americans are dehydrated either because they do not drink enough pure, clean water or because they are dehydrating themselves with coffee, soda, and processed foods.

Treatment of DDD starts with good nutritional support for the discs. Proper protein digestion ensures that amino acids will be available to build the collagen matrix of discs. Therefore, first see that the patient's stomach and pancreas, both intimately involved in protein digestion, are functioning properly. Correcting this area of digestion will require taking a digestive enzyme with pepsin, pancreatin, and betaine hydrochloride, at each meal. Reducing stomach bloat from maldigestion will also reduce the overstretching of the abdominal musculature (see diagram). In turn, this will reduce the need of the lumbar spine to increase its lordosis (concave curve) out of compensation for the convexity of the bloated abdomen. This creates balance and removes sheering strain from the discs of the thoraco-lumbar region of the spine.

Secondly, vitamin C is crucial to ensure the production of collagen needed by the discs. As noted earlier, vitamin C is an increasingly common deficiency. This is primarily due to the destruction of vitamin C by heating, canning, radiating, pasteurizing and other forms of processing of food. Canning is estimated to reduce between 70% and 80% of the vitamin C content of food. When we learn to soak whole grains properly, we *increase* the vitamin C of these foods.

Lastly, we must ensure proper hydration by encouraging patients to drink pure, filtered water throughout the day. Water, however, should never be consumed in large amounts with meals. Doing so dilutes the stomach acid and makes digestion sluggish and incomplete. I advise my patients to purchase a good quality water filter to remove volatile organic compounds, chlorine, and more. Radiant Life has different water filters for any budget. Their website at www.radiantlifecatalog.com offers several excellent options for water filtration. (See Appendix F p. 362 for more information on water filters.)

My most important suggestion to help a patient restore the health of their discs is not a new breakthrough or modern miracle. It is to recommend making an old-fashioned food our grandparents knew as bone broth. Simmering bones in an acidic medium extracts vital minerals and gelatin (collagen proteins). Sally Fallon's masterpiece *Nourishing Traditions* has a wonderful section on broths, their importance and recipes for everything from fish stock to beef stock. Consult her book *Nourishing Broth* for an in-depth discussion of broth's health benefits and for additional recipes.

Proper back exercise is also important. Since each person is unique, a well-trained physician, physical therapist, or trainer is needed to work with you on a one-on-one basis. I have used many different types of exercises and I recommend learning the Gokhale Method developed by Esther Gokhale. She recently published a book called *8 Steps to a Pain-Free Back* which has excellent information, pictures and explanations to guide you. The exercises are easy to learn, can be done by patients of all ages and, most importantly, are safe.

Sciatica

Sciatica is a very painful condition whose hallmark is sharp, shooting low back pain associated with the sciatic nerve. This nerve runs from the lower part of the spinal cord, including lumbar and sacral nerve roots from L4-S4 down the back of the leg, to the foot. Injury to an intervertebral disc can place pressure on the sciatic nerve causing the characteristic pain of sciatica: a sharp or burning pain that radiates from the lower back or hip following the path of the sciatic nerve.

People suffering with very bad cases of sciatica have come to my office. In most cases, using proper adjustments and care they respond well without pills or costly surgeries, since pills and surgery do not address the cause of sciatica. In fact, medications and surgery can be even more dangerous and harmful to the body. I have never seen a case of sciatica cured with drugs. Sciatica is a mechanical/structural and nutrition-based problem. And although this may not be the viewpoint of the conventional medical establishment, chiropractic has always been more effective with sciatica and other back and neck conditions.

When a patient presents with sciatica and other serious back issues, we first look at their posture and structure to see what stands out regarding posture, positioning, muscle tension, and joint position. We work backwards starting with the feet, and working up to the neck and skull to trace these problems back to a cause. We must do this. Knowing where normal posture should fall, we compare the patient to this norm and work from there (diagrams pp. 156, 157).

Two common structural problems contributing to low back pain and sciatica are pes planus (flat feet/misaligned feet) and weak abdominal musculature due to weight and bloating/distension of the abdomen. Pes planus is very common. Nearly everyone would benefit from custom made orthotics to correct hip and spinal misalignment. For over 30 years we have relied on a company called Foot Levelers to custom make orthotics for our patients. By addressing this one simple structural problem, I have helped patients with back pain and sciatica more than with any other method except the chiropractic adjustment. These orthotics eliminate flat feet, one of the main causative factors of back pain. Furthermore, the orthotics help hold the chiropractic adjustment for the patient far longer by maintaining postural balance, something that adjusting alone cannot accomplish.

To make the orthotics we use a 3D laser scanner made by Foot Levelers. With the scanner we take a 3 dimensional image of the feet which shows where the patient is putting pressure, and any asymmetry from left to right. The software also allows us to evaluate the percentage of weight being placed on the left side of the body versus the right and how this affects the spine. We then have a pair of custom orthotics made which will rebalance the patient's posture while standing, walking and running. Ultimately, this relieves the uneven stress being placed on one side of the body (including the foot, ankle, knee and spine) and enables better balance and healing.

The second common factor involved in sciatica is abdominal distension and overstretching of the abdominal wall. The patient with this structural problem will present with a bloated and overstretched abdominal wall with a reactive hyperlordosis of the lumbar spine and anteriorly tilted pelvis (diagram p. 157). These conditions create a wedging of the low back vertebral segments and concomitant weakening of the structural integrity of the lumbar intervertebral disc(s). Over time, this opens the door for disc degeneration, arthritis and uncovertebral sclerosis (arthritic change in the joints where two vertebrae meet) as well as nerve root impingement. Nerve root impingement will cause inflammation and is at the center of sciatica.

Next we must ask what causes this postural abnormality? Quite simply, the answer is diet. People consume processed foods, mostly carbohydrates, all day long. What most are never taught is that our digestive system, including the stomach, pancreas, gallbladder and liver, must work with the intestines to coordinate digestion of our food. When one or more of these organs is damaged, digestion suffers. Over time, the digestive system wears down until it can no longer handle the abuse. Food sits too long in the digestive tract and, as a result, begins to rot (ferment) instead of breaking down and being assimilated by the body. Combined with the overuse of antibiotics, aspirin, Tylenol and prescription medications (which almost all invariably damage the digestive tract) this creates a recipe for digestive disaster.

Whether it is fat, protein, carbohydrate, or a combination of all three, this lack of complete digestion results in the build-up of caustic waste products in the intestinal tract. As a result, bacteria and yeast begin to overgrow in an attempt to complete the digestive process which the body has failed to do. This fermentation produces gases, like hydrogen sulfide and methyl mercaptan that bloat the abdominal wall, as well as organic acids that can lead to many other health problems. This overstretching of the abdominal wall combined with anterior weight gain (especially belly weight) creates a tightening of the lumbar musculature. These hypertonic lumbar back muscles then create the wedging of the lumbar vertebra, eventually leading to sciatica and many other low back and spinal problems.

A more complete discussion of digestion is found in Section III on the Importance of Proper Digestion.

Osteoporosis/Arthritis and Calcium

The vast majority of people over the age of 50 develop hypochlorhydria, a decrease in production of hydrochloric acid in the stomach. (Refer to Section VI beginning on p. 93 on digestion and GERD.) I believe this is key in effectively treating osteoporosis, and should be addressed before any calcium supplement is given. This decrease in stomach acid causes many problems for the body. These include increased risk of parasitic infection (our stomach acid, normally around a pH of 1.5–3.0, is our first line of defense against any ingested pathogen), incomplete digestion of food, especially protein, and lack of absorption of many key vitamins and minerals including vitamin B12, iron and others.

This is where the absorption of calcium becomes a problem for many people. Calcium needs strong acid to be properly converted

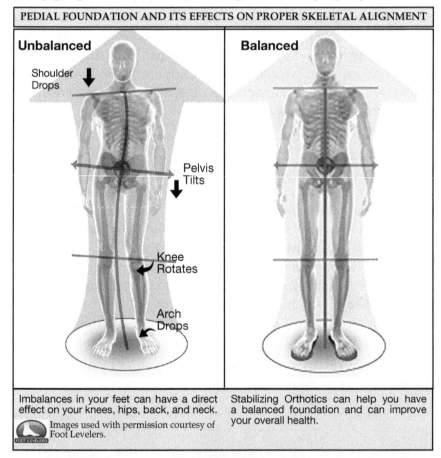

PEDIAL FOUNDATION AND ITS EFFECTS ON PROPER SKELETAL ALIGNMENT

Imbalances in your feet can have a direct effect on your knees, hips, back, and neck. Stabilizing Orthotics can help you have a balanced foundation and can improve your overall health.

Images used with permission courtesy of Foot Levelers.

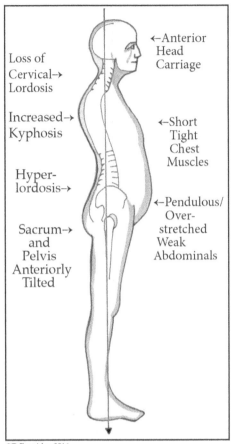

KYPHOTIC/LORDOTIC POSTURE

to its bicarbonate form and absorbed. Without adequate stomach acid, the body's pH will tend to be more acidic, as organic acid wastes from improperly digesting (fermenting) foods build up. This creates a need for calcium, an alkaline ash mineral, to leach out of the storage house that is our bones and into the bloodstream to act as a buffer. Therefore it is paramount that the doctor first examine and correct any stomach problems that are likely to exist in the osteoporotic patient. Typically, this can be accomplished with a simple digestive enzyme containing betaine hydrochloride. In our office we use Zypan® from Standard Process and recommend that the patient first perform the Zypan Test (to confirm hypochlorhydria see Appendix B p. 343 for instructions on how to perform the Zypan Test). Other digestive enzymes may also be needed to aid in the complete digestion of food, including fats and carbohydrates. However, we are only focusing on the hydrochloric acid production as it pertains to calcium absorption and utilization. For a more detailed explanation see the discussion of hypochlorhydria in Section VI p. 93 on stomach disorders.

We next consider the eating habits of the patient. Weston A. Price is quoted as saying on his death bed, "You teach, you teach, you teach!" We instruct our patients with osteoporosis to eat a diet of 80% alkaline whole foods to 20% acid whole foods. This will ensure a properly pH balanced body chemistry which maintains alkaline minerals like calcium in the bones and teeth where they belong.

A Legacy of Healing

Earlier peoples ate a diet entirely composed of whole, unadulterated, chemical-free foods likes organ meats, connective tissue, nuts, seeds, fruits and vegetables. Over the last 150 years we have so altered our diet that it has become predominantly processed, refined, and extruded foods of convenience. In the process, we have lost many of the key nutrients our bodies need to function optimally. Some of these nutrients include enzymes, cofactors, vitamins like D and K and even B vitamins. These are just a few. There are many more. We lose most of vitamin C through canning; we lose enzymes through pasteurization and cooking; we lose B vitamins through the milling process.

Appendix D #28 gives a website that provides a list of alkaline-based and acid-based foods. James Baroody's book *Alkalize or Die* gives a complete list of foods and their acidity/alkalinity. We recommend that patients maintain their alkalinity by following the guideline of eating roughly 80% from the alkaline foods list. It is also important to consider the source and processing of the food we eat. A good goal is to eat 1/3 of one's foods raw. This includes, but is not limited to, nuts and seeds (which must be properly soaked), salads, vegetables, fresh raw dairy and even pastured, organic eggs and wild-caught fresh fish.

Where osteoporosis and bone health are concerned, consuming processed grains can pose a problem. Over the last quarter century, the American public has been led to think that whole grains should be a dietary staple. This oversimplification of a very complex subject has done more harm than good. Products masking themselves as health-giving "whole foods" may be nothing more than junk food in disguise. One example is Whole Grain Cheerios. They are marketed as a health food in magazine advertising and television commercials. They are portrayed as having the "heart healthy" stamp of approval from the American Heart Association and can even lower cholesterol. (This book's section on the cholesterol myth reveals another story.) In reality, Cheerios undergo processing which removes many of the important B vitamins, minerals, and enzymes crucial to good health. That is why they can last in a cardboard box for months without going bad and do not have to be cooked. Yet what we have here is really a dead food. What do I mean by dead? A food devoid of health-giving, life-sustaining enzymes and a full complement of unaltered nutrients in the form nature provided. In contrast, we have "real" cereal, for example, steel cut oatmeal. Steel cut oatmeal is still in its whole form. It must be soaked and prepared properly, the nutrients in the seed liberated and anti-nutrients like phytates eliminated. Then cooking is required.

What has this to do with osteoporosis? Grains need to be soaked properly according to traditional methods in order to remove certain compounds that are detrimental to digestion and overall assimilation. Specific to osteoporosis, soaking eliminates most of the phytate present in grains and other foods. The Mayans knew this fact 2,000 years ago. They learned to soak their corn in lime juice to prevent the loss of minerals and even vitamins like niacin (vitamin B3), thus preventing the disease pellagra. Phytates are a plant's way of storing phosphorus. Unfortunately, phytates bind quite easily with any positively charged minerals, like iron, zinc, calcium and magnesium, in the intestinal tract, preventing their absorption. So when we eat grains (or nuts, seeds, legumes, and beans, all of which contain phytates) that are not soaked properly, we lose these important bone minerals and upset the mineral balance of our body. This in turn forces the body to recruit calcium and other minerals out of the bone for use in other places in the body that are temporarily more important. Obviously this is not a good recipe for bone health. Our diet is largely based on the inclusion of large amounts of processed, unsoaked grains, especially whole grains. These phytate-laden whole grains are everywhere. They are in your morning bagel, your cereal, and your whole grain bran muffin. Phytates are even in those "heart healthy" nuts you bought last week at the local market and the beans and rice you cooked for dinner, all the while robbing your bones of the vital minerals you need to build a strong skeleton.

Furthermore, the SAD contains other foods which demineralize bone, thereby robbing our bodies of the important alkaline-ash minerals like calcium and magnesium. Soda, for example, is laden with phosphoric acid. It and other "energy" beverages demineralize bone and hasten osteoporosis and arthritis. Coffee, tea and other acidic beverages (especially when sugar is added) are also culprits in causing osteoporosis. Almost any food that has been processed will have an acidifying affect on the body and therefore will drive alkaline minerals like calcium out of the bone.

My point is two-fold. First, to build strong bones, food must be properly prepared. This means soaking grains — including rice, beans, legumes, nuts, seeds — before cooking. Second, one's diet needs to be on a strong foundation of unprocessed whole foods that nourish the body with the key nutrients needed to build a healthy skeleton. The result of proper preparation is healthier bones.

Another recipe for strong bones and teeth is preparing stocks from bones of meat, chicken and fish, thus providing important minerals for maintaining a healthy skeleton. As Fallon Morrell in *Nourishing Traditions* p. 116 states, "Properly prepared, meat stocks are extremely nutritious, containing the minerals of bone, cartilage, marrow and vegetables as electrolytes in a form that is easy to assimilate." The gelatin of meat broth is beneficial for numerous health conditions, including protecting the gastric mucosa. Gelatin is also rich in the amino acid glycine which, with the help of the amino acids cysteine and glutamic acid, stimulates the production of glutathione. Glutathione is one of the most potent antioxidants ever discovered. It aids the liver in the detoxification of some drugs, and is a cofactor in many cellular enzyme reactions.

Fish broth is important because of its health benefits for the thyroid gland. Thyroid disease has been on the increase in America. In many cases it is subclinical, never showing up on routine bloodwork. Stock made from the heads and therefore the thyroid glands of the fish, supplies the thyroid hormone, iodine and other substances that nourish the thyroid gland. Since the thyroid and parathyroid glands are critical in regulating calcium balance in the body, soup stock made from fish is a critical component of the diet for anyone wishing to avoid or lessen osteoporosis. *Nourishing Traditions* includes recipes and detailed explanations regarding stocks, the cornerstone of any bone-building lifestyle.

Patients concerned with osteoporosis often ask, "But can't I just drink milk to get my calcium and build my bones?" On the surface, this sounds logical, but actually it may cause more harm than good. When conventional milk is subjected to pasteurization (typically 160°F), and increasingly more common ultra-pasteurization (temperature 280°F for 2 seconds) critical nutrients, vitamins and enzymes are destroyed, including one very important enzyme known as phosphatase. Without this enzyme we cannot properly digest and utilize the calcium in milk. This is only the tip of the iceberg on what makes pasteurized milk so bad for our bodies. Milk is also almost universally homogenized, creating unnatural fats recently linked to heart disease. For those looking for more information, *The Untold Story of Milk* by Ron Schmid has a detailed discussion on the dangers of pasteurized/homogenized milk and the benefits of fresh raw milk.

When it comes to calcium and building strong bones, because of the problems with pasteurization, the only milk we recommend for our patients is fresh, raw milk from grass-fed, healthy cows, preferably as Morrell says, "from old-fashioned Jersey or Guernsey cows (or from goats), tested free of tuberculosis and brucellosis and allowed to feed on fresh pasturage." For sources of fresh, raw milk in your area, visit the Real Milk website at www.realmilk.com.

Now that we have provided a foundation for building strong bones, we will discuss some of the critical osteofactors that work with calcium to accomplish this building task. The most crucial nutrient is vitamin D, which may not be a vitamin at all. Many experts consider it a hormone in the steroid family known as secosteroids. Deficiency of this vitamin is common in our country because people do not consume the most common sources of real, active vitamin D — organ meats including animal and fish liver. Our bodies can also convert 7-dehydrocholesterol (a form of modified cholesterol in the skin) to vitamin D by exposure to UVB radiation thus making the chemical conversion. The problem with this is that most people who work all day indoors are not exposed to adequate sunlight to build up their vitamin D levels in any substantial way. Furthermore, not everyone lives in a climate where the sun is strong enough all year long to prevent deficiencies. A final factor to consider is the overuse of sunscreen for fear of getting skin cancer from sun exposure. This unfounded view has grown out of a media-driven "sunphobia."

When looked at in total, it is clear why so many of our patients test low or sub-optimal for vitamin D levels. We routinely check blood levels of 25-OH vitamin D in our patients and consider anywhere in the range of 50ng/mL–80ng/ml to be optimal. When a patient is shown to be deficient, we supplement with Green Pasture™ Fermented Cod Liver Oil at a dosage ranging from 1 teaspoon to one tablespoon per day depending on the patient and the time of year. For children under the age of three, we use a few scant drops in their food each day; from ages 3–5, ¼ teaspoon to one teaspoon per day; for 6 years and older ½ teaspoon to two teaspoons per day; and for adults anywhere from two teaspoons to a tablespoon per day. Recognize that in some more severe cases of deficiency, a larger dose may be necessary. Always work with a trained holistic physician to ascertain the correct dosage for you or your child.

The next critical osteofactor that we use to treat osteoporosis is calcium. However, not all calcium is created equal. Therefore, we recommend that our patients use only Standard Process calcium lactate or their whole bone complex called Calcifood® which comes in wafers or powder. Calcifood® is made from ground bovine and veal bone carefully handled so as to preserve the efficacy of the nutrients and minerals. I often recommend that patients take one heaping tablespoon full of Calcifood® and add it to a whey protein shake or smoothie daily. In more severe cases of osteoporosis, it may be necessary to give the patient both Calcium Lactate and Calcifood® together.

Regarding calcium, be aware that product lines differ. When taking calcium, a crucial consideration must be whether or not the form being used is easily ionized. Ionization refers to the ability of a compound to carry a charge, either negative or positive. The ionization of minerals is achieved through our body's enzyme system and these are the only forms of minerals functional in our body tissue. This is important because the only form of calcium that the body can ionize in the bloodstream is calcium bicarbonate (NOT calcium carbonate). Calcium lactate requires only one chemical reaction in the body to produce the ionized bicarbonate form, so it is the best form of supplemental calcium.

A quick chemistry lesson regarding choosing the proper form of calcium may help. Most cheap brands of calcium use the carbonate form, which is the same as limestone, or chalk. You are being sold an inorganic rock as a supplement. This form of calcium mandates that the body perform no fewer than a dozen changes for it to become the usable, ionized bicarbonate form. Calcium bicarbonate is the form of calcium you find in spring water. If you take that spring water and heat it in a tea kettle, the soft organic calcium bicarbonate changes to the hard inorganic calcium carbonate, which is insoluble. It precipitates to the bottom of the tea kettle. In our bodies, if calcium is not ionized, it will stay in the fluid where it can build up in the plaque of clogging arteries or other areas where it does not belong. As a result, choosing the wrong form of calcium can actually harm your body.

For the shake or smoothie mentioned above, we recommend adding good quality flaxseed oil to both the shake and the general diet. Flaxseed contains unsaturated fatty acids that help the body get calcium from the blood into the bone, whereas vitamin D helps take the calcium from the intestinal tract into the blood. Several tablespoons per day of flaxseed oil is recommended. Some of the better brands include Udo's Choice® Perfected Oil Blend and Omega Nutrition's Hi-Lignan Flax Oil.

Once you have created a balanced, whole food alkaline diet rich in meat and fish stocks combined with the basic supplements mentioned above, you have a far better remedy for brittle, osteopenic bones than any drug can offer. Many of the osteoporosis drugs, especially the bisphosphonate class (think Boniva and Fosamax), are extremely dangerous. In rare cases they can cause irreversible rotting of the jaw bone. More commonly they leave a patient with brittle, old bones because they prevent the breakdown of old bone for remodeling by the body. They will never help a patient build stronger bones.

For women, one final consideration regarding osteoporosis is the hormonal connection. Hormonal balance is critical for women, and when menopause comes into the picture there can often be problems, especially if a weak-functioning thyroid (hypothyroidism) is present. Typically, the medical profession handles this with hormone replacement therapy, HRT, or by telling women that estrogen is necessary to keep them from developing osteoporosis. A very popular drug given to women for many years was known as Prempro or Premarin®. It was essentially estrogen made from horse's urine and it eventually was linked to an increased risk for stroke and cancer. Women were told that these drugs would protect their bones with the added benefit of shielding them from cancer. Unfortunately, the reverse proved to be the case.

Instead of giving hormones, we need to enable the body to create its own balance between the major female hormones progesterone and estrogen. This will ensure a much stronger bone structure and can correct degenerating bones. First, our practice with a patient is to test the female hormones using salivary hormone testing. Then corrections can be made using wild yam cream (known as Progest E) to elevate progesterone if necessary (see Appendix A, p. 328 for directions). High estrogen levels can be lowered using a product called Cruciferous Complete™ by Standard Process. Typical dosage is three to six capsules per day. Vitex is an herb which is extremely helpful in balancing these hormones.

It must not be overlooked that many women are suffering from undiagnosed hypofunctioning of the thyroid (subclinical hypothyroidism). Without proper thyroid function, the female system cannot process calcium properly. Whether this is due to iodine deficiency, vitamin A and D deficiencies, overproduction of cortisol blocking the proper formation of the T3 hormone, or some other environmental factor, is up for debate. In my opinion, it is a bit of many of these things. The use of birth control pills, smoking, alcohol, fluoride, soy and soy products are just a few of the many contributing factors to thyroid damage. All of these factors will be taken into consideration by an astute physician. Therefore, a good thyroid examination must be performed when examining and treating any female patient for osteoporosis. Section VII, Menopausal Arthritis beginning on p. 141, and Section VIII, Osteoporosis beginning on p.156, contain more information on the steps necessary to achieve thyroid balance.

SECTION IX
CONDITIONS OF THE MALE AND FEMALE REPRODUCTIVE TRACT

Erectile Dysfunction (ED)

Erectile dysfunction (ED) is a multifaceted condition which cannot be solved with a cookie cutter approach. ED can have psychogenic, hormonal, vascular, iatrogenic (side effects from other medications) and even neurogenic causes. Because they are commonly the cause, the vascular and hormonal components of ED are what I will focus on. In my opinion you cannot separate these two components with regard to ED. Judging from the amount of literature on the subject, you would come to find that ED is overwhelmingly associated with diabetes and cardiovascular disease including hypertension (HTN). I will discuss this first.

To treat ED, we must first understand the complex physiology behind achieving and maintaining an erection. In 2002 researchers at Johns Hopkins discovered that release of nitric oxide (NO) from nerve endings in the penis caused erection. These scientists found that after an initial burst of NO, blood vessels release more nitric oxide to harden and maintain the erection. The erection is maintained as more NO causes relaxation of the blood vessels, resulting in greater blood flow. Greater blood flow results in further NO production to maintain the erection. This cascade of events is initiated when the man has erotic thoughts or physical sensations. Nitric oxide, a relaxant, allows blood vessels to open up or dilate, thus increasing blood flow and swelling of tissues. The flow of blood creates a stress on the blood vessel wall activating the release of more nitric oxide, this time from endothelial cells in the wall of the blood vessel rather than from nerves. Endothelial nitric oxide causes more tissue to relax and the process repeats until the penis is fully erect.

Diabetes, the condition most closely related to ED, has become an epidemic in the United States over the last 25 years. Since we have covered a detailed discussion of diabetes in a later section in this book, here I will explain only its relation to ED. Diabetics have high levels of insulin circulating in the bloodstream. In fact, as diabetes progresses, more and more insulin is secreted from the pancreas to try to force the sugar into the cells. Often the patient will develop insulin resistance despite these high levels of insulin in the blood. However, something rarely ever explained to people is that this high circulating level of insulin, combined with high levels of glucose in the blood, inhibits nitric oxide (NO) gas production by the endothelial cells of the blood vessels in the penis. (De Vriese AS, Verbeuren TJ, Van de Voorde J, Lameire NH, Vanhoutte PM. Endothelial dysfunction in diabetes. British Journal of Pharmacology 2000;130(5): 963-74) As explained previously, NO is the gas released by the nerve endings and endothelial cells of the blood vessels to help enlarge the penis and achieve the erection. When this gas is inhibited by poor circulation and high insulin levels, both common in diabetics, achieving an erection or maintaining it becomes very difficult. Therefore, the first course of action we take with patients presenting with symptoms of ED is to check for dysglycemia or diabetes. This can be done by performing a standard blood test for fasting glucose, glycosylated hemoglobin (HbA1c) and fasting insulin levels. If dysglycemia or diabetes is found or suspected, we implement the dietary and nutritional strategies outlined in the segment on Diabetes in Section XI of this book.

Several important vitamins involved in the biochemical pathway that produces NO gas must be considered as well. The adjacent diagram clearly shows that the amino acid arginine is broken down by the enzyme NO synthase and releases citrulline and NO gas in the endothelial cell (Harper's Biochemistry. 25th ed. McGraw-Hill Companies; 1999. p. 730).

"NO synthase is a very complex enzyme, employing five redox cofactors: NADPH, FAD, FMN, heme and tetrahydrobiopterin." (Ibid) What this complex biochemistry is really saying is that the enzyme which enables the endothelial cells to produce the NO gas necessary for an erection, requires five specific nutritional factors. They are:

1. Nicotinamide Adenine Dinucleotide Phosphate (NADPH) – vitamin B3 is the precursor for this coenzyme.

2. Flavin Adenine Dinucleotide (FAD) – vitamin B2 (riboflavin) is the precursor for this coenzyme.

3. Flavin Mononucleotide (FMN) – vitamin B2 is also the precursor for this coenzyme as well.
4. Heme – an iron containing group that carries oxygen.
5. Tetrahydrobiopterin (BH4) – an essential cofactor whose deficiency has been linked to cardiovascular disease as well as ED.

Therefore it is important to consider a deficiency of some or all of these five vitamins, especially the B vitamins, niacin (B3) and riboflavin (B2), as a causative factor in ED. Interestingly, it is many of these same B complex vitamins which are deficient in the SAD, a diet rich in processed wheat and sugar products as well as altered, processed fats. We will normally perform a urinary organic acids test to further assess the B complex vitamins. For this we use the Genova Diagnostics Labs urinary organic acids test called the Organix® Profile as well as the Amino Acids profile. These profiles can help eliminate the guesswork by identifying a deficiency in the B vitamin family as well as the possibility of amino acid deficiency, specifically L-arginine.

Another area of concern for those with ED is adequate vitamin D status. The typical cutoff for blood levels of vitamin D sufficiency (measuring the 25-OH vitamin D) is currently defined as 30 ng/mL. In our office, we consider the optimal blood range of vitamin D to be between 50-80 ng/mL. Unfortunately, today the overwhelming majority of patients do not even come close to this optimal range. In fact, most patients are below the sufficiency level of 30 ng/mL. And low levels of vitamin D have a role in blood glucose levels and diabetes. In a 2011 study, a 4-week program of high-dose vitamin D supplementation (10,000 IU daily) in subjects with impaired fasting glucose was associated with an improved insulin sensitivity and a decreased acute insulin response to glucose, both risk factors for Diabetes mellitus (DM) (Nazarian S, St. Peter JV, Boston RC, Jones SA, Mariash CN. Vitamin D3 supplementation improves insulin sensitivity in subjects with impaired fasting glucose. Translational Research. 2011 Nov; 158(5):276–81). A 16-week randomized, placebo-controlled study indicated that 2,000 IU of vitamin D_3 daily increased b-cell function, as shown by a 37% improvement in insulin secretion (Mitri J, Dawson-Hughes B, Hu FB, Pittas AG.

Effects of vitamin D and calcium supplementation on pancreatic b cell function, insulin sensitivity, and glycemia in adults at high risk of diabetes: the calcium and vitamin D for diabetes mellitus (CaDDM) randomized controlled trial. Amer J Clinical Nutrition 2011 Aug; 94(2):486-94). Therefore it is very important to check patients with ED for low levels of vitamin D, and if they are at suboptimal levels, supplement with Blue Ice™ Fermented Cod Liver Oil. Generally we use one to two teaspoons per day or three to six capsules depending on how low the individual's levels are.

Hypertension (HTN) is also commonly found to be associated with ED. In a study published in the *Journal of the American Geriatrics Society*, the authors found that close to 50% of men with hypertension also had ED. One study published in *The Journal of Urology* found the rates even higher with 68% of men with hypertension having some degree of erectile dysfunction. Complicating this issue is the fact that diuretics and beta-blockers, common drugs prescribed for hypertension, can also cause erectile dysfunction by causing decreased blood flow to the penis or by interfering with nerve impulses. Furthermore, diuretics decrease the body's zinc supply, and zinc is needed for producing testosterone. Testosterone is a vital male hormone involved in sexual arousal and the production of an erection (WebMD.com - http://www.webmd.com/hypertension-high-blood-pressure/guide/high-blood-pressure-erectile-dysfunction). Therefore it is very important that, when addressing a patient with ED who is also being treated for HTN, we take into consideration the possibility of drug side effects. In fact, a good

Nitric Oxide Biochemistry in ED

clinician should always rule out drug side effects first before considering other likely causes. A review of the medical literature shows that over 200 medications can cause erectile dysfunction as a side effect. In reality, that number is probably far greater. I have seen patients suffering with complications from medication side effects that had not been considered by their physicians. To understand the causes and holistic treatment of HTN and how it relates to ED, refer to this book's Section XI on Diseases of the Circulatory System.

Finally, with regard to ED, I would like to discuss the importance of exercise and the role a sedentary lifestyle may play in this disease. It is a well known fact that a sedentary lifestyle is a huge risk factor for all cardiovascular diseases. And as we have shown earlier, ED has cardiovascular implications related to insulin balance, diabetes, and even hypertension. All of these illnesses can be ameliorated to some degree by exercise.

Why does exercise play an important role in such a seemingly unrelated condition as ED? The answer is simple: blood flow and tissue oxygen capacity. As pointed out earlier, the ability of the body to achieve an erection is directly related to the blood vessel's ability to produce NO gas and to increase blood flow. These depend on blood sugar balance and proper circulatory function. A sedentary lifestyle weakens the body in these two regards because it causes a loss of tone in the muscles, as well as the vasculature, decreasing overall circulatory capacity. Furthermore, being sedentary has been linked to increased risk of HTN and diabetes, both of which were discussed earlier as major players in ED. Therefore, implementing a simple exercise routine which includes slow burn exercises as well as light to moderate cardiovascular activity is the key, not only to mitigating ED, but to overall cardiovascular health. *The Slow Burn Fitness Revolution* by Fredrick Hahn, et al. gives a simple and effective way to exercise in order to improve overall cardiovascular health. Implementing rebounding (trampoline exercise) for 15 minutes per day with walking and/or elliptical training are just a few of the many simple and safe ways to get your blood pumping and improve your body's circulation. A knowledgeable physician or trainer can assist you in designing an appropriate program. A final note: smoking has been linked to problems with ED. This should be self-evident because smoking is well known to cause circulatory damage including high blood pressure. Implementing a smoking cessation plan would go a long way to lessen ED by improving overall cardiovascular health.

The last factor I will touch on, one seldom discussed as being related to ED, is the psychological component. Psychological factors including stress, depression, fear, anxiety, and nervousness are estimated to cause approximately 10% of ED cases. Many of these symptoms are often related to hypothyroidism (low thyroid function) which is often subclinical and undiagnosed. Since these psychological factors can be related to hypothyroidism and to ED they must be evaluated in a patient presenting with ED. The relationship between hypothyroidism and sexual dysfunction, including a lack of libido, has been well documented in medical literature (Arem R. The thyroid solution. New York: Random House Publishing Group, Ballantine Books; 1999; p. 140–44). Therefore treatment of the thyroid may be crucial to helping the patient with ED. Furthermore, stress causes a release of adrenaline as well as cortisol from the adrenal glands. These hormones can inhibit an erection both by raising blood sugar levels and reducing blood flow to the penile tissue in order to shunt it to other parts of the body. Refer to Appendix B p. 338 for the appropriate blood tests and self-screening thyroid assessment to identify if you have a thyroid issue. Work with your physician to address this appropriately.

Conditions of the Prostate

Benign Prostatic Hypertrophy (BPH)

In today's world there is a growing problem among men regarding prostate health. Benign prostate hypertrophy (BPH) and prostatitis occur when the prostate gland swells and even becomes inflamed. BPH can happen to 40% of men over the age of 50 and is believed to be present in 80% of men at the time of death. The prostate is a walnut-sized gland located between the bladder and the penis and just in front of the rectum (diagram on page 173). The urethra passes through the center of the prostate, from the bladder to the penis, letting urine flow out of the body. The prostate gland secretes fluid that nourishes and protects sperm. During ejaculation, the prostate squeezes this fluid into the urethra, and is expelled with sperm as semen.

When the prostate gland becomes swollen it can pinch the urethra, closing the lumen and obstructing the flow of urine. This can lead to symptoms including: nocturia (having to get up during sleep to urinate one to several times); weak urine flow/incontinence; and even difficulty starting a urine stream (hesitancy and straining); an urge to urinate again shortly after urinating; dysuria (painful urination) and low back pain. Unfortunately, symptoms are not always a direct reflection of the severity of the condition. Some men with BPH have no symptoms at all. However, when symptoms do arise, they can often disrupt sleep and have deleterious effects on a person's overall wellness.

Most often this is related to poor dietary habits and a lack of specific foods and therefore nutrients in the diet. Most men in today's world do not eat a basic, healthy diet of whole foods. The more processed carbohydrates and rancid, man-made fats a man consumes the more he will deprive his body of the nutrition needed to keep the body functioning at its best. In my experience, a diet too high in fats, refined sugars, cakes and other sweets, and processed conventional dairy (laden with hormones, antibiotics, etc.) and pasta is to blame.

The fats one consumes influence the levels of testosterone and estrogen in the body, causing them to become imbalanced, which can lead to prostate enlargement. Fat was recently found to be an endocrine organ with the ability to release hormones, including leptin. Leptin research is showing that it is intimately related to obesity, diabetes and even endocrine and hormonal problems (Richards BJ, Richards MG. Mastering leptin: your guide to permanent weight loss and optimum health. Minneapolis MN: Wellness Resources; 2009. p. 85). Therefore it is important to eliminate all processed, rancid fats from the diet. This includes the typical offenders: vegetable oils including corn and soybean oil; safflower, sunflower, cottonseed oils; and any hydrogenated/partially hydrogenated or interesterified oils found in processed foods, including margarine and spreads. (For a simplified guide on fats, see Appendix C p. 353–54.) Of special note here is the fact that most, if not all, conventional farms use soy and corn to feed their chickens, cows and other animals. Therefore, the animal's fat profile will be altered accordingly. When we eat an animal, we are eating what they ate in a sense. If they are being fed unnaturally, then we too are doing the same when we consume them. The best way to avoid this is to purchase organic and pastured meats.

The typical diet we would recommend for treatment of this condition is as follows:

Breakfast – Whole grain cereals which must be soaked and cooked. Examples include brown rice, millet, oats and oat bran. See soaking instructions in Appendix C. You may also have nuts and seeds but they MUST be purchased raw and organic and then soaked and dried according to the directions in Appendix C. Some excellent choices which benefit the prostate are pumpkin seeds, almonds, walnuts, sunflower seeds, macadamia nuts, brazil nuts.

Lunch – Eat plenty of the cruciferous vegetables like broccoli, Brussels sprouts, cabbage; also have pumpkin, carrots, yams, squash. Mixed green salads with extra virgin olive oil, lemon, avocado, organic raw apple cider vinegar, and sea salt are also permitted. Do not use store-bought dressings of any kind. Try to consume lacto-fermented vegetables as well. Make soup stocks each week and use them with lunch and dinner for making soups or to consume as a cup of broth tea. Soup stocks and broths are crucial to patients with BPH because they provide a rich source of well-assimilated minerals. Especially important to the patient with BPH are the minerals zinc and calcium. Do NOT have meat of any kind with lunch.

Dinner – Fish (see the list of clean/safe fish in the Food Quality segment of Section III), organic pastured chicken, lamb, or turkey with two green (non-starchy) vegetables, lacto-fermented vegetables and/or a salad.

Fruits – Apples, cantaloupe, all berries, cherries, grapes, plums. These can be used for breakfast as well. Do not mix different fruits at one time. Wait 45 minutes before having a different type of fruit.

Legumes – Chickpeas, red beans, lentils, fava beans, kidney beans, black beans, etc. Since they are starchy, limit the portion to ½ cup a day. Legumes are seeds and so should always be soaked properly prior to eating. See Appendix C p. 344-46 for directions on soaking.

NOTES: If you combine any bean with brown rice it becomes equal to a complete protein, but you should never put beans and rice with meat. This digestive mistake is done so often in our society and there is no mention of it at all. When you go to almost any restaurant in the United States you will see starches and animal proteins put together on the same plate. This poor combination is a common cause of bowel trouble. Refer to the section on proper food combining for a more detailed discussion.

One of the more common nutritional components involved in BPH and prostatitis are poor vitamin and mineral status and balance. Typically, low levels of zinc and vitamin B6 are involved. A high level of copper in the body warrants examination as well as it can cause the release of zinc and vitamin B6. This examination can be done via hair analysis and blood testing as well as organic acid testing. Most of the problem involving prostatic enlargement comes directly from the lack of these specific nutrients. Research has repeatedly found correlations between calcium, zinc, and even testosterone to be involved. Calcium balance and utilization are intimately related to pH and a properly functioning stomach. What

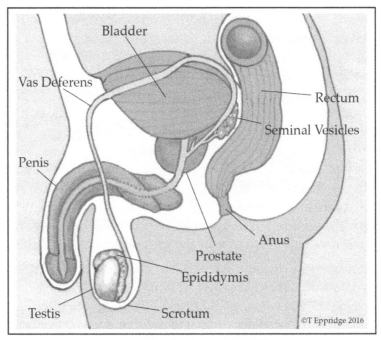

MALE REPRODUCTIVE SYSTEM

I have found over the years is that many men with prostate issues tend to have low stomach acid (hypochlorhydria) and an inability to utilize calcium properly. Calcium supplementation alone will not help this problem. See the section on the stomach in Section VI to learn how to rectify a stomach problem involving hypochlorhydria.

Thyroid dysfunction has also been implicated in the process leading to BPH. This is not surprising since the thyroid/parathyroid glands work to control calcium balance. Unfortunately the standard blood tests for PSA (prostate specific antigen) and thyroid hormones are neither reliable nor accurate. The tests lack what we refer to as sensitivity and specificity. Refer to Appendix B p. 338 regarding thyroid problems for appropriate diagnostic tests and work with a qualified holistic practitioner to correct any dysfunction.

Chiropractic Treatment Procedure

To treat BPH and prostatitis appropriately, we must take a holistic approach. This begins by examining structure, and that is where chiropractic comes into play. Chiropractic care of the spine in the sacral and lumbar regions where the prostate is neurologically connected must be treated. The human prostate gland receives dual autonomic innervation from both parasympathetic (cholinergic) and sympathetic (noradrenergic) nerves in the prostatic nerve plexus, a part of the pelvic autonomic plexus that lies adjacent to the prostate gland. The pelvic plexus receives its parasympathetic input from the sacral segments of the spinal cord (S2–4) and sympathetic fibers from the hypogastric presacral nerves (T10–L2). (Kirby RS, McConnell JD, Fizpatrick JM, Roehrborn CG, Boyle P. Textbook of benign prostatic hyperplasia. New York: CRC Press/Taylor & Francis Group. 2001. p. 7.) Therefore, chiropractic care must be given to both the thoracolumbar region of the spine as well as the sacral region. Lumbar vertebrae L3 and L4 are particularly important to adjust; therefore it is important to work with an experienced chiropractor to treat this area of the spine appropriately.

In examining a patient with BPH, another important test to perform is a digital rectal exam. Although this may also be normal depending on where the gland is swollen, an astute physician can often identify the problem. A second test that must be performed in order to evaluate the thyroid is the axillary temperature test. This is a test performed by taking a thermometer (preferably non-digital) and measuring the temperature under the armpit first thing in the morning (See Appendix B p. 338, Instructions on Taking Axillary Temperature and for the Thyroid Survey to assess your thyroid function). The thyroid gland influences proper calcium balance as well as the entire body's metabolic functioning and is therefore very important to prostate health. Iodine, vitamin A, and even certain fats are crucial for proper thyroid function and must be tested for by the doctor. In some cases, a gluten sensitivity/allergy may be related to a thyroid condition known as Hashimoto's Thyroiditis. Work with a qualified holistic physician who can run the appropriate bloodwork mentioned in the Thyroid Survey in Appendix B. From there, he or she can guide you on supporting the thyroid nutritionally if needed.

The patient's nutrition must be looked at holistically as well. To accomplish this in our office we use Genova Diagnostics organic acid testing, fat soluble vitamin testing, and even salivary hormone panels and hair analysis to identify nutrient imbalances at the center of the problem. We recommend finding a holistic physician in your area who offers this type of testing.

Typical supplementation in our prostate protocol includes Super EFF (3–6 per day), Calcium Lactate (6–9 per day), Cataplex® F (3–6 per day), Prost-X™ (3–6 per day) and Prostate PMG® (3–6 per day) all by Standard Process (dosage varies from 3–9 per day); Udo's Flax Seed Oil/Perfected Oil Blend at a typical dose of 2 tablespoons a day; Green Pasture™ Cod Liver Oil for active vitamin D at a dose of 1–2 teaspoons or 3–6 capsules per day; and zinc at a dosage of 50 mg per day. The key is to look at the whole body. Test nutritionally as mentioned above and make corrections where deficiencies and problems exist. Combining custom nutrition with improved diet, exercise, and chiropractic care will go a long way in curing your BPH.

Herbal treatment is also a crucial factor in helping treat prostate inflammation and BPH. The herbs I have used with the greatest success are saw palmetto, african pygeum, pumpkin seed extract, and even stinging nettle. It is important to use only standardized herbs from a reputable company. As mentioned previously, we use herbs from the MediHerb company. You can also find these herbs combined into one formula usually including zinc as well. We have also used pau d'arco, suma, and golden seal in the form of teas. We recommend alternating the teas on a routine basis.

A final consideration in treatment of the prostate involves certain exercises as well as reflexology treatment. Sitting for long periods of time at work, combined with a sendentary lifestyle have been directly linked to prostate dysfunction. Therefore, Kegel exercises are a wonderful adjunct in prostate treatment. Reflexology treatment of the prostate involves treating reflex points on the foot/achilles tendon as well as other parts of the body. You can rub the achilles tendon on both legs for about 2 minutes, going up and down on the tendon. We advise finding a well trained reflexologist to assist you in this treatment. See exercise for the prostate in Appendix A p. 337.

Here I will present two different case studies involving prostate hypertrophy which I feel are important to mention. The first patient, José, presented with the BPH symptom of nocturia with concomitant GERD. We began our evaluation of this patient with Genova Diagnostics Labs Ion Test. The test identified several deficiencies in this patient, the minerals zinc and magnesium as well as several B-vitamins. During our history and physical examination of José, we identified upper gastric tenderness and bloating symptomatic of gastritis. The patient noted a history of reflux and indigestion. At the time he presented to our office, José complained of having to get up from bed to urinate between 4–6 times per night.

Our treatment plan began by putting José on a blended/liquid diet specifically to heal the stomach first. The only supplements given to him at that time were for healing the stomach and for aiding in food digestion. After several weeks on this protocol, outlined in Section VI, José was doing much better, with drastically diminished bloating, little to no reflux and even slight improvement in his prostate symptomatology. A key factor was eliminating the processed dairy products which José consumed regularly, as noted in his food diary. Once completely off of all dairy, José noted that he was no longer getting up at night at all to urinate. Interestingly, when he strayed and would have dairy, his symptoms would return slowly. This was affecting his energy levels and ability to concentrate.

Dr. Angelo Rose; Dr. Christopher Amoruso

The last phase of our treatment plan for José, after his diet was improved and he was given education on nutrition and food, involved prostate-specific nutritional support. This involved using Prostate PMG® to provide nutrients needed to help rebuild the prostate gland at the nuclear level, as well as Palmettoplex and Prost-X™ to provide nutritional and herbal support to aid the prostate in functioning more efficiently. All three products are made by Standard Process.

At the six month re-evaluation José continues to enjoy a complete absence of gastric reflux and minimal prostate symptoms. He also managed to lose over 35 pounds of excess weight as a benefit of his improved eating habits. We made sure to educate José according to the rules discussed in Section III of this book and gave him a base of supportive/maintenance vitamins to stay on moving forward. They included a digestive enzyme, cod liver oil, multi-vitamin and multi-mineral, and the prostate support mentioned above. If José maintains consistency with his improved eating habits and basic nutritional support, he will never have to worry about his prostate or his stomach again. Of important note is the fact that, even when José attempted adding back raw dairy with our guidance, his prostate symptoms returned, though never to their original severity.

This second case study is the most unique I have ever encountered. It involves a long-time patient we will call Dave. Dave is a thin man in his mid-thirties with severely thinning hair and long-standing digestive difficulty including heartburn. He presented to our office with a chief complaint of pain into his testicle and blood in his ejaculate, as well as occasional problems with nocturia. Upon examination, his stomach was found to be inflamed and tender to palpation. We immediately placed him on the blended/liquid diet with digestive enzyme support. The diet removed all of the common food allergies like conventional dairy, wheat, corn, soy, etc. Within a few weeks his gastric complaints were eliminated; however he still complained of blood in his ejaculate and pain in the testicle and low back. To this point his doctor had only been treating his condition with broad spectrum antibiotics.

When Dave presented to the office for his follow-up visit, we found a notable subluxation of L3 and L4 with a concomitant positive prostate reflex at the ankle. When a digital prostate exam was performed, the patient had notable tenderness in the left prostate lobe with a desire to urinate upon palpation of the gland. The situation was discussed further with the patient, upon which he disclosed that he had participated in anal sex with his wife on many occasions, asking if it were possible that this might have something to do with the problem. As a result, we decided to have Dave submit a sample of his ejaculate to a lab for evaluation. As suspected, the ejaculate tested positive for infection with Streptococcus faecalis, a bacterium typically found in the feces and colon.

We immediately began treatment for the infection of the prostate with a multi-pronged attack which included the following:

1. Argentyn 23 Silver Hydrosol (Natural Immunogenics) – taken orally in intensive doses multiple times a day at first, followed by a graduated decline to a maintenance dosage. The purpose of the Argentyn 23 is to act as a potent, natural antibiotic without the side effects of pharmaceutical antibiotics.
2. ProBio 225 (by OrthoMolecular) – one packet a day on an empty stomach for one month. This potent probiotic helps re-establish the gut flora which in turn influences the flora of the urinary tract and therefore the prostate gland.
3. Prostate PMG®, Palmettoplex®, and Prost-X™, all three by Standard Process – taken three times per day. These provide the necessary nutrients to support prostate function and healing. Consult with your physician.
4. Routine enemas using organic coffee and repeated several times per week for a few weeks. Enemas help to cleanse the colon and intestinal tract, supporting the rebuilding of the probiotic bacteria.
5. Chiropractic adjustment to the corresponding lumbar and sacral areas twice per week for 3 weeks to stimulate the innervation of the prostate gland.
6. Reflexology treatments to the prostate at the ankle and foot twice a week for 3 weeks.

Within a few weeks, Dave returned to our office with good news – the blood he was seeing in his ejaculate was gone, and he was no longer having symptoms of pain in the testicle and nocturia. At his

3 month follow-up, Dave continued to see improvement, with no return of his symptoms. He told us that he felt the ProBio 225 and the Argentyn 23 made an immediate difference, steadily reducing the blood present in his ejaculate and pain in his testicles.

I have included these two case studies to illustrate the unique presentation and individuality in each patient. Every case must be handled differently, using critical thinking, logic and different holistic applications to achieve healing. Patients will often present in a very different manner from that which is taught in text books. An astute physician should not get frustrated and should be patient, taking a thorough history, listening to the patient carefully. The patient will often guide the physician as to the appropriate direction for treatment and course of action.

In cases where there is cancer of the prostate, the above information on testing, diet, supplementation and care all apply. However, there would be some added considerations regarding supplementation. First and foremost, we recommend seeing a qualified holistic physician who will work with you in using these treatments. They include: shark cartilage, MGN3 made by Lane Labs, pectin, MMS, and Silver Hydrosol.

Ovarian Cysts and Menopausal Symptoms

Female ovarian problems include small cysts or even enlargement of the ovaries, often without overt symptomatology. The most frequent cause is an imbalance in the estrogen and progesterone hormones related to poor diet, often with concomitant thyroid dysfunction. Many cases of hypothyroidism are subclinical and will not show up on the less-than-accurate standard blood tests. Therefore we recommend that anyone testing the thyroid use the axillary temperature test as well as a complete panel of thyroid bloodwork (see Appendix B p. 338 for which thyroid blood tests to have performed). These test results identify possible iodine and nutrition deficiency. It is also important to note that most women who have menstrual trouble also have an imbalance in their thyroid function and are vitamin and mineral depleted.

To properly address this issue we take our examination of the patient a step further. A palpatory exam of the thyroid is a helpful starting point because the gland will often be tender, usually more on one side, and even nodular. Most doctors do not screen the patient's condition with this simple physical examination. Rather they rely completely on a less-than-reliable blood test. If the blood test is normal, the patient is told that their thyroid is not a factor. When palpating the gland, if the thyroid is tender, there will also be a subluxation at C4 or C7, the location of the recurrent layrngeal nerve (parasympathetic) as well as sympathetic fibers which are distributed from the superior, middle, and inferior ganglia of the sympathetic trunk, all of which serves to innervate the thyroid gland. Therefore, chiropractic examination and adjustment at this region of the spine are important.

Salivary hormone testing (Diagnos-Techs Lab for salivary testing as well as an Estronex panel from Genova Diagnostics Labs) is an important step in evaluating the balance of the patient's hormones. Occasionally a temporal cortisol test is also necessary to evaluate adrenal dysfunction. The adrenals can play an important role in affecting the female hormone system. Some women in their earlier years develop cysts because of a lack of estrogen or estriol or an imbalance with progesterone. These hormone imbalances may cause an egg to come to the surface of the ovary and not rupture out so that it can be released to travel down the fallopian tubes and into the uterus.

Unruptured eggs remaining in the follicle can grow and become cysts. They can remain dormant or they can grow and cause a great deal of pain, leaving no other option but surgery. However, in many cases there are natural things one can do to avoid surgery. The natural approach involves trying to balance the hormone levels and stimulate better functioning of the ovaries. We use a three-pronged approach using diet, natural hormone replacement and reflexology.

Most women suffering with cystic ovaries run a pH below 6.8 which is too acidic. Therefore our first goal dietarily is to get the patient more alkaline by quite simply doing the following:

1. Remove all processed and refined foods as much as possible from the diet, especially wheat products, sugar, caffeine-containing beverages and foods including chocolate, wine and

other alcohol, and in some cases even dairy. The goal of the diet is to consume 80% alkaline foods and 20% acid foods.

2. Fruit – include various kinds, preferably organic and in-season, eating every 30 minutes or so throughout the morning.
3. Purified water (filtered or reverse osmosis) – drink at least two 8 ounce glasses prior to each meal.
4. Fresh vegetable and pure, unsweetened, fresh-squeezed fruit juices are allowed, but only 3–4 ounces at any one time.
5. Lunch should consist of all raw or partially cooked vegetables using only those vegetables that grow above the ground (they tend to have less starch); vegetable soup made with homemade bone broth is also a good option.
6. Dinner should be organic, pastured meats, including lamb, chicken, turkey, cornish hen, or wild-caught fish including shell fish. Have two green, non-starchy vegetables steamed and/or salad with the meat either lightly sautéed or grilled.
7. Increase the patient's intake of green and non-starchy vegetables. Include sea vegetables like nori, dulce, and kelp, very nourishing to the thyroid gland and excellent sources of iodine. Use liberal amounts of raw, pastured butter on your vegetables.
8. Maintain a moderate intake of animal protein, preferably organic and pastured. Try to include in this organ meats like calf's liver. The thyroid gland needs the fats and vitamin A from these foods to function.
9. Fish stocks made from the carcass of the entire fish should be a staple in the diet.

Other foods that you may choose from, but only 3 times per week are as follows:

Cereal: cooked or dry cereal including homemade granola (preferably soaked – see recipe in *Nourishing Traditions*), millet, quinoa, amaranth, barley or steel cut Irish oatmeal. All grains must be soaked overnight. See Appendix C for soaking instructions.

Dairy: should preferably be *raw, organic* and include full fat milk, cream, buttermilk, butter or plain yogurt. Goat's milk is generally the easiest to digest. Eliminate pasteurized/homogenized cheeses as much as possible. Feta or goat cheese is best, preferably raw.

Bread – the best breads are sourdough or sprouted versions and made in small batches. These can be found in the freezer of health food stores, Trader Joe's, Whole Foods, etc. Ezekiel, spelt, and sourdough rye are just a few of the more nutritious breads now available commercially. I recommend using the Weston A. Price Foundation's Shoppers Guide for a complete list of breads. Of course, if you test postive for gluten sensitivity, or your physician suspects you may be gluten sensitive, it will be necessary to exclude all gluten-containing grains. Gluten testing, although much improved, is still not 100% reliable in identifying sensitivities.

Potatoes – baked, steamed or mashed; sweet or yams with skins best served as a lunch.

Spices and Condiments – use them sparingly if not fresh; use fresh cilantro often as it is one of the best herbs to cook with or put in salads. Salt should only be unrefined sea salt like Himalayan or Celtic brand sea salt.

Nuts – must always be purchased raw and in sealed packages and soaked prior to eating. Refer to *Nourishing Traditions* by Sally Fallon and see Appendix C for directions on proper soaking of the different nut types.

Eggs – 3 minute egg or soft-cooked, poached or scrambled is fine. Purchase only organic omega-3 eggs, preferably pastured organic.

The supplement approach we use to treat ovarian dysfunction including menopausal symptoms:

1. Ovex® (Standard Process) – chew one to two tablets per meal for a minimum of one month.

2. Vitamin D – (preferably taken as Blue Ice™ Fermented Cod Liver Oil) three to six capsules per day based on patient's vitamin D level. If below 25 ng/mL take six capsules per day until your level is within the optimal level of 50–80 ng/mL. If your vitamin D level is above 25 ng/mL but not in the optimal range, take three capsules per day until blood levels are rechecked. The proper blood test for vitamin D is known as the 25-OH vitamin D (or hydroxy vitamin D).

3. Calcium Lactate (Standard Process) – six to nine tablets per day on an empty stomach. Warning: if you are taking thyroid medication it is important to know that you must NOT take calcium with your medication, as this will block the medication from working. Talk with your physician about this if you have any concerns.
4. Prolamine Iodine – see the Iodine Test in the Appendix B p. 344 to determine if supplementation is necessary. Work with your physician on how much to take.
5. Wheat Germ Oil (Standard Process) – a rich source of vitamin E which is known as the fertility vitamin because it has long been known to nourish the ovary (tocopherol, the name for vitamin E is derived from the Greek word *tokos* for child birth/offspring).
6. Utrophin (Standard Process) – chew one with each meal
7. Organic Minerals (Standard Process) – four per day
8. Udo's Perfected Oil Blend – two tablespoons per day with food.

As a side note to the information above on supplements, I have had success in certain cases using a product known as IP-6 (which stands for Inositol Hexaphosphate). This product has, in some cases, had excellent results with reducing tumors and cysts. I recommend reading the book entitled *IP6: Nature's Revolutionary Cancer Fighter* by Abulkalam M. Shamsuddin, MD.

Reflexology treatment should be done by a trained reflexologist familiar with the reflex points just below and above the malleoli of each ankle. Stimulate these regions for approximately 2 minutes on each side several times per day.

Many women suffer their whole lives with erratic periods without ever being properly examined and guided by their physician. Very few physicians relate this to progesterone deficiency. In fact, most women have this problem because of an imbalance between estrogen and progesterone, not from too little estrogen. So the physician will give these women synthetic (man-made) estrogen, which causes the thyroid to slow down by blocking thyroid hormone receptors, and also disrupts the adrenal glands. In menopausal women, there is usually an imbalance of one of the two hormones, and therefore it is crucial that we perform a salivary hormone panel. Panels for premenopausal, perimenopausal, postmenopausal women are available through many quality labs such as Diagnos-Techs (see Appendix D p. 357 #16 for information).

Most menopausal women have abnormally low progesterone levels. This combined with often subclinical hypothyroidism (low functioning thyroid) is a recipe for osteoporosis and other problems like hot flashes and night sweats. Women who take estrogen will have a problem with weight-gain or difficulty keeping weight off, typically around the hips and thighs if estrogen dominance is severe, or around the chest and abdomen if estrogen dominance is not severe. As long as these women stay on estrogen they may see poor bone scan results continue while increasing their risk for cancers, strokes and more. Over the years many doctors prescribed Premarin thinking it was better because it contained both progesterone and estrogen, only to find decades later that it too caused cancers and other severe problems.

If there is more serious thyroid involvement, further supplementation may be necessary to support the thyroid gland. See Appendix B p. 338 for information on thyroid assessment and work with a qualified holistic physician to treat this gland naturally.

Sexual and Reproductive Dysfunction

Painful Intercourse (Dyspareunia)

Painful intercourse, dyspareunia, afflicts more women than most people realize. In my experience, the three most common causes are: lack of flexibility in the tissue of the vaginal opening, chronic inflammation from endometriosis and prolonged use of the birth control pill.

First and foremost it is important to understand that the Standard American Diet (SAD) is responsible for much of the lack of tissue flexibility seen in dyspareunia and for arthritis and other degenerative conditions. The overconsumption of processed grains has led to an ever-increasing deficiency of minerals and the concomitant epidemic of arthritis and osteoporosis. Therefore, it is important to refer to Section III, pages 17 through 47 of this book.

Dr. Angelo Rose; Dr. Christopher Amoruso

Dr. Weston A. Price, a Cleveland dentist, has been referred to as the "Charles Darwin of Nutrition." He travelled the world studying primitive cultures and meticulously catalogued the health and diet characteristics he encountered. In doing so, he discovered an additional fat soluble vitamin which he called "Activator X" and which was also referred to by others as the "Price Factor" or "X Factor." Activator X is now believed to be vitamin K2. Some 60 years after its discovery, vitamin K2's role in human health is just beginning to be fully understood. One place that it is known to play a significant role is in the flexibility of the connective tissue.

To increase the flexibility of the connective tissue, key nutrients are required. Most important, though often deficient, is the X-Factor, or vitamin K2. It is a powerful catalyst which, like vitamins A and D, helps the body absorb and utilize minerals. Present in the diets of healthy population groups studied by Dr. Price, it has almost vanished from our western diet. Sources of K2 include organ meats from pastured cows, fish eggs, and shellfish. Butter is a rich source of Activator X/vitamin K2 when it comes from cows eating rapidly growing grass in the spring and fall, but disappears in cows fed cottonseed meal or high protein soy-based feeds. Fortunately, Activator X/vitamin K2 is not destroyed by pasteurization.

A second consideration regarding the flexibility of the tissue is the Wulzen Factor. High-vitamin butter oil contains the "Wulzen Factor," or "anti-stiffness factor," discovered by researcher Rosalind Wulzen. Present in raw animal fat, this compound provides the tissue with flexibility as well as protects against degenerative arthritis, hardening of the arteries, cataracts, and calcification of the pineal gland. *The Wulzen Factor is not present in the dairy products available in supermarkets, as it is destroyed by pasteurization.* Therefore, good, clean sources of raw, organic, pastured dairy are crucial as a source of vitamin K2 and the Wulzen Factor for our diet.

To insure tissue flexibility, it is important to eat many foods that contain the complete vitamin C complex. Vitamin C is found in citrus fruits, dark berries, sprouted grains and leafy green vegetables. Collagen cannot be produced in the body without vitamin C. One must also include foods that contain a lot of zinc, such as shellfish, fish, lean meat, and raw, organic dairy products. Zinc helps maintain collagen and elastin fibers and links together with the building blocks of protein to form new collagen. Lastly, silica is a crucial mineral needed in maintaining elastin and therefore the flexibility of the tissue. A great way to supply silica, and many of the other vitally important minerals is through preparing your own bone broths and soup stocks. For recipes, consult *Nourishing Traditions*, by Morell, pp. 116–126.

The second consideration in resolving dyspareunia is determining if there is endometriosis involved. Endometriosis occurs when cells lining the uterus begin to grow in areas outside of the uterus. This can lead to irregular bleeding, pain, and infertility. In my experience this condition is directly related to a low functioning thyroid (hypothyroidism) and an imbalance in female hormones including progesterone, estradiol, estrone, and estriol. Therefore it is crucial to support and heal the thyroid in order to resolve endometriosis and therefore dyspareunia.

The main nutrients critical to the thyroid gland are the minerals iodine and selenium, vitamin A and the amino acid tyrosine. Therefore a patient presenting with this problem needs fish stock. "Fish stock, made from the carcasses and heads of fish, is especially rich in minerals including all-important iodine. Even more important, stock made from the heads, and therefore the thyroid glands of the fish, supplies thyroid hormone and other substances that nourish the thyroid gland."(Fallon S. Nourishing Traditions. p. 117) High vitamin fermented cod liver oil is a rich source of active vitamin A, and is a critical supplement needed by these patients. Turkey, eggs, and beef are rich in the amino acid tyrosine. However, since stomach dysfunction is so common due to the SAD, one must ensure proper hydrochloric acid production to enable the breakdown and absorption of amino acids from protein. See Section VI on Conditions of Poor Digestion for further details.

To rebalance the female hormone system we first conduct a non-invasive saliva test, The Female Hormone Panel (the lab we use is DiagnosTechs™; see Appendix D p. 357 #16 for information and website.) Then we make the necessary hormonal adjustments via nutritional supplementation. For example, if estrogen levels are too high, which they commonly are, we use a product from Standard Process called Cruciferous Complete™ at a dosage of 6 per day. This product is a concentration of phytonutrients from the cruciferous vegetable family (think broccoli) and is highly effective at helping the liver remove excess estrogen from the body. If progesterone is too low we use a product called Progest E which is made from the wild yam plant. Work with a qualified holistic physician to address these nutritional and hormonal imbalances.

Lastly, I have found that use of the birth control pill has played a significant role in dyspareunia. This may be due to the fact that prolonged use of the "pill" has been proven to cause several serious nutritional deficiencies. Aside from the long list of potential side effects, birth control pills can deplete vitamin B2, vitamin B6, vitamin B12, folic acid, vitamin C, magnesium and zinc. (Pelton R. Drug-induced nutrient depletion handbook. Natural Health Resources Inc. 1999. p. 172.) Of these, zinc, vitamin C and vitamin B6 play a crucial role in maintaining tissue flexibility. Vitamins B6, B12 and folate are crucial in the metabolism of the harmful amino acid homocysteine, which has been implicated as a major causative factor of cerebrovascular disease, stroke and myocardial infarction (heart attack). Young women need to be advised about the dangers of birth control pills and educated about the options they have regarding contraception.

Menopausal Bleeding

Some patients start bleeding between their periods. This is often the body's signal that hormone levels are dropping and/or becoming imbalanced. It is not necessarily something to worry about. One needs to work with an alternative doctor and start taking some of the supplements mentioned above on menopause and arthritis. The patient may also need to temporarily supplement with iron due to the excess blood loss. For this I recommend Ferrofood® by Standard Process or Floradix with iron. When supplementing with iron, always use the heme or ferrous not ferric form and have your levels checked (Wright J, Lane L. Why stomach acid is good for you: Natural relief from heartburn, indigestion, reflux & GERD. Lanham MD: M Evans & Co; 2012. p. 61). Your physician can run tests if necessary to examine hormone levels. Salivary tests are more accurate in this case than the blood tests for female hormones. For iron, one needs a simple blood test. Beware of unnecessary D&C or hysterectomy. First explore the options available holistically/

naturally. In 95% of all cases, this problem can be corrected by using safe, natural supplements and herbs. For more reassurance, consult *The Hysterectomy Hoax* by Stanley West, MD; *Confessions of a Medical Heretic* by Robert S. Mendelsohn, MD; and *What Your Doctor Won't Tell You About Menopause,* by John Lee, MD. All three of these books explain the dangers behind birth control pills, hormone replacement, and the surgical procedures used unnecessarily. Educate yourself first. This situation can be frightening, but keep a cool head. Do not be frightened into one of these procedures or pills without exploring other avenues.

The diet for this problem revolves around eliminating industrial fats, refined sugars and the excess carbohydrate of the SAD. Refer to the dietary guidelines discussed in Section III. Women with menopausal bleeding should use bone stocks, particularly fish stock as it is very healing to the thyroid gland which is involved in these cases. Regular flushing of the liver and gallbladder is recommended as outlined in the book *The Amazing Liver and Gallbladder Flush* by Andreas Moritz. This enables better flow of bile, and cleanses the liver as well, allowing for detoxification and elimination of excess hormones. For maximum benefit, work with a physician familiar with alternative procedures such as these.

Chiropractic Adjustment

Chiropractic treatment for this area centers around the manipulation of the pelvic area to stimulate the nervous input to the ovaries and uterus. Ovarian innervation comes mainly from the superior hypogastric plexus of nerves located at the L4 and L5 lumbar vertebrae. The uterus sends neurological connections to the spine via sympathetic nerves from the lower thoracic and lumbar splanchnic nerves. Parasympathetic nerve supply is derived from pelvic splanchnic nerves whose origin is from ventral rami of sacral spinal nerves at S2, S3, and S4. Therefore, the lower lumbar and sacral regions of the spine must be examined and any subluxations corrected so as to influence the neural input to the ovaries and uterus.

A small percentage of women will always need special attention for their female problems. It is best, however, to question one's doctor and seek counsel from an alternative professional trained in nutrition and the holistic approach before drastic steps are taken.

DR. ANGELO ROSE; DR. CHRISTOPHER AMORUSO

Fibroids

Fibroids are benign, muscle-based tumors originating in the wall of the uterus; they grow under the influence of estrogen, the hormone all women produce every day of their reproductive lives (West S. The hysterectomy hoax. New York: Main Street Books: Doubleday Publ; 1994. p. 71). Under most conditions, fibroids do not cause any pain or discomfort. However, if they get quite large they can cause problems like blocking the fallopian tube, thereby making getting pregnant difficult. They sometimes cause acute pain, severe menstrual pain, and severe pressure creating tugging and pulling sensations. The approach of conventional medicine in these situations is often a quick move toward surgery — almost always hysterectomy (removal of the uterus). In my professional opinion this is almost always a foolish mistake that can lead to a lifetime of problems.

It is best to work with a doctor who has the experience of removing just the fibroids without removing the uterus, a procedure known as a myomectomy. In the words of Stanley West, MD, in *The Hysterectomy Hoax* p. 113:

> The argument here is that there is no reason to keep a uterus that has outlived its childbearing function. I discussed this useless-uterus attitude earlier in this segment. I can only repeat here that hysterectomy can do you more harm than good and should be reserved for life-threatening situations. But the most frightening argument a doctor can use against myomectomy is not an argument at all. It is a scare tactic, namely the suggestion that you may have cancer. Let me repeat again: a woman with fibroids is at no more risk for any kind of cancer than any other woman. Any time a doctor suggests the possibility of malignancy to justify hysterectomy, your best course of action is to find another doctor. Don't let yourself be frightened into an unnecessary hysterectomy. If you have fibroids and you need surgery, the appropriate operation is myomectomy, not hysterectomy.

There are also some natural approaches that may help to reduce or even eliminate fibroids. The first is a product known as IP-6, or Inositol hexaphosphate. It is made by Enzymatic Therapy and is explained in *IP6: Nature's Revolutionary Cancer-Fighter*, a fascinating book on tumors by Abulkalam M. Shamsuddin MD, PhD. Research has found that IP-6 will protect the body from cancer of the breast and colon as well as reduce cholesterol and triglycerides. Hormonally, an inexpensive saliva test examines the estrogen levels in the body. If they are high as we would suspect, then we use a Standard Process product called Cruciferous Complete™. It contains concentrated extracts from cruciferous vegetables and has the ability to reduce excess estrogen in the body by enhancing the liver's detoxification of excess estrogen from the blood. A study was done on this by The Metametrix Institute showing a 500% reduction in estrogen. (West B. Health Alert. 2008 Nov;25(11)3.) It can be taken at a dose of three to four capsules daily.

I have successfully treated fibroids by using protomorphogen supplements made by Standard Process. If the fibroids are occurring in the breast, we add Mammary PMG® to the protocol at a dosage of three to six per day in most cases. Fibroids occurring in the uterus require Utrophin PMG® at a dosage of three to six per day. Lastly, if we palpate the fibroid and find it to be painful, we include Zymex® at a dosage of two to six per day.

Many of my patients' cases of fibroids have shown a concomitant yeast infection (candidiasis). A good physician will always consider this and rule it out as part of the examination and treatment. For more information on what to do in cases of candidiasis, see Section IV p. 72 on Candidiasis/Yeast Infection.

Lastly, there are dietary implications. First, reduce intake of alkaloids like nicotine and caffeine from all sources. This means cigarettes, tobacco, coffee, chocolate, teas, sodas, stimulants and energy drinks. These compounds (and alkaloid compounds in general) are believed to stimulate further growth of fibroid tumors. Dietarily, avoid refined sugars which stimulate the increase of estrogen in the body. Work with a nutritionist if you are unsure about some of the main and hidden sources of refined sugar, or read the section in this book on creating a healthy and balanced diet. Lastly, avoid using birth control, hormone replacement and other external sources of estrogen like common plastics. These all contribute to fibroid tumor growth which is stimulated by excess and exogenous etrogens.

Ovarian Cysts

Ovarian cysts are often caused by the incomplete rupture of the follicle. As an egg develops in the ovary, a hormone deficiency leads to improper release of the egg from the follicle. A good analogy is to think of it as having a pimple that comes to a head but never bursts open. If the cyst forms and does not get reabsorbed by the body, the follicle swells and grows larger and pain may be experienced. The first course of action in conventional medicine is often to operate. Surgery only gets at the immediate problem; it never addresses the conditions that started the cyst in the first place. And so the real underlying problem continues unresolved. Many doctors neglect to look at the patient's history and lifestyle. It may go unobserved that women with a history of cysts, difficult and painful periods, scanty periods, prolonged/heavy bleeding, have previously been put on some form of the birth control pill by a doctor.

I have used chiropractic combined with sensible nutritional advice to resolve these problems. For chiropractic we have to look to the lumbar and sacral regions as outlined above in the Section on menopausal bleeding. These regions of the spine are where the ovaries receive their nerves from. I often find tight gluteal and piriformis muscles surrounding the sacrum which must be stretched and retrained. Soft tissue work, stretching and adjusting these areas of the spine will help to remove any impedence to the neurological connections of the ovaries.

Adjusting alone is not enough. We must take a history from the patient of pertinent dietary habits, birth control use, and consider hormonal testing. There is often an underlying undiagnosed thyroid problem, due to an iodine deficiency. This can be tested through bloodwork as well as use of the Axillary Temperature Test. (See Appendix B p. 338 for instructions and for recommended blood tests.) Since conventional thyroid blood tests can be very inaccurate, if you have been told your thyroid is fine, yet you still suffer from menstrual problems, you should consider further testing as outlined in the Axillary Temperature Test found in Appendix B.

Good, solid supplement support for the ovaries nutritionally comes from Ovex®, made by Standard Process. One tablet chewed with each meal (3/day) can be enough, but can be increased in more severe cases. For those patients needing thyroid support, Thytrophin PMG® and Cataplex® F also made by Standard Process are very helpful. Cataplex® F supplies iodine as well as unsaturated fatty acids needed for proper thyroid hormone production and function.

Diet advice includes the removal or severe limiting of alcohol (especially wine), pasteurized/homogenized dairy products, soy of all kinds and chocolate/caffeine. These women must also be taken off of all refined sugars and be given a restricted amount of carbohydrate until their sugar and insulin levels can be brought into better balance. When insulin levels in the blood rise with rising sugar levels, estrogen levels tend to follow suit, laying the groundwork for cysts and other hormonal problems. Refer to Section III for general dietary guidelines.

Lastly, making use of castor oil compresses over the area of the ovaries (in the pelvic region in the front of the body) can also be of great assistance. Compresses should be applied for one hour duration and repeated as much as possible in the initial phases of treatment. (See Appendix A p. 324 for instructions.) Reflexology work on the feet and at the ovarian points in the pelvic region can facilitate a more rapid recovery as well. Work with a qualified reflexologist for help with this.

Birth Control Pill

The subject of birth control demands discussion. Research has shown that the synthetic hormones used in birth control pills (BCPs) are directly related to breast cancer, a fact denied for years by the drug companies. Early in the development of the "pill", strokes, phlebitis, and cancer were some of the problems occurring from its use. As early as 2002, more information was brought forth from other countries that the pill did not stop heart attacks, strokes, cervical cancer, and osteoporosis as was claimed. Finland and Denmark did long-running studies on the subject of the birth control pill and came out with similar results. Now, some 50 years later, the drug companies are putting on packaging labels the warnings of cancer and stroke, the very side effects they denied for so long.

For young women today, birth control is an easy, obvious choice. The commercials on television encourage women by saying "It isn't medically necessary to have a period every month," and "You can have only four periods a year!" Not surprisingly, when we circumvent Mother Nature we pay a price. Weston Price was quoted as saying, "Life in all its splendor is Mother Nature obeyed." We are quietly encouraging our young women to live for today and simultaneously encouraging them to have unprotected sex. Over the years I have heard all kinds of excuses from young women — their medical doctors told them it would clear up their skin; their boyfriend doesn't want to use a condom; it would help their periods; they don't want to get pregnant. What these young women aren't being told are the risks they are taking. Several I have treated had strokes as a result of their birth control efforts. Some even developed cancer. Aside from these serious side effects, there are other consequences to consider. Since they are on birth control and are having sex without protection, they are leaving themselves open to vaginal herpes, Chlamydia, gonorrhea, yeast infections and HIV. Many young patients do not give these conditions a thought. When you mention it to them, they say "Oh, I only have one boyfriend" or "I'm not worried, I'm careful."

When taking "the pill", the body is depleted of the crucial vitamins C, E, B6, B12, folic acid, magnesium and zinc. (Pelton, R. Drug-induced nutrient depletion handbook. Cincinnati OH: Natural Health Resources 2001. p. 172.) These are just the main vitamins, but there are others. I have not met one woman who was told this by her doctor or even advised to supplement with vitamins to counter these side effects. Craig K. Comstock, in the article "The Nutritional Cost of Birth Control Pills," written for the Huffington Post, notes the following:

> Scientific researchers have known for years that the birth control pill depletes nutrients, but to what extent have women been told this information and guided to supplements that will supply what's lost? Browsing in a used book shop, I found a copy of the "Drug-Induced Nutrient Depletion Handbook," by pharmacist Ross Pelton and his colleagues. (A revised and updated edition will appear next year. Meanwhile, Pelton has a chart and much other free information on his website.) "Many drugs deplete nutrients," explains Pelton, "but oral contraceptives are the worst." The depletions may increase

a woman's risk of: depression, a weakened immune system, heart disease, cancer, and having a child with birth defects. Pelton is not arguing that pharmaceuticals are useless. (He's a pharmacist.) He's saying that people taking prescription medicine should also ingest supplements to deal with side effects, which may otherwise cause great and possibly irreparable harm. "An ounce of prevention is worth not a pound of cure," he says, "but a ton." (http://www.huffingtonpost.com/craig-k-comstock/the-pill-and-what-else_b_877875.html)

For several patients, their periods did not return after coming off "the pill". One had to be given injections, and it took over a year before her monthly cycle returned. Gastrointestinal problems, though seldom mentioned, are common with BCP use. Doctors routinely fail to tell women that "the pill" damages the thyroid and adrenal glands. Fortunately, these glands can be tested through bloodwork, salivary hormone testing and axillary temperature. My advice is to avoid BCP, and if you are using it, get off ASAP. Work with a holistic physician, chiropractor, naturopath, or medical doctor who is knowledgeable in functional medicine to correct glandular problems and nutrient deficiencies caused by the BCP.

Feminine Hygiene

Hygiene is the most important aspect regarding the female vaginal opening and reproductive tract. Few young women are taught about this subject and how to use a bidet/douchette or douche to maintain good hygiene. Throughout Latin America, East Asia, China and many European countries use of a bidet/douchette and douches are common and are commonly found in bathrooms. The purpose is to maintain good hygiene after going to the bathroom as well as during and after having your period. It is certainly always a good practice to clean out the vagina after having your period. If your bathroom is not equipped with a bidet (as it probably is not) you can simply use a douche bulb. A simple solution to make is two tablespoons of white vinegar mixed in a quart of sterilized water (do so by boiling the water and allowing it to cool down to room temperature). You can use a douche bulb while simply lying down on your back in your bathtub or shower. By placing the tip of the douche into the vagina and squeezing, the solution effectively cleans the vagina and cervix.

SECTION X
CONDITIONS OF THE URINARY TRACT

Bladder and Urinary Tract Infections

Over the course of their lives, most women will experience a bladder or urinary tract infection (UTI). Most allopathic physicians will prescribe a medication, usually a strong course of antibiotics. Many times, the symptoms will disappear, but sometimes they return shortly. Here again the symptoms of the problem are being treated, not the cause. Furthermore, the patient is often unaware of the damage these drugs, especially antibiotics, cause. In my experience, almost all bladder infections start in the intestinal tract. As yeast over-grow, they travel through the wall of the colon and plant themselves into the bladder wall. Here they cause inflammation, irritation, and oftentimes bleeding and burning upon micturition (the proper terminology for voiding of urine). Yeast, especially one type known as candida albicans, can be tested for with a simple stool or urine test through Genova Diagnostics Laboratories.

There is help for this condition naturally without the use of antibiotics. First, restrict dietary intake of sugar, as sugar feeds the yeast that is causing the symptoms. Secondly, drink two 8 oz. glasses of water before every meal. Water helps to keep the body hydrated and is necessary for proper body homeostasis. Next, use concentrated cranberry extract mixed with water and made into a drink. Also, Progressive Labs makes a product called U-tract which my patients have used successfully. Take all supplements under the supervision of a trained physician and according to directions.

Interestingly, female children commonly develop a problem if they are playing and wait extremely long to go to the bathroom (because they do not want to stop what they are doing). Some urine may leak out onto their underwear and can lead to irritation of the urethra. If this repeatedly occurs without being addressed, it can lead to inflammation and burning upon urination, making the child afraid to urinate. When treating these types of cases in children, it is best to have the child pass the urine in a warm tub; this will allow the child to pass the urine without much pain. Then put castor oil on the external opening of the urethra. (See recommended brands in Appendix D p. 356 #13). If this is not enough to give relief, use plain organic yogurt placed onto a pad and put in the underwear up against the urethra. The yogurt is extremely soothing to the area and should be replaced twice a day until the inflammation abates.

Acidophilus supplementation should be used every day to keep the healthy, predominant intestinal bacterial count up. More importantly, the patient should be taught the importance of lacto-fermented foods. Using lacto-fermented foods on a regular basis can help restore the natural bacterial flora so important to the health of the intestinal tract, and therefore, the health of the entire body. This applies to children and adults developing this type of UTI. This will help restore balance in the intestinal tract which will influence the urinary tract. I have also taught my patients to douche with sterile water with a few acidophilus capsules emptied into it. Douching like this regularly can be a big help to patients with UTIs.

Many women experience repeated urinary tract infections, treating them over and over with antibiotics, only later to find out that the antibiotics left them vulnerable to yeast infections and repeatedly damaged the flora of the gut. Eventually, a UTI can spread from the bladder up the ureters (tubes connecting each kidney to the bladder) to either kidney, where more serious damage to the kidneys can occur. In *The Yeast Syndrome*, Dr. James Trowbridge, MD discusses the common connection between antibiotic-overuse and yeast infection, and its relationship to cystitis and UTIs.

My protocol to resolve UTIs and protect a person in cases where the kidneys may be involved, begins with a natural, food-based vitamin C, a powdered product from The Synergy Company called Pure Radiance C. It tastes good and is easy to administer even to children. The dosage in severe cases is one teaspoon 6 times a day; in less severe cases only 3 times per day. The product also comes in capsules and can be dosed at three capsules 3 times a day in severe cases and two capsules 3 times daily in less severe cases. Secondly, we use parsley tea (see Appendix A p. 320 for recipe). This can be sipped 2–3 times daily. Thirdly, we use a fermented cod liver oil for its active vitamin A content at a dosage of three to four capsules a day. Finally, we use a Standard Process product called Renatrophin® PMG. It is a protomorphogen (extract of the nucleic acids of the cell) which supplies the necessary nuclear components to help rebuild the kidneys and keep them strong. Use a dosage of six to nine tablets per day, chewed, as it is very important to taste the product. Tasting allows the brain to know what nutrients are present, and to use innate intelligence to affect the cure.

Chiropractic Treatment

Chiropractic treatment of cystitis (bladder infection) and UTIs is geared to the area of the pelvis and sacrum. Sympathetic nerve supply to the bladder and urinary tract is via lower thoracic and lumbar splanchnics. Parasympathetic innervation is from pelvic splanchnics with their origin from branches of ventral rami of the sacral spinal nerves from levels S2, S3, and S4. Therefore, a chiropractor must examine the areas of the lower thoracic (T10–T12), lumbar (L1–L5) and sacral (S2,3,4) levels of the spine for subluxations and make the appropriate corrections. It is important to stretch the muscles that correlate to these areas as well, using soft tissue and stretching. Spasm of the gluteal and piriformis muscles as well as the sacral ligaments must be considered. Consult with a good chiropractor in your area for this treatment.

Further treatment of the bladder can be done externally through reflexology. I use a form of reflexology where a contact is made on the bladder just above the pubic bone. This helps to relax the detrusor muscle of the bladder, enabling the restoration of normal function. A reflexologist can help you to do this.

SECTION XI
DISEASES OF THE CIRCULATORY SYSTEM

"Theorists almost always become too fond of their own ideas, often simply by living with them for so long. It is difficult to believe that one's cherished theory, which really works rather nicely in some respects, may become completely false." Francis Crick, Nobel Prize Laureate for discovering the structure of DNA.

Should Cholesterol Be Our Main Focus?

Ever since the infamous *TIME Magazine* cover from March 26, 1984, cholesterol has been regarded as the villain behind cardiovascular diseases. The cover showed a plate with two sunny-side up eggs arranged as eyes and a slice of bacon arranged as a frowning mouth. It read: "And Now the Bad News." The article accused cholesterol of being the cause of atherosclerosis and cardiovascular diseases. From that point on, the pharmaceutical-medical-government hegemony waged a war on fat, including eggs and bacon. It is safe to say that the American diet has not been the same since.

To understand that infamous study, we quote a passage from Gary Taubes' book *Good Calories, Bad Calories* regarding the findings:

> In January 1984, the results of the trial were published in *The Journal of the American Medical Association*. Cholesterol levels dropped by an average of 4 percent in the control group — those men taking a placebo. The levels dropped by 13 percent in the men taking cholestyramine. In the control group, 158 men suffered non-fatal heart attacks during the study and 38 men died from heart attacks. In the treatment group, 130 men suffered non-fatal heart attacks and only 30 died from them. All in all, 71 men had died in the control group and 68 in the treatment group. In other words, cholestyramine had improved by less than two percent the chance that any one of the men who took it would live through the next decade. To call these results "conclusive," as the University of Chicago biostatistician Paul Meier remarked, would constitute "a substantial misuse of the term." Nonetheless, these results were taken as sufficient by Rifkind, Steinberg

and their colleagues [those who had been searching for 'proof' for decades that cholesterol causes heart disease] so they could state unconditionally that Ancel Keys had been right and that lowering cholesterol would save lives.

Regarding the conclusions drawn concerning diet despite the fact that diet intervention was not a part of the study, Taubes states:

> Pete Ahrens [a cholesterol researcher at Rockefeller University] called this extrapolation from a drug study to a diet "unwarranted, unscientific and wishful thinking." Thomas Chalmers, an expert on clinical trials who would later become president of the Mt. Sinai School of Medicine in New York, described it to *Science* as an "unconscionable exaggeration of the data." In fact, the Lipid Research Clinics (LRC) investigators acknowledged in their JAMA article that their attempt to ascertain a benefit from diet alone had failed. (New York and Canada/Alfred A. Knopf, Division of Random House, Inc. 2007. p. 57)

Over time research has repudiated the claims of that fateful study. Well-respected doctors, scientists, researchers and even a NASA astronaut have written books on the topic. Pseudo-science and statistical manipulation have gone into making cholesterol the cash-cow villain for the pharmaceutical industry. I recommend Anthony Colpo's book *The Great Cholesterol Con* or Uffe Ravnskov's book *The Cholesterol Myths*. They dissect the facts and expose the truth about cholesterol. Ancel Keys, the man responsible for advancing the diet-heart-cholesterol hypothesis, manipulated findings in his infamous Seven Countries Study, begun in 1958, to portray cholesterol and saturated fats as the cardiovascular villains.

In 1997, years later, he reversed himself and stated:

> There's no connection whatsoever between cholesterol in food and cholesterol in the blood. And we've known that all along. Cholesterol in the diet doesn't matter at all unless you happen to be a chicken or a rabbit.

Uffe Ravnskov, MD, in an article entitled "The Benefits of High Cholesterol," perceptively states, "It is difficult to explain away the fact that during the period of life in which most cardiovascular disease occurs and from which most people die (and most of us die from cardiovascular disease), high cholesterol occurs most often in people with the lowest mortality." (Wise Traditions. Heart Disease Issue. p. 54)

It is warranted here to mention the Masai and Samburu people of Kenya. The Masai and Samburus, shepherd people for thousands of years, daily walk or run many miles with their cattle searching for food and water. Their diet consists of mainly raw milk (sometimes over a gallon a day), meat and blood. Essentially, their consumption of animal fat is far above that of western cultures. Taking this information into account, George Mann (a researcher/professor from Vanderbilt University) took a mobile laboratory to Kenya to study the Masai. Uffe Ravnskov remarks, "If the diet-heart hypothesis were correct, coronary heart disease would be epidemic in Kenya. But Professor Mann found that the Masai do not die from heart disease — although they might die from laughter if they heard about the campaign against foods containing cholesterol and saturated fat."(Ravnskov U. The cholesterol myths. Washington DC: New Trends Publishing; 2014. p. 32–33.) Professor Mann writes "The cholesterol of the Masai tribesmen was not sky-high as Mann had expected; it was the lowest ever measured in the world, about 50% lower than the value of [that of] most Americans."

Where does this leave us? Let us start with *the real facts that every person should know about cholesterol*. Cholesterol is actually a repair substance. In an article entitled "What Causes Heart Disease?" co-authored by Mary Enig, PhD and Sally Fallon they write that "when your arteries develop irritations or tears, cholesterol is there to do its job of patching up the damage." Cholesterol is responsible for providing the cell membrane with the flexibility and rigidity it needs to function. Malcolm Kendrick, MD points out that "cholesterol is absolutely essential for life . . . . It is not some alien chemical that we can remove from our diets, or our bodies. . . . Cholesterol is so vital that all cells, apart from neurons, can manufacture cholesterol, and one of the key functions of the liver is to synthesize cholesterol. We also have an entire transportation system dedicated to moving cholesterol around the body."(Kendrick M. The great cholesterol con. London: John Blake Publishing, Ltd; 2008. p. 11–12.) Furthermore, cholesterol is also a powerful antioxidant, protecting us against cancer and aging (Fallon S, Enig M. The dangers of statin drugs: what you haven't been told about popular cholesterol-lowering medicines. Wise Traditions. Heart Disease Issue WAPF:54.)

There is more. Cholesterol in our skin is converted to vitamin D by the action of the sun's ultraviolet rays. In this way and through diet the body obtains vitamin D. Maybe the reason vitamin D deficiency has become such an epidemic is because so many people have been trying to drive their cholesterol levels down with statin drugs. Combine this with a fear of eating fat and a fear of skin cancer, and therefore a fear of being in the sun and you have a potent recipe for a vitamin D deficiency epidemic. As pointed out in *The Great Cholesterol Con*, cholesterol is also needed for brain synapses. This explains why statin drugs often cause memory loss and other brain issues like violence, anger and aggression. Cholesterol is also needed for making our steroid hormones which include testosterone, progesterone, estrone, estradiol, pregnenolone, aldosterone and others. It is also a key component of bile. Cholesterol, a critical component of our body's endocrine system, is needed for cellular integrity where it acts as a building block of vitamin D.

There are more benefits of cholesterol. Many studies have shown that low levels of cholesterol open the door to an increased likelihood of infection. After following more than 100,000 people in the San Francisco area for 15 years, researchers found that those who had low cholesterol at the study's start had more often been admitted to the hospital because of an infectious disease. (U. Ravnskov, "The benefits of high cholesterol," from Wise Traditions Heart Disease Issue p. 46) The famous Framingham Study showed that the more saturated fat one ate, the more cholesterol one ate, the more calories one ate, the lower people's serum cholesterol. (Ibid p. 35) The study also showed that the higher the person's cholesterol level was, the longer he or she lived. Many studies have actually shown that *lower cholesterol levels are associated with a much greater risk of death from cancer, cardiovascular disease, and other causes.*

If you are sceptical, do the research. It's all there in black and white. Malcolm Kendrick points this out, reminding us that:

> . . . statins may not be quite as super-wonderful as you may have thought. You may also be wondering how it is

that, despite their almost complete lack of any real benefit — i.e. actually saving lives — statins have been hyped to the very skies. There is a very simple reason for this. It's called money. Crestor was launched a couple of years ago, or so. In the first year of its launch, $1 billion was spent on sales and marketing.... Positive findings can then be hyped relentlessly, and the health editors of newpapapers wined and dined. Ghost authors can then be found to write up the findings of trials, ensuring that the correct marketing spin is applied to the data. (Kendrick. p. 169)

This type of deceptiveness goes on in research, advertising, marketing and in the medical field itself. In Melody Petersen's book *Our Daily Meds* we learn how common this type of falsification and manipulation of research is. Doctors and researchers are enticed to manipulate drug safety and efficacy records with the purpose of getting specific medications used solely for financial gain. The real dangers involved in using these medications are often ignored.

For more facts on cholesterol, and to make informed decisions, visit Chris Masterjohn's website *www.cholesterol-and-health.com*.

If cholesterol is not the real villain behind the heart disease epidemic, then what is? I will introduce my thoughts on this in the coming sections. One interesting hypothesis mentioned by Thomas Cowan, MD is the *Myogenic Theory*. He writes:

> The major etiologic (cause and effect) factor in a myocardial infarction (MI) is a destructive chemical process; specifically, in situations of stress on the myocardial (heart muscle) tissue, often as a result of small vessel disease, the myocardial tissue gets insufficient oxygen and nutrients. This leads to destructive lactic acidosis in the tissue, which, if unchecked, leads to death of the myocardial cells. This process is largely unrelated to coronary artery disease. (Cowan T. What causes heart attacks. Wise Traditions. WAPF. Heart Disease Issue:35.)

This means that there seems to be no relationship between the "clogged arteries" and actual heart attack incidence. Published in 1988, "Twenty Years of Coronary Bypass Surgery" the conclusion based on two studies, one by the Veterans Administration (VA) and the other by the National Institute for Health (NIH) concluded that surgery to bypass blocked arteries did not improve the chances of patient survival. This is not what we would expect if the answer to what was causing heart disease was blocked arteries. The truth is, we've known for a long time that collateral circulation develops around blocked arteries to the heart. And what the myogenic theory hypothesizes is *"that, as a result of disease in the small vessels — the capillaries and small arterioles — which is a consequence of such factors as stress, diabetes, smoking and nutritional deficiencies, heart cells, which are very active metabolically, suffer from inadequate oxygen and nutrient supply."* This oxygen and nutrient deficiency forces myocardial (heart) cells to use anaerobic metabolism, which ultimately leads to a build-up of lactic acid. If oxygen and aerobic metabolism is not restored, stress reduced, and nutrients replenished, myocardial cells begin to die. As a result, Cowan notes, "inflammatory debris collects in the tissues, and it is this debris that is the actual source of the coronary artery blockages seen in death from acute MI. (Ibid p. 37)

That people with low cholesterol become just as sclerotic as people with high cholesterol is, of course, a devastating blow to proponents of the diet-heart idea. (Ravnskov U. The cholesterol myths. p. 135.) In fact when you investigate the body of research available, examine the studies that have used sound scientific method, there is only one conclusion. People with high levels of cholesterol circulating in their blood should have, on average, greater sclerosis in their arteries than people with low blood cholesterol — *but they do not*. And this theory conflicts with many long-term angiographic studies of the coronary arteries as well.

Saturated Fat and Cholesterol – Real Facts about Fats

In *Good Fats, Bad Fats: Separating Fact From Fiction*, author Chris Masterjohn writes "the myth that saturated fatty acids are 'bad fat' while polyunsaturated fatty acids (PUFA) are 'good fat' emerged in the 1950s as the diet-heart hypothesis. This hypothesis stated that the saturated fat found in animal fats and tropical oils would contribute to heart disease by raising blood cholesterol levels while the PUFA found in vegetable oils would do just the opposite."

A Legacy of Healing

Chris Masterjohn explains a very important point about research and traditional diets regarding fats, and I think it is important to note the following excerpt from *Good Fats, Bad Fats* by Enig:

> If the nutritional and medical establishments had taken the approach of Weston Price and endeavored to begin unraveling the causes of heart disease by studying the diets and lifestyles of populations that were immune to the disease, it is unlikely the diet-heart hypothesis would ever have emerged. The traditional diets of Pacific Islanders free of heart disease, for example, vary widely in their proportions of fat and carbohydrate, but as can be seen in the chart below, they are all rich in saturated fat and low in PUFA when compared to the standard American diet. Each of these traditional diets is based primarily on starches, fruits, coconut and fish, so the PUFA comes mostly from fish rather than from vegetable oils.
>
> The foundation of the establishment's approach to the riddle of heart disease featured no such investigation of traditional diets, and the result of this negligence was the diet-heart hypothesis. Advocates of this hypothesis supported it in the early 1950s with two key pieces of evidence. The first was that blood cholesterol levels were statistically associated with heart disease risk. The second was that, in highly controlled laboratory experiments, replacing saturated fats like butter, lard or coconut oil with polyunsaturated oils like corn or safflower oil would lower blood cholesterol levels. Playing a game of connect the dots, they argued that

	TOKELAU	PUKAPUKA	KITAVA	USA
Protein	12	12	10	15
Carbohydrate	34	50	69	50
Total Fat	54	38	21	33
Saturated	49	30	17	11
Monounsaturated	3	6	2	12
Polyunsaturated	2	2	2	7

MICRONUTRIENT INTAKES IN THE TRADITIONAL DIETS OF THREE PACIFIC ISLAND POPULATIONS FREE OF HEART DISEASE AND IN THE STANDARD AMERICAN DIET AS A PERCENTAGE OF TOTAL CALORIES.

substituting vegetable oils for traditional animal fats and tropical oils would lower the risk of heart disease.

In 1957, the American Heart Association called the hypothesis "highly speculative," and concluded that "the evidence at present does not convey any specific implications for drastic dietary changes, specifically in the quantity or type of fat in the diet of the general population, on the premise that such changes will definitely lessen the incidence of coronary or cerebral artery disease." Four years later, the state of the evidence remained the same but three members of the committee were dropped and replaced by four new members, including Ancel Keys, a leading proponent of the hypothesis. The updated report recommended that men who are overweight, have high blood pressure or high cholesterol, lead "sedentary lives of relentless frustration," or have a strong family history of heart disease should replace part of the saturated fat in their diets with PUFA.

The hypothesis nevertheless remained controversial in the scientific community for decades. The tide turned in 1984 when the Coronary Primary Prevention Trial showed that cholestyramine could prevent heart attacks. Cholestyramine is a drug that binds bile acids in the intestine and causes their excretion in the feces. As a result, the liver takes cholesterol in from the blood in order to make more bile acids and the concentration of cholesterol in the blood falls. *TIME Magazine* hailed the trial as a vindication of the American Heart Association's twenty-three-year-old stance against animal fats. Butter, eggs, and bacon were all conspicuously absent from the treatment protocol of this trial, but TIME nevertheless ran a cover story entitled "Hold the Eggs and Butter," which artfully featured a frowning face with eyes of sunnyside up eggs and a downturned mouth of a slice of fried bacon. The article declared, "cholesterol is proved deadly, and our diet may never be the same. (Wise Traditions Spring 2012, Vol 13 # 2 p. 17)

It is hard to believe but true that there *has never been one single double-blind, randomized, placebo-controlled study performed to show that cholesterol in the diet raises cholesterol in the blood.*

We are told to cut back on the eggs and red meat. I remind my reader of a basic physiologic fact. Udo Erasmus points it out in his book *Fats That Heal, Fats That Kill*, p. 35: "Part of the metabolic breakdown products of simple sugars from dietary carbohydrate is the formation of a 3-carbon acetate (think vinegar) molecule. Normally, our cells will further break these acetates down to produce energy ... unless, of course, the acetates are produced faster than they can be burned (think consumption of more sugar than can be burned at any given time). In this case, our cells pressure enzymes to link the acetates end-to-end to form saturated fats and cholesterol." What does this mean to us? It means we should be asking, *"Why aren't doctors explaining this to patients?"* and *"Shouldn't we be more concerned with all of the sugar we are consuming instead of vilifying eggs and red meats?"* Since our bodies have a failsafe way of making saturated fats and cholesterol from sugar, might that not indicate how important these fats really are? Are people consuming excess sugar or excess eggs and steak (Here I am referring to organic, pastured meats and eggs which are superior in nutrient quality and density to the typical CAFO product). Sugar is a far more pressing problem where our major health issues like diabetes and cancer, are concerned. Remember, CAFOs are feeding poultry and cattle with soy, corn and other cheaper forms of carbohydrate to fatten them more quickly and keep cost at a minimum. This practice excessively raises the levels of polyunsaturated fatty acids in their diet and therefore in their tissues, which we consume.

Secondly, *the majority of fat found in the atherosclerotic plaques associated with cardiovascular diseases is actually polyunsaturated fat, not cholesterol.* The common belief is that it is the cholesterol that clogs up the artery. Yet Thomas Cowan, MD notes that his "only issue with the theory (Ancel Keys' theory from the 1950s that excess cholesterol in the blood built up as plaque in the arteries) centered on the material in the plaque, which research subsequently revealed to be mostly inflammatory debris, not cholesterol."(Cowan T. What causes heart attacks. Wise Traditions. Heart Disease Issue:34.) In fact, oxidized polyunsaturated fats (found in processed vegetable oils like corn and soy) are a far greater component of the plaque than cholesterol. Natasha Campbell-McBride, author of *The Gut and Psychology Syndrome* and *Put Your Heart in Your Mouth!* (Cambridge England: Medinform Publishing. 2007. p. 34), points out that "the average composition of an advanced atherosclerotic plaque is as follows: 68% fibrous tissue (tissue of repair mainly made out of collagen), 8% calcium, 7% inflammatory cells, 1% foam cells and 16% lipid-rich necrotic core. In that lipid part of the plaque most fats are unsaturated — 74% of total fatty acids." Focusing on reducing saturated fat and cholesterol is misguided when you consider that the most fat composing the plaque in the arteries is unsaturated. Where does this unsaturated fat come from? The answer may surprise you.

Since Ancel Keys' pronouncement, clinical trials have failed to support the hypothesis that replacing saturated animal fats with polyunsaturated vegetable oils would prevent heart disease. They have shown instead that vegetable oils may promote both cancer and heart disease. It is reasonable to assume that this is in large part due to the processing of these oils. Masterjohn further notes that "Arachidonic acid in animal fat is not 'deadly,' but is necessary for our bodies to initiate, suppress, or resolve inflammation as needed. These are all vital processes that allow us to respond appropriately to our environment. 'Solid fats' do not 'dilute' the nutrient density of our food. On the contrary, they carry fat-soluble nutrients and provide for their absorption."

Our fats of choice should come in the form nature provided, not from industrial fats found in packaged, processed foods. Good fats include: extra virgin olive and coconut oil, palm oil, pastured animal fats for cooking, organic raw dairy including raw butter, and unprocessed cod liver oil.

Here are a few additional points I would like to make about fat and cholesterol. Mary Enig, PhD, internationally known in the field of lipid bio-chemistry and author of the book *Know Your Fats*, wrote in her paper "The Oiling of America," "Scientific literature clearly delineates a number of vital roles for dietary saturated fats — they enhance the immune system, are necessary for healthy bones, provide energy and structural integrity to the cells, protect the liver and enhance the body's use of essential fatty acids."(Wise Traditions.

Heart Disease Issue. 106.) She further emphasizes the importance of saturated fats by pointing out that "stearic acid (a saturated fat), found in beef tallow and butter, has cholesterol lowering properties and is preferred food for the heart. As saturated fats are stable, they do not become rancid easily, do not call upon the body's reserves of antioxidants, do not initiate cancer, do not irritate the artery walls."

In the Section XI, Diseases of the Circulatory System, we presented cholesterol's nutritional importance which is highlighted in the listing below from *What Causes Heart Disease?* by Fallon and Enig:

• Cholesterol is the body's repair substance, found in high levels in scar tissue. When arteries develop irritations or tears, cholesterol is there to repair the damage.

• Along with saturated fats, cholesterol provides our cell membranes with necessary stiffness, flexibility and stability. When the diet contains an excess of polyunsaturated fatty acids (clear processed vegetable oils like corn, soybean), these replace saturated fatty acids in the cell membrane so that the cell becomes flabby and the membranes leak.

• Cholesterol is a precursor needed for the production of vital corticosteroids which regulate blood sugar and mineral metabolism. These hormones help us deal with stress and protect the body against heart disease and cancer. Furthermore, our sex hormones, including androgens, testosterone, estrogen, and progesterone are all made from cholesterol.

• Cholesterol is a precursor to make vitamin D.

• Cholesterol is a critical component of bile salts, which enable us to digest and assimilate fats in the diet.

• Recent research shows that cholesterol is an antioxidant. It actually protects us against the free radical damage that leads to heart disease and cancer.

• Serotonin receptors in the brain require cholesterol for proper function (one reason why cholesterol medications can cause mental sequelae; low cholesterol levels are linked to aggressive and violent behavior, depression and even suicide).

- Mother's milk is especially rich in cholesterol which is crucial for the developing brain and nervous system.

- Dietary cholesterol plays an important role in maintaining the health of the intestinal wall. This is why low-cholesterol vegetarian diets can lead to leaky gut syndrome and other intestinal disorders.

- Men who have cholesterol levels over 300 mg/dL are at a slightly higher risk for heart disease. For women, there is no greater risk for heart disease, even at levels as high as 1,000 mg/dL. In fact, mortality is higher for women with low cholesterol than for women with high cholesterol.

- Cholesterol readings are highly inaccurate. They vary with the time of day, time of the patient's last meal, levels of stress and the type of test used. Tests for HDL and LDL are especially subject to inaccuracies. (Wise Traditions. Heart Disease Issue. p. 24.)

It is clear from the aforementioned list that blaming saturated fats and cholesterol for causing cardiovascular disease is too simplistic. What does make sense is that there are multiple contributing factors to cardiovascular disease, many known and some still unknown. The best way to avoid cardiovascular disease, and other illnesses as well, is to stop worrying about the level of your cholesterol on bloodwork, and concentrate on creating a healthier lifestyle. To do that, start with the following **Ten Basic Principles of a Healthy Heart:**

- Eat a traditional foods diet rich in bone broths, sea food, whole, raw dairy including raw butter, pastured eggs, pastured meats, fats and organ meats from organic pastured animals.

- Study the Weston A. Price Foundations (WAPF) guidelines and implement them into your lifestyle one at a time. Use this link to see the characteristics of the WAPF diet in more detail: http://www.westonaprice.org/traditional-diets/differences-between-the-weston-a-price-foundation-diet-and-the-paleo-diet.

- Exercise regularly: yoga, dance classes, pilates, slow burn weight training, using a trampoline, or other forms of exercise. Do something you enjoy and do it regularly. There are many excellent and healthy ways to get your body moving as nature intended. This is especially important if you work in a sedentary job as a sedentary lifestyle has been linked to increased risk of cardiovascular disease.

• Never consume packaged, processed foods, especially those labeled "low-fat" or those which contain preservatives, artificial sweeteners, hydrogenated fats, white flour, refined sugar, or other artificial additives.

• Eat copious amounts of fresh, organic vegetables and salads every day. Include small amounts of organic fruit as well.

• Do not smoke.

• Avoid excessive stress whenever possible. When stress levels rise, counter them with paying extra care to eating a nutrient-dense, whole food diet like the WAPF diet. To balance the stress, participate in something relaxing that you enjoy like transcendental meditation. Visit www.tm.org to learn more on transcendental meditation.

• Limit exposure to chemicals, pesticides, toxins, pollutants, etc. Read Walter Crinnion's book *Clean, Green and Lean* to learn how to eliminate common household toxins.

• Supplement regularly with whole-food vitamins and minerals. Work with a qualified doctor or nutritionist to identify your specific needs, one who is well versed in whole food vitamins and supplements.

• Get adequate sleep, preferably as close to the sun going down as possible and in dark, quiet surroundings.

Nutrition and Cardiovascular Disease

It is a fact that Cardiovascular Disease (CVD) kills more Americans than any other disease. The Center for Disease Control, CDC, states this on their website and points out that CVD does not discriminate. It strikes people of all ages and backgrounds. It is of great concern that between the years 2007 and 2008 the cost of CVD increased by over 11 billion dollars. (http://www.heart.org/idc/groups/ahamah-public/@wcm/@sop/@smd/documents/down-loadable/

ucm_434592.pdf). According to the American Heart Association (AHA), less than 1% of U.S. adults meet the definition for "Ideal Healthy Diet" and essentially no children meet the goal. If so few meet the basic standards of a healthy diet, perhaps this is a primary area we should examine in order to correct our health problems, especially regarding the number one killer. At the same time we need to eliminate two other indisputable culprits – smoking and a sedentary lifestyle. The AHA states that 19.8% of boys and 19.1% of girls in grades 9–12 report being current smokers. Among adults, 21.2% of men and 17.5% of women over the age of 18 years are smokers. That tells us that if you start smoking early in life, you tend to keep smoking into adulthood. Those numbers do not bode well for our heart health. In addition, the 2012 AHA update on CVD states that only 20.7% of adults meet the federal guidelines for physical activity and among 9th–12th graders, only 37% meet the recommendations. This means that over 60% of high school students are not meeting federal guidelines for a healthy, active lifestyle and approximately 20% of these are habitual smokers.

Could these three factors of inadequate diet, a sedentary culture and smoking be the main reasons why Americans have such a high level of circulatory disease? To better understand how to cure heart disease and diabetes naturally, let us consider key nutritional components for circulatory health, ones I have found effective in reversing circulatory damage.

The first component is diet. We have been told that the way to a healthy heart is through a low-fat, high-carbohydrate diet. This is not true. In fact, this one recommendation has led to more circulatory damage and death than any other cause, even smoking. Let us look at the nutritional basics of why this is so.

1. The Standard American Diet persuaded the public to fear fats and laud carbohydrates as heart healthy. But as Gerald Reaven, MD notes in *Syndrome X The Silent Killer*, p. 19, "the culprit with Syndrome X (or Metabolic Syndrome, aka Insulin Resistance) isn't red meat or butter, it's carbohydrates." He goes on to explain, "Excess insulin in the bloodstream prompts the damage associated with Syndrome X. Unfortunately, excess insulin is the first in a series of events which triggers damage to arteries that may precipitate a heart attack." A final emphasis is made when he writes "the more

carbohydrate an insulin-resistant person eats, the more the liver will increase its production of triglyceride-rich VLDL and release it into the bloodstream (Reaven G. Syndrome x: the silent killer. New York, London, Sydney, Singapore: Simon & Schuster; 2001. p.49). Dr. Reaven concludes that we should ignore the "best" medical advice and shun the low-fat, high-carbohydrate diet everyone "knows" is good for the heart (Ibid p. 17–18). Read the dietary guidelines in the next section on diabetes to learn more.

2. Current recommendations by the most knowledgeable lipid researchers and biochemists suggest an intake of no more than 3 to 4 parts omega-6 fatty acids to one part omega-3 fatty acids. The best sources of omega-3 fatty acids include grass-fed or wild game meats, organ meats, and cold-water, wild-caught fish such as Alaskan salmon, herring, sardines, and mackerel (Gedgaudas N. Primal body, primal mind-beyond the paleo diet. 2nd ed. Rochester VT: Healing Arts Press, Inner Traditions/Bear & Co; 2011. p. 129). Maintaining a proper ratio of omega-3 to omega-6 fatty acids is crucial for controlling inflammation in the body as well as the arteries.

3. The third nutritional cause is deficiencies in both vitamin P and vitamin C as a result of the SAD and stressors from both environmental and social behavior, including smoking, stress, and prescription medications. Vitamin C cannot be made by the human body so we must get it from our food. Unfortunately, most vitamin C is destroyed by canning and other processing methods. Vitamin C plays a very important role in the production of collagen which provides strength and stability to all of the body's tissues including the arteries.

> Linus Pauling believed that whilst humans normally obtain sufficient vitamin C to prevent full-blown scurvy, we do not consume enough to maintain the strength of the walls of the arteries. He suggested that of all the structural tissues in the body, the walls of the arteries around the heart are subject to the greatest continual stress. Every time the heart beats the arteries are flattened and stretched, and this has been likened to standing on a garden hose thousands of times a day. Many tiny cracks and lesions develop and the artery

walls become inflamed. (Orthomolecular Medicine News Service. 2010 June 22; 1)

Hypoglycemia

Hypoglycemia is a condition of low blood sugar and can be the beginning of many problems. Not surprisingly the culprit is sugar. In *Deep Nutrition* by Catherine Shanahan, MD and Luke Shanahan they state:

> Hypoglycemia is a commonly recognized problem of low blood sugar. But it may be the earliest sign that a person is on their way to developing insulin resistance. The symptoms of hypoglycemia include feeling tired, hungry, shaky, or nauseated before lunch or dinner. These feelings come from adrenaline, which helps the liver pump out more sugar but also makes us shaky, nauseous, even panicky. Because sufferers often figure that their symptoms are due to "low" sugar, they often self-medicate by eating more sugar which, as we'll see next, only makes the problem worse. (p. 210)

The precipitous drop in blood sugar familiar to hypoglycemics comes partially from the fact that their cells become starved of the normal amount of glycogen (sugar stored in muscle and the liver) as a source of sugar, leaving the patient feeling weak, confused, tired, moody, shaky, and with headaches. If their blood sugar drops below 40 mg/dL, the patient risks going into a coma. When this happens an emergency procedure involving adrenaline injection is necessary to keep the heart pumping until the sugar can be restored to normal levels. All this can be tied to the overconsumption of refined sugars ("garbage carbohydrates" or "garbohydrates" as I call them) and the greatly imbalanced Standard American Diet. The chart on the next page reveals the evolution of our sugar addiction.

Many people with hypoglycemia do not realize that years of eating sweets and sugar-spiking garbohydrates wear away at the endocrine system, including the pancreas, thyroid, and adrenal glands, eating up crucial minerals like magnesium and B vitamins until depletion. With stress, lack of sleep and exercise, consuming coffees with sugar to "push through" the day on a daily basis,

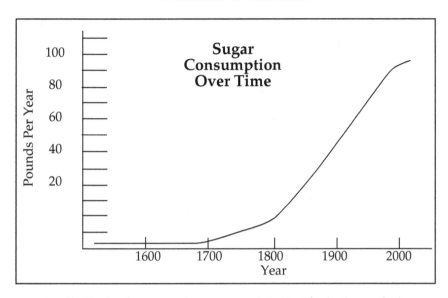

eventually the body can no longer regulate itself. The hypothalamus in the brain is taxed trying to keep up. When there is an overload of these *refined sugars* the pancreas must work harder to produce a high amount of insulin to shuttle the sugar out of the blood and into the cells. This eventually precipitates the sharp drop in blood sugar associated with hypoglycemia. This in turn uses up enzymes, chromium and other nutrients which the body can only replace by eating wholesome foods. Unfortunately, because the hormone system is affected, adrenaline is activated, cravings and moodiness are common, and as a result, the person usually reaches for the sugar-fix that initiated the problem. Eventually, for most people, hypoglycemia will no longer be the problem because the body will give out and hyperglycemia or diabetes will have come to stay.

The body, however, needs *some* sugar, the primary fuel source of the neurons in the brain and in red blood cells. In fact, glucose deprivation causes stress on the liver forcing it to manufacture glucose from protein. This can also increase toxicity and reduce longevity. Conversion of protein to glucose generates ammonia as a toxic by-product. The high protein intake associated with this strategy is associated with shortened lifespan, impaired immune function, and deficiencies of nutrients primarily found in edible plants (Jaminet P, Jaminet SC. Perfect health diet: regain health and lose weight by eating the way you were meant to eat. New

York: Scribner: 2013. p. 32–33). I am not advocating a very low carbohydrate or overly high protein diet. However, it is essential to avoid the refined sugars found in candy, cake, and commercial breads. I agree with Paul and Shou-Ching Jaminet who state that ".. . for most people, we would suggest . . . about 400 carbohydrate calories per day (or 100 grams per day)." (Ibid p. 45) It is important to note that mitochondria, the energy producers in most human cells, prefer to burn fat as the primary fuel. (Ibid p. 29)

I diverge from these authors' opinions in that I do not think these calories should come only from white rice, taro, sweet potatoes, fruits and berries. In fact, I use only *whole grain rice, not white rice*, which should be soaked in the traditions of the cultures extolled by Dr. Weston A. Price. Furthermore, I would modify their position on the source of carbohydrate calories so that they come from whole grains and legumes prepared by soaking, sprouting or sour leavening to neutralize phytic acid, enzyme inhibitors and other anti-nutrients. Most fruits, especially organic ripe fruits from the acid and sub-acid groups are acceptable as long as they are eaten in season, preferably in the earlier part of the day either for breakfast or as snacks approximately three hours after a meal. This is an important point as it is not good to mix fruits in the stomach with protein and fat. Other carbohydrates to include in your diet are sweet potato, beets, yam, parsnips, jicama, rutabaga, turnip, carrots, radish, daikon and others. For pregnant women, the total caloric carbohydrate intake per day can be increased to 600 calories without a problem. We are not counting non-starch vegetables in this calculation because they are more of a fiber and so are broken down by bacteria in the intestinal tract and processed more as fats.

I also recommend all of the healthy fats discussed throughout this book and the nutrient-dense organ meats and protein from pastured, organic animals. For more information on balancing blood sugar control and optimal health, read the next section on diabetes. After all, hypoglycemia is the precedent to diabetes.

Diabetes and Cardiovascular Diseases (CVD)

According to the American Heart Association (AHA) an estimated 18.3 million Americans around 20 years of age have physician-diagnosed diabetes. An additional 7.1 million adults have undiagnosed diabetes and about 81.5 million adults have prediabetes. Diabetes is affecting children as much as adults and seniors. We are even seeing early signs of heart disease in children. Diabetes statistics from the International Diabetes Federation for 2015 indicate that 1 in 11 adults has diabetes. By 2040 it is projected that 1 in every 10 will be diabetic. The Centers for Disease Control (CDC) states that for the year 2014, 29.1 million Americans or 9.3% of the US population have diabetes with another 8.1 million people undiagnosed (27.8% of people with diabetes are undiagnosed). (Taken from the CDC's national diabetes statistics report, 2014. Further data can be obtained from the CDC website at www.cdc.gov/diabetes/pdfs/data/2014-report-estimates-of-diabetes-and-its-burden-in-the-United-states.pdf)

Diabetes and CVD go hand-in-hand. A study published in the medical journal *The Lancet* stresses the importance of preventing diabetes amid rising rates worldwide. The disease is now linked to 1 out of every 10 cardiovascular deaths. That translates to roughly 325,000 deaths each year. In this significant study, researchers reviewed data from almost 700,000 people who had been studied for 10 years in 25 different countries. They found that diabetes appeared to double the risk of coronary disease, stroke and other vascular deaths and they estimated that diabetes accounts for 10–12% of all vascular deaths. Source: "Diabetes Mellitus, Fasting Blood, Glucose Concentration, and Risk of Vascular Disease: A Collaborative Meta-Analysis of 102 Prospective Studies" *The Lancet*, Vol. 375, No 9733, pp. 2215–22, June 26, 2010.

In general there are two types of diabetes. One, a juvenile form characterized by a malfunctioning of the pancreas at birth or shortly thereafter. The other is called adult onset and is divided into Type I and Type II. In Type I diabetes or Insulin Dependent Diabetes Mellitus (IDDM) there is an autoimmune reaction to the beta cells that produce insulin in the pancreas, leaving the patient unable to produce sufficient amounts of insulin. As there is no known cure, this condition must be treated with insulin and other medications. Type II diabetes, or Non-Insulin Dependent Diabetes Mellitus (NIDDM) now commonly called insulin resistant diabetes, is characterized by the body's cells becoming unresponsive to insulin. More specifically, the cells become desensitized to the effects of insulin, leaving the body unable to pull sugar out of the blood for use in energy production. I am omitting a less common form of diabetes known as diabetes insipidus because its root cause is completely different. It is a problem involving the pituitary gland in the brain. There is also a nephrogenic form which involves a malfunction in the kidneys and is congenital.

In recent years, a condition known as Metabolic Syndrome, or Syndrome X, has come to replace adult onset diabetes(Type II) as the central health topic. Syndrome X is defined by The International Diabetes Federation as ". . . central obesity combined with any two of the following four factors: raised triglyceride levels ≥ 150 mg/dL, reduced HDL-cholesterol ≤ 40 mg/dL in males ≤ 50 mg/dL in females, raised systolic blood pressure ≥ 130 mm Hg or diastolic blood pressure ≥ 85 mm Hg, raised fasting plasma glucose of ≥ 100 mg/dL or previously diagnosed Type II diabetes." (International Diabetes Federation — www.idf.org/webdata/docs/MetS_def_update2006.pdf) "Syndrome X is characterized by these risk factors: impaired glucose tolerance, high insulin levels, elevated triglycerides, low HDL cholesterol, slow clearance of fat from the blood, smaller, more dense LDL cholesterol, an increased propensity of the blood to clot, decreased ability to dissolve blood clots, and elevated blood pressure. Lifestyle factors that worsen syndrome X are obesity, poor diet, lack of physical activity, and smoking." (Reaven G, Strom T K, Fox B. Syndrome X: the silent killer: the new heart disease risk. New York : Simon & Schuster; 2000. p. 220.) Researchers are now finding a link between all of these factors and overall health. Complex pathophysiology plays a role in the development of cardiovascular disease and diabetes, and often we cannot separate them. They seem to be intimately related.

Syndrome X is the most prevalent form of diabetes today. Paul and Shou-Ching Jaminet note in their book *Perfect Health Diet* p.42, " . . . either glucose or insulin can convert human vascular smooth muscle cells to osteogenic (bone secreting) cells. When this happens . . . cells secrete calcium phosphate into the vascular lining of the arteries." Hardening of the arteries does not bode well for cardiovascular health. It makes the arteries rigid and unable to expand and contract with changes in blood pressure. This may seem harmless at first, but that pressure has to go somewhere. As a result, the heart must work harder and harder to pump blood through these "noncompliant" passageways. Over time, this takes its toll on the heart muscle. Like any other muscle in the body that is worked harder and harder, it will first hypertrophy (grow in size). This seems benign but remember, the valves of the heart have to function just right to keep blood moving in the right direction, opening and closing to control the pumping of the blood and the timing of the beats. However, as the heart enlarges the valves will eventually become stenotic and compromised. Blood pressure rises to try to compensate for this lack of function and efficiency. Eventually, this leads to regurgitation of blood backward from the atria into the ventricles and reduces the cardiac output (oxygen-rich blood being pumped to the body).

Dr. Bruce West notes on p. 90 in *The Encyclopedia of Pragmatic Medicine* "For most Americans, it is about insulin. Both the *Journal of the American Medical Association* (May 16, 2007) and *TIME Magazine* (June 11, 2007) agree. If you consume lots of conventional, processed wheat, grains and processed foods (which all contain gluten), your pancreas secretes higher than normal amounts of insulin." Insulin, as mentioned above, is irritating to your blood vessels, creating a hardening of the artery through calcium deposition as well as inflammation to the endothelium (inner lining of the blood vessel wall). This sets the stage for atherosclerotic plaque and, unless dietary/nutritional and exercise intervention are put in place, eventual clogging of the artery. This initiates a spate of problems including myocardial infarction (heart attack), cerebrovascular accident (stroke), thrombosis (clotting) and impending death.

Let us take a slight detour to explain where most problems with vascular damage originate. In the past, the medical community has blamed dietary cholesterol for this plaque build-up and clogging of the arteries. This has made cholesterol-lowering statin drugs the number one money-maker among all classes of drugs. However, research has shown that the main fats that are found in the atherosclerotic plaques are not cholesterol but are oxidized (damaged) polyunsaturated omega 6 fats which come from rancid industrial vegetable oils, corn oil and soybean. Susan Schenck notes, " . . . in reality only 26% of the fat clogging the arteries is saturated.

Most, 74%, is unsaturated, of which 41% is polyunsaturated, the kind found in vegetable oils that were supposed to make our arteries healthy."(Schenck S. Beyond broccoli: creating a biologically balanced diet when a vegetarian diet doesn't work. Concrete WA: Awakenings Publications; 2011.85) In fact, Ancel Keys who put forth the cholesterol-diet/heart disease hypothesis in the 1960's, decades later admitted it was flawed. Susan Schenck Lac, in her book *Beyond Broccoli*, notes: "Interestingly, Keys himself recanted the theory decades later, stating, 'There's no connection whatsoever between cholesterol in food and cholesterol in the blood. None. And we've known that all along.'"(Beyond Broccoli. p. 82)

In the Heart Disease Issue of *Wise Traditions*, Sally Fallon and Mary G. Enig, PhD have an article entitled "What Causes Heart Disease." In order to separate myth from truth, they discuss the many different factors involved in cardiovascular disease. Aside from the aforementioned plaque that builds up in the arteries, they state that "Inflammation may also cause blockages. In fact, a new view considers coronary artery disease to be an inflammatory process, characterized by cycles of irritation, injury, healing and re-injury inside the blood vessels. The inflammatory response is actually a defense mechanism that helps the body heal but when the inflammatory process goes awry, plaques may rupture, provoking clots that lead to heart attacks." (Ibid p. 23)

Many researchers now believe that cholesterol is acting as an antioxidant in a desperate attempt by the body to heal the damage to the endometrial lining. After all, cholesterol is necessary for a myriad of bodily functions including making male and female hormones, building vitamin D, and even making up part of the cell membrane of all cells. To further understand the truth about cholesterol the following resources may help. (Also consult the database at www.westonaprice.org)

1. *The Great Cholesterol Con: The Truth About What Really Causes Heart Disease and How to Avoid It*, by Malcolm Kendrick, MD.

2. *The Great Cholesterol Con: "Why everything you've been told about cholesterol, diet and heart disease is wrong,"* by Anthony Colpo.

3. *How Statin Drugs Really Lower Cholesterol and Kill You One Cell At a Time*, by James B. Yoseph and Hannah Yoseph, MD.

4. *Put Your Heart in Your Mouth*, by Natasha Campbell-McBride.

5. www.cholesterol-and-health.com (Chris Masterjohn's website devoted to the truth regarding cholesterol.)

Since cholesterol is not the real villain wreaking havoc in our bloodstream, we must discuss the true culprits — poor blood sugar control/levels and insulin deregulation. Though there are other contributing factors, controlling the amount of glucose and insulin that we secrete into our bloodstream on a daily basis is the key to avoiding diabetes and therefore the key to avoiding cardiovascular diseases. Control is achieved by avoiding common offenders: refined sugars; wheat and wheat products like bagels, pretzels and pasta; sugary soft drinks and other beverages; candy, etc. Instead, replace these altered, processed, and in some cases completely man-made foods with wholesome, organic green vegetables and healthy unrefined fats from olive, coconut, flax as well as pastured animal fats (suet, tallow, lard). Follow a traditional whole foods diet as espoused by the Weston A. Price Foundation.

Let us explore diabetes, cardiovascular disease and diet a little further. As Dr. Bruce West writes, "A healthy meal of whole-grain cereal is not the breakfast of champions. It is the breakfast of diabetics." (West B. How to cure diabetes, heart disease, high cholesterol and obesity. Encyclopedia of Pragmatic Medicine. Monterey CA: Health Alert & Bruce West;91.) For those who want more information on the effects of wheat, read renowned cardiologist Dr. William Davis' book *Wheat Belly*. Davis explains how eliminating wheat from our diets can prevent fat storage, shrink unsightly bulges, and reverse many health problems including diabetes and cardiovascular disease. Also read *Grain of Truth: The Real Case For and Against Wheat and Gluten* by Stephen Yafa to learn about the differences between modern industrial wheat products and properly-prepared traditional grains.

A second dietary consideration is the prevalence of processed, rancid fats in our diet: corn oil, soybean oil, safflower oil, cottonseed oil, margarines, shortenings and more. In "What Causes Heart Disease?" Wise Traditions. Heart Disease Issue. 28, Sally Fallon and Mary Enig write ". . . it is the type or quality of the fat that matters. Ninety years ago, Americans consumed mostly animal fats — lard, butter, tallow from pasture-fed animals. These fats were stable and provided many important fat-soluble nutrients. Today most of the fats in the American diet are derived from plants — as liquid vegetable oils or oils that have been hardened through the process of partial hydrogenation." The authors warn that "large amounts of calories from polyunsaturated vegetable oils are new to the human diet and should certainly be examined more fully for their effects on health." The message here is that we shouldn't be fearful of wholesome, unadulterated fats from healthy, pastured animals. Nor should we avoid good quality, unprocessed, unheated, unfiltered flax seed oil, olive oil, coconut oil, palm oil, and even walnut and sesame oils. What we need to avoid are the "newfangled" fats as Sally Fallon puts it, which are found in corn, vegetable, soy, cottonseed, safflower, margarines, shortenings and other industrially processed oils. Trans fats are "hardened fats created from liquid vegetable oil by a process called partial hydrogenation, and much evidence supports the theory that these manufactured fats contribute to heart disease and diabetes." (Wise Traditions. Heart Disease Issue. 29.) I urge my patients to use raw, organic pastured butter especially from animals grazing on rapidly growing, pesticide-free grass, to cook with lard and tallow and to use unrefined flax and olive oils as a drizzle on salads, vegetables, or for dipping. One good rule of thumb is this: solid fats are better for cooking with higher heats (their chemistry is more stable under heat so they do not damage as much). Liquid oils like olive and flax are best as drizzles on salads and vegetables, although light sautéing in olive oil with low heat is permissible.

Several specific nutrients are crucial to controlling diabetes and heart disease. Not surprisingly, many of these nutrients are lacking in our diet due to the industrial processing and milling of foods. Two vitamins very seldom spoken of with regard to heart health are vitamins A and D. "Heart disease researchers have largely ignored the possible role of vitamins A and D in protecting the heart, probably because these fat-soluble vitamins are found only in the foods they have demonized — animal fats."(*Wise Traditions*, Heart Disease Issue, p. 25.) Vitamin A is needed for maintaining the integrity of the blood cells as well as conversion of cholesterol into steroid hormones. Vitamin D, an integral part of normal blood clotting, prevents arrhythmias via its action with calcium, and is helpful in controlling blood pressure. The vast majority of my patients present with low levels of this vitamin. I am not sure whether this is due to avoidance of or inadequate exposure to the sun, overuse of sunscreen, lack of natural vitamin D in the food supply, or a combination of all three.

Vitamin E is also a crucial heart healthy vitamin for many reasons. First, it is a natural blood thinner and antioxidant. It protects the body from the inflammation and oxidation that wear away at the blood vessels and cause clotting. Second, it promotes the dilation of blood vessels and "plays an essential role in cellular respiration, particularly in the cardiac muscles."(Wise Traditions. Heart Disease Issue 26) The lack of vitamin E in the diet is partially due to the milling process which eliminates the highly perishable wheat germ, a significant source of vitamin E (Ibid p. 26). When purchasing vitamin E, keep in mind that our bodies need the complete whole food complex which includes selenium, and several other compounds including tocopherols and tocotrienols.

Vitamin C and vitamin P are two of the most heart and blood vessel friendly vitamins. Vitamin P, or the bioflavonoids as they are more commonly known, is almost always found in foods alongside vitamin C. "Found in a variety of citrus fruits, vitamin P enables our bodies to absorb vitamin C properly. Its bioflavonoid properties impact the condition of our blood as well, by helping to ensure that our red blood cells and the blood platelets do not clump together. The vitamin also promotes capillary health, aiding in the proper function of the capillaries and also helping to prevent capillary bleeding. It is also helpful for anyone who is prone to bleeding gums, as the vitamin helps to prevent and also heal weak blood vessels located in the gums." (www.wisegeek.org) Vitamin P also lowers blood pressure, acts as an anti-inflammatory, and is important in wound healing. This is particularly important to diabetics, who often do not heal well.

With regard to heart health and controlling inflammation, in *The Heart Revolution*, Kilmer McCully notes the importance of the B vitamin family: particularly folate, B6 and B12. He found that deficiencies of these vitamins correlated with hardening of the arteries as well as plaque build-up. The author also brought to light the inflammatory effects the amino acid homocysteine has on the blood vessels if it builds up in the blood. Furthermore, he shows the importance of these three B vitamins in the metabolic pathway that reduces homocysteine by converting it back to methionine or into cystathionine.

Another important nutrient is Coenzyme Q10, or CoQ10. This coenzyme is crucial for providing the heart muscle with oxygen as well as acting as an antioxidant in its reduced form. Since CoQ10 is only helpful supplementally in its reduced form known as ubiquinol, avoid cheaper brands that sell the ubiquinone form. (Williams LL. Radical medicine: cutting edge natural therapies that treat the root cause of disease. Rochester VT: Healing Arts Press, Inner Traditions/Bear & Co; 2011.337) CoQ10 has been shown to be helpful in treating congestive heart failure, diabetes, and for patients who are taking statin drugs which deplete this crucial nutrient. (http://lpi.oregonstate.edu/infocenter/othernuts/coq10/)

Finally we consider magnesium. We typically draw blood on our diabetic and cardiovascular patients to measure red blood cell magnesium. In *Heart Frauds,* Charles T. McGee observes that adequate red blood cell magnesium is an important protector from the ravages of coronary artery disease and may be one of the most important indicators of cardiovascular risk (pp. 118–20). "Magnesium operates as a natural calcium channel blocker and is responsible for relaxation, counter to calcium's contraction, making magnesium pivotally important to the healthy functioning of our parasympathetic nervous system."(Czapp K. Magnificent magnesium: the neglected mineral we cannot live without. Wise Traditions. WAPF. 2010 Fall;11(3):35.) It is magnesium's partnership with calcium in a proper balance which helps prevent calcium precipitating out of the blood and depositing in the lining of the arteries causing arteriosclerosis.

Surprisingly, magnesium is one of the most common mineral deficiencies. In her article "Magnificent Magnesium," Czapp states that magnesium deficiency is endemic in the U.S. and that it is in fact one of the most depleted minerals in farm soils. She further states that "Unfortunately, it is difficult to reliably supply our bodies with sufficient magnesium, even from a good, balanced whole foods diet. First of all, modern agricultural methods favor the universal use of NPK fertilizers (nitrogen, phosphorus, and potassium). Both potassium and phosphorus are antagonists of magnesium in the soil, and on calcareous soils create a relative magnesium deficiency."

Diabetes Protocol

That brings us to diabetes and our healthy heart protocol. Not everyone with diabetes or CVD receives the same protocol. There will always be unique strengths and weaknesses to each person. As part of a lifestyle change, some people will have to quit smoking (and will probably need extra vitamin C as a result). Others may be sedentary and in need of regular exercise. Still others may need a complete dietary overhaul. Many, if not most, will need to make changes in several of these areas. Listed below is the foundation of a good vitamin and supplement protocol for diabetes that has been very effective:

1. Cataplex® GTF (Standard Process) – This combination of the trace mineral chromium with B complex vitamins known as the glucose tolerance factor (GTF), enables insulin to pull sugar out of the blood into the cells to be burned for energy. Dosage is 3–6 per day with meals.
2. Diaplex® (Standard Process) – Dosage of 6–9 per day with meals. This combination product includes B vitamins, pituitary extract (protomorphogen) and pancreas extract to support rebuilding of these important glands. It also contains kidney supporting nutrients taken from beets as well as betaine from beet leaf for converting harmful homocysteine.
3. Cardio-Plus® (Standard Process) – This may be the single most important supplement for the heart and it is five products in one. It contains vitamin E2 (the oxygen-sparing portion of the vitamin E complex); vitamin C complex (whole food of course); the calming side of the B vitamin complex; heart extract; and calcium lactate. It also contains selenium, CoQ_{10} and more.
4. Cataplex® B (Standard Process) – It is rich in vitamin B4 which helps to conduct nerve impulses to the heart and is especially important for diabetics who suffer from neuropathy.
5. Fermented Cod Liver Oil, either Green Pasture™, Dr. Ron's, or Radiant Life brand – Dosages vary based on nutritional testing

of fatty acid balance and vitamin D levels but typically range from one teaspoon to two tablespoons per day.

If there is a more serious heart condition involved, or if the diabetes is longstanding, the following supplements would be added to our protocol:

6. Berberine – 500 mg 3 times daily. Taken from ncbi.nlm.nih.gov: Compared to metformin, berberine exhibits an identical effect in the regulation of glucose metabo-lism, showing significant ability to decrease HbA1c levels. Authors: Jun Yin, Huili Xing and Jianping Ye. Source: *Efficacy of Berberine in Patients with Type 2 Diabetes Mellitus.*

7. Min-Tran® (Standard Process) – nine capsules per day with meals.

8. Calcium Lactate (Standard Process) – nine capsules daily.

Next we attend to diet. We start by removing the biggest offender of blood sugar control, wheat and wheat products. As mentioned earlier, wheat does more to deregulate blood sugar and insulin levels in some cases, than refined white sugar. The book *Wheat Belly* by Dr. Willam Davis is very informative and goes into great detail about the effect of modern wheat on blood sugar.

Second, we remove *refined sugars*. These are hidden under many guises on labels and popular health products. Avoid products that contain the following:

1. Fructose or any variation including high fructose corn syrup, corn syrup, corn syrup solids, corn sugar, sucrose or crystalline fructose.

2. Granulated, invert, brown, cane, beet, palm, date, coconut, raw cane sugars.

3. Fruit juice concentrate and fruit juice (these seem harmless but are not so).

4. Honey *(although small amounts of raw, unheated/unfiltered honey are healthy for most people).*

5. Evaporated cane juice.

6. Dextrose, maltose and maltodextrin (breaks down into glucose and is high glycemic).

7. Malt syrup, rice bran syrup, brown rice syrup.
8. Muscovato, succanat, turbinado sugar.
9. Maple syrup.
10. 1Barley malt extract and barley malt syrup.

For an overview of the various forms of refined sugars and their benefits/detriments, see pages 536-537 in *Nourishing Traditions* by Sally Fallon Morrell.

There are many reasons to avoid these ingredients. Most if not all of these forms of sugar come from what was once a whole food. For example, maltodextrin is a starch (complex carbohydrate) that can be taken from barley, wheat, rice, corn, or even potato. However, all of the other nutrients that were once there have been destroyed by the processing, leaving the sugar behind. This imparts the "high glycemic effect" on these types of refined sugars. They spike blood sugar and therefore insulin resulting in damage to the cardiovascular system, weight gain, dyslipidemia and other detrimental health consequences. The graph on the next page represents the difference between the effects processed sugars have versus whole food carbohydrates.

As you can see from the Hyper/Hypo Glycemia graph, once your blood sugar spikes beyond the ideal range (shown on the y-axis) of 75-90 mg/dL, a rapid response for insulin to be secreted into the blood is initiated. This leads to a cascade of events including signaling to store fat, elevation of triglycerides and dysglycemia (improper regulation of blood sugar levels) — essentially, the characteristics which define Syndrome X. The sharp drop in blood sugar resulting from high levels of insulin secretion by the pancreas creates the "crash" so many Americans are familiar with on a daily basis. Symptoms from this crash can be headaches, hunger, fatigue, lack of concentration and even cravings.

Therefore, diet needs to include the carbohydrates with the least impact on blood sugar and which are loaded with wholesome vitamins and minerals. I call them the green vegetable group, although many are not green. They are more accurately the non-starchy carbohydrates, vegetables like broccoli, zucchini, peppers, kale, beet tops, collard greens, salads, asparagus, and Brussels sprouts. Many charts showing the carbohydrate content of vegetables are available. Vegetables containing 10% starch or less can be eaten with impunity. Anything between 10-15% should only be eaten in moderation, and those vegetables with over 15% should be strictly avoided. As a reference, fruits like banana and dried fruits are much higher in sugar concentration and would be contraindicated for diabetics and those looking to improve cardiovascular function. In the same light, starchier vegetables like potato, beans, beets, corn and yams should be strictly limited or avoided altogether, not because starchy vegetables are inherently unhealthy but because a diabetic is already poor at handling sugar and is better off limiting these foods.

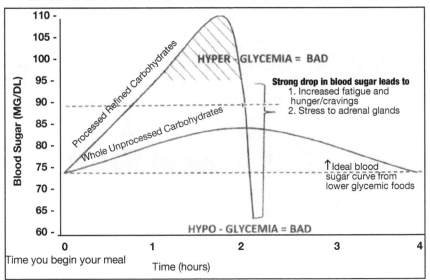

GUIDELINES:
1. Limit/Avoid processed white flour products and grains (ex. boxed cereal, breads, baked goods, pasta). Familiarize yourself with refined sugars like high fructose corn syrup, corn syrup, fructose, sucrose
2. Limit starches to one per day and do not include more than one starch per meal.

Hyperglycemia Causes:
1. Increased/Sustained insulin output weight gain damage to cardiovascular system
2. Estrogen imbalance for women
3. Feeds yeast
4. Stress to adrenal glands

High insulin output leads to:
1. Slowing of metabolism
2. Storage of fat
3. Dysglycemia/diabetes
4. High triglycerides

Missing from processed refined carbohydrates:
1. Fiber 2. Vitamins 3. Minerals 4. Enzymes

Liquid fats/oils in the diet should be from unrefined flax and olive oil primarily. They can be used as drizzles, dips, or added to shakes or smoothies, dressings, etc. They should never be cooked with any significant amount of heat as this will damage their delicate chemical structure. Cod liver oil should be taken as a supplement. As for the much maligned saturated fats, I believe that their danger to our health is grossly overstated. In fact, I believe it to be the contrary. As long as the saturated fats are from unrefined, organic and pastured sources, they are crucial to our health. Here is just a quick look at some of the important roles played by saturated fats:

- Saturated fats constitute over 50% of the cell membrane structure, providing stiffness and integrity to the cell.
- Fallon and Enig cite a study showing 50% of our dietary fats need to be saturated in order for calcium to be effectively incorporated into the skeletal structure. (*Beyond Broccoli*, p. 85)
- Coconut and palm oil as well as animal fats are the richest source of dietary saturated fats. Protein cannot be utilized without these fats.
- Without the fat soluble vitamins A, D, E, and K we cannot absorb water-soluble vitamins and cannot utilize minerals. (Schenck, p. 85)
- Fats are a great fuel, providing more energy per gram (9 cal/gram) and thought to be the primary fuel used by Paleo-man.

The goal must be to eliminate the "wrong" carbohydrates and fats from what we eat. We need to make enlightened choices about our food. Avoid anything man-made, genetically modified, processed, refined, spray-dried, homogenized, pasteurized, hydrogenated, etc. If food is not the way it would be found in nature or on a farm, resist it. It is almost assuredly harmful to our health.

A very important point regarding diabetes and CVD is the importance of exercise. Perhaps the most effective, efficient, and least time-consuming way to do it is with slow burn exercising. *The Slowburn Fitness Revolution* by Frederick Hahn, Michael Eades, MD and Mary Eades, MD explains the benefits of this type of exercise.

At the least, get moving. Go for walks regularly, bike, swim, move around. Most importantly, find something that you enjoy. It will improve your circulation, help your joints, increase your energy and change your outlook on life.

Chiropractic treatment of the spine with regard to the heart is critical to ensuring proper neurological communication from the brain to the heart, and back from the heart to the brain. The heart receives its parasympathetic innervations from the vagus nerve, a cranial nerve which helps slow the heart. "Sympathetic innervation to the heart occurs from spinal levels T1–T5, with T2 contributing the most."(American Osteopathic Association. Foundations of Osteopathic Medicine. Chila A. ed. Philadelphia US: Lippincott Williams & Wilkins; 2010. p. 24.) Therefore, proper cervical adjustment as well as adjustment to the thoracic spine is critical, with special attention given to the T2 vertebra. Make sure you work with a qualified chiropractor who understands this.

My final recommendation to everyone struggling with diabetes and CVD is the book *The Great Cholesterol Con* by Anthony Colpo. The closing section on page 307 (after Chapter 30), entitled *The Twelve Commandments for a Healthy Heart*, gives excellent guidelines.

Juvenile Diabetes

In discussing juvenile diabetes, we need to look at probable causes. Eating habits are front and center. School lunches may be laden with processed carbohydrates from pizza, white bread sandwiches, sodas and candy/ice cream. Convenience junk food disguised as healthy food is fed to children and marketed to parents. The home environment is often at fault. There are bagels in the morning or cold processed and extruded breakfast cereals followed by microwave dinners, pasta, refined white flour products and seldom a green vegetable. I see these children frequently. Fortunately, when and if parents willing to make changes are educated about food and nutrition, the children quickly get better.

Eliminate refined sugars and flour products and you are well on your way to recovery. Parents need to replace the empty, processed carbohydrates with green vegetables, salads, fresh fruit, and plenty of raw pastured dairy products and meats along with

A Legacy of Healing

fish. *Nourishing Traditions* by Sally Fallon is a priceless resource for parents making these changes. It contains recipes and provides information regarding sources of healthy, traditional foods. In addition, *Nourishing Traditions* gives the novice an introduction that explains the problems with modern, processed foods and how to recognize and avoid them.

An important dietary consideration in juvenile diabetes and in heart disease is the overconsumption of bad fats. We are told that saturated fats and cholesterol found in animal products, eggs, and tropical oils are what are causing our arteries to clog with cholesterol. In fact, we need these fats. They are now and have always been good for us. The fats destroying the vitality of children are trans fats, the result of the industrial processing of oils. Hydrogenated and partially hydrogenated oils from soy, corn, and vegetable sources are the real culprits. Coupled with the ubiquity of polyunsaturated fats in processed and fasts foods, we have a recipe for disaster. Hydrogenated fats damage the arteries, promote an imbalance toward inflammatory prostaglandin production and cause membranes to become "leaky." I recommend reading *Real Food* by Nina Planck and *Know Your Fats* by Mary Enig. These books present the truth about fats rather than the selective nutritional information offered on packaging. A further resource for this information is the Weston A. Price Foundation's website at www.westonaprice.org.

Also, children need exercise. As recently as 40 years ago, children walked to school and were outside physically exercising and playing much of the day. Today's children play at video games. When not doing this, they are on the internet or texting. They have lost the physical exercise that comes with play. I advocate that children have at least one hour of physical exercise each day.

The final consideration that compounds the problem for children is the lack of proper vitamin supplementation. Proper vitamin and mineral supplementation tailored to the individual is more important now than ever. Children in this country are not getting the nourishment they need. It starts with birth. Children may not be breast fed. Instead they are raised on soy and milk-based formulas that are sugar-laden, processed and just a slight step above poison. Is it any wonder that juvenile diabetes is on the rise?

We must consider the consequences of genetic engineering as well as the severity of soil depletion. Studies have shown that conventional fruits and vegetables are far inferior to organic produce in terms of vitamin and mineral content. Pesticides, herbicides and chemical fertilizers degrade the soil and damage vitamin and mineral content. If the soil isn't healthy, how can anything that is grown in it be healthy?

When considering vitamins, be aware that not all vitamins are created equal. Through years of experience, I have found that vitamins and minerals should be produced from organically grown food, and be carefully handled without heat or preservatives which damage their chemical properties. Adherence to this philosophy regarding supplements has shown the best results in my patients.

One company providing excellent products is Standard Process, established in 1927. The company has its own organic farms and when they produce vitamins, they do so in whole food forms. This means that you consume them with their entire complex of complementary cofactors still present and their enzymes intact.

As a side note, any time I have taken synthetic vitamins, I have noticed a bright greenish-yellow color to my urine almost immediately after consuming them. I took this to mean that my body was excreting the vitamins because it could not use them. This never occurs with Standard Process vitamins.

If you are the parent of a diabetic child, what are you to do?

1. Get your child into a program of some form of exercise. Exercise is the one constant that has repeatedly been shown to help diabetics, especially a type of exercise known as Slow Burn which was developed by Dr. Eades and is highlighted in the book *The Slow Burn Fitness Revoltion*.

2. Proper diet is the key. This means cutting back on white sugar, white flour, trans fats, artificial sweeteners, processed foods and sugary drinks. Introduce more fresh fruits, vegetables, raw milk and dairy, pasture-raised chickens and eggs, grass-fed beef, and wild-caught fish. Include coconut and palm oils in the diet as well as pastured, organic animal fats. Learn to soak grains, nuts, seeds, beans and legumes to make them easier to digest and more

nutritious. To become more familiar with these foods and with recipes, use these resources: The Weston A. Price Foundation website (www.westonaprice.org); *Nourishing Traditions* cookbook by Sally Fallon; *Real Food* by Nina Planck and the website www.realmilk.com.

3. Children should be taught to drink 1½ glasses of water *before* each meal. Drinking water in large quantities during the meal is not advisable as this will dilute the acid in the stomach and therefore hinder digestion.

4. Most diabetics need the trace minerals selenium and chromium as well as alpha lipoic acid, calcium and vanadium. These are helpful in enabling insulin to work properly. This helps the body utilize sugar for energy instead of having it accumulate in the blood where it can wreak havoc.

5. Standard Process makes four very important products which I use with great efficacy in my diabetes protocol. They are: Catalyn (multivitamin), Cataplex® GTF (stands for glucose tolerance factor-contains chromium), Diaplex®, and Min Tran. All four are extremely effective in aiding the diabetic condition.

6. Lastly, all children should be given a high-vitamin fermented cod liver oil supplement. See sources in the back of the book for recommendations.

One final note on juvenile diabetes bears mention — the possible link between it and mercury in vaccines. Read this book's section on vaccines before you decide to have your child vaccinated. My wife and I raised our entire family of 6 children and 10 grandchildren without any vaccines. It can be done. Check the resources listed and do your research. Find a doctor who will work with you without vaccinating your child. Their number is growing as more and more people become aware of the inherent dangers of vaccination. Better yet, go to see the movie "Vaxxed."

Congestive Heart Failure

Congestive heart failure (CHF) is a condition resulting from long-standing nutritional neglect. (Read this book's section on Diabetes and Cardiovascular Disease, pp. 210–229, to learn the basic causes, physiology and nutrition involved in most cardiovascular cases.) When one has been eating poorly over many years and does not put into the body the necessary elements that the heart requires, it begins to fill with fluid and to fail. As the heart loses its ability to function and pump blood, the body begins to starve for oxygen. Something very few doctors know about the heart is that it is incredibly regenerative. It is able to repair itself cell for cell every 90 days.

Conventional treatment of CHF is centered on medications to either slow or increase the heart rate. If coronary arteries (the arteries that supply blood to the heart) are clogged, stents will often be put in to force the blood vessel open. If that does not work, a bypass may be performed. All of these procedures have two things in common: they are reactive not preventative, and they ignore the causative deficiencies that weakened the heart to begin with. Conventional medicine never tries to improve the function of the heart from within using proper vitamin supplements or with dietary changes/suggestions. Weston A. Price's dying words were, "You teach, you teach, you teach!" In our office this is exactly what we do. We teach the patient how to heal the body from within, and the heart is no exception.

Not too long ago (perhaps no more than 100 years) Americans ate a diet rich in fresh fruits, vegetables, nuts, seeds and animal products, including fats from pastured animals. Fruits and vegetables were free from pesticides and herbicides, and were not genetically modified. Animals grazed on pasture, were not fed hormones and were not crowded into small pens on factory farms. People had a connection to the earth, to life and death, and a respect for the animals that provided us with food. Now children don't know what an avocado is let alone where it comes from while most adults don't know that a chicken is an omnivore, not a vegetarian. We have become disconnected from our food sources, consuming excessive quantities of processed sugar, eating laboratory-made fats which extend the shelf life of a product; and consuming fast foods which are available everywhere. As a result, our nutrition has degenerated and heart disease has risen to become the number one killer. How did this happen so quickly?

After the turn of the 20th century, milling of flour became more ubiquitous and with it so did heart disease. Unfortunately the processing of wheat removes a large portion of the B-complex vitamins found in the outer sheath of the wheat kernel. B vitamins are crucial to heart health, especially B4 and B1 (thiamine). A deficiency of each of these can lead to a condition Dr. Bruce West refers to in his Health Alert publication as beri-beri of the heart. The heart muscle weakens, becomes incompetent and begins to fill with fluid. Soon the person cannot walk more than a block without getting out of breath. Walking up a flight of stairs becomes nearly impossible without stopping to rest and catch a breath.

A change in diet is a crucial step in correcting CHF and regenerating the heart. The changes, for the most part, should be common sense: eliminate refined sugars found in processed and packaged foods like cereals, soda, and cookies; eliminate all man-made and processed fats including clear vegetable oils like soybean, corn, canola, and cottonseed; eliminate trans fats found in hydrogenated oils, margarines, and shortenings. Be aware that even if a label reads "No Trans Fats" it can still contain up to 0.5 grams. No amount of trans fat is safe to consume.

Instead fill the refrigerator with fresh, organic fruits and vegetables. Rather than buying homogenized/pasteurized dairy, find a local farm to purchase fresh, organic, raw milk and dairy. Two Weston A. Price Foundation websites, www.westonaprice.org and www.realmilk.com can be helpful in this search. Purchase grass-fed meats and pastured chicken if possible. When one eats the product of mistreated, unhealthy animals, animals forced into confinement and fed GMO soy and corn which produce inflammatory eicosanoids (hormone-like messengers that control inflammation), one consumes their inflammation. Also one does not get the fats, vitamins, minerals and enzymes one would if the animals were pastured and properly tended. Cheap food comes with a cost. Consuming nutrient-depleted foods results in a decline in health and a rise in healthcare bills. A further discussion of farming and animal husbandry can be found in *Nourishing Traditions* by Sally F. Morrell and *Folks This Ain't Normal: A Farmer's Advice for Happier Hens, Healthier People and a Better World* by Joel Salatin.

Recommended Treatment

Vitamin supplementation for CHF must be centered upon using whole-food supplements. Synthetic, fractionated supplements do not work, nor do synthetic, fractionated vitamins. You cannot reproduce wholesome, organic foods in a lab. Wholesome, whole-food supplements give good results.

Vitamin supplementation for CHF begins with Cardio Plus made by Standard Process (dosage between six to nine per day depending on the severity of the case). These tablets contains the extract of organic animal heart muscle and extract of yeast, sprouted grain and calf brain. This supplies enzymes to make cholinesterase to perform with acetylcholine at the neuromuscular junction. It also contains the entire vitamin E complex as well as Coenzyme Q10 which helps to protect the heart from oxidation and provides more oxygen to the heart muscle.

Separate supplementation with Coenzyme Q10 is often necessary and begins at a dosage of 300 mgs per day with breakfast. I use a product made by Designs for Health known as Q-Avail which contains the fat soluble form Ubiquinol. The third crucial supplement necessary in treating CHF naturally is fish oil. There are many different viewpoints on what type of fish oil to use and at what dosage. I use Green Pasture™ Fermented Cod Liver Oil, one teaspoon a day up to one tablespoon twice a day depending on the severity of the disease. Not only do you get the benefit of the EPA (eicosapentanoic acid) and DHA (docosahexanoic acid) fish oils, you also get the natural vitamin D and vitamin A rich in the fish liver as well as many other nutrients. I typically use a dosage of between one to three teaspoons (between five to eight capsules) a day of the high vitamin fermented cod liver oil. Be wary of most fish oil products found on the store shelf. Most fish oils are made by boiling the fish oil at temperatures in excess of 200 degrees Fahrenheit for several hours. This causes irreparable oxidative damage to the delicate omega-3s. As noted in the Caustic Commentary section of *Wise Traditions* Fall 2013 edition, a new study from the National Cancer Institute showed that those with high concentrations of elongated omega-3s (the kind found in fish oil) in their blood had a 43 percent higher risk of developing cancer than those with the lowest levels (Brasky TM, Darke AK, Song X, et al. Plasma phospholipid fatty acids and prostate risk in the select trial. J Nat Cancer Inst. 2013 Aug 7;105(15):1132-41). I concur with the Weston Price Foundation recommendation to use only fish liver oils, especially those processed at low temperatures to protect the delicate structure of the oil.

Another crucial vitamin for treating CHF is Cataplex® B from Standard Process. This vitamin contains the B complex vitamins crucial for proper heart function, including Vitamins B4 and B1. This whole food complex consists of bovine liver, nutritional yeast, extracts from beet and carrot root among others. Cataplex® B will provide the heart with the important B factors needed for proper electrical conduction of the heart muscle as well as supporting its ability to contract efficiently.

Finally, one herb that I have used over the years to complement my nutritional protocol is hawthorne. I prefer to use only standardized herbs prepared by MediHerb, producers of quality herbal products. Work with a qualified holistic practitioner when taking herbs, especially if you are taking medication.

The last consideration in treating CHF naturally is exercise. A study released in 2012 confirmed that people who spent most of their day at work sitting, whether at a computer or on the phone, had a far greater risk of dying from a cardiovascular event. Therefore, we counsel patients to begin a program of light cardiovascular training at least 3–4 times a week. The exercise protocol has to be tailored to the individual, and entered into slowly and comfortably. I prefer to begin with a technique called "exercise with oxygen therapy" (EWOT). This involves providing portable oxygen to the patient while he or she performs cardiovascular exercise. The purpose of this exercise is to increase the oxygen supplied to the body, especially the heart, to help strengthen and improve its function.

For patients with a less severe case of CHF, using a different form of exercise called Slow Burn exercise may be more appropriate. Slow Burn was developed and espoused by Frederick Hahn and Drs. Michael and Mary Eades (authors of the bestseller *Protein Power*) in their book *The Slow Burn Fitness Revolution*. Anyone with CHF, diabetes, or any serious illness seeking to bring exercise into their lives would do well to read this book. Once read, speak directly with your physician on the best and safest way to introduce EWOT and Slow Burn exercise into your new lifestyle.

For the patient who really wants to understand these concepts and learn about heart health and nutrition I suggest *Put Your Heart in Your Mouth* by Natasha Campbell-McBride. Below is a list of the "Twelve Commandments for a Healthy Heart" from Anthony Colpo's book *The Great Cholesterol Con*. Anyone with a heart problem would do well to print this list and display it prominently as a reminder.

Twelve Commandments for a Healthy Heart

1. Do your best to *keep a handle on stress*; be especially conscious of avoiding stress during and after eating.
2. *Exercise regularly;* at least 30 minutes on most days of the week.
3. *Get to bed as soon as practical after darkness* falls and sleep in the darkest, quietest possible surroundings.
4. *Keep your fasting blood sugar level well within the normal range (ideally 70mg/dL–90 mg/dL).* Eat a low glycemic load diet (i.e. avoid high carbohydrate intakes and the consumption of highly refined carbohydrates).
5. *Maintain a healthy weight.* You can easily find Body Mass Index Charts online to find the healthy range for your height. If you are overweight, utilize a program incorporating increased activity and/or calorie restriction to reduce your body fat mass.
6. *Avoid processed, packaged foods and eat fresh, pastured and organic meats, organic vegetables, fruits, nuts and seeds regularly.* Remember to soak all your nuts, seeds and grains. Ask the doctor for directions if you are unfamiliar with the soaking procedure.
7. *Consume omega-3 fats like flax seed oil, extra virgin olive oil.*
8. *Skip the low fat fad: enjoy animal and tropical fats but avoid omega 6 rich vegetable oils and trans fat-rich margarines.*
9. *Take your supplements every day.*
10. *Avoid high bodily stores of iron.*
11. *Avoid cigarettes and passive or second hand smoke.*
12. *If you drink, consume no more than 1–2 glasses of alcohol per day.* Drink alcohol at mealtimes only. Never binge at night.

SECTION XII
NEUROLOGIAL DISORDERS

Multiple Sclerosis (MS)

Multiple sclerosis is a disease that more commonly affects women between the ages of 20 and 40 (WebMD.com). According to WebMD.com, multiple sclerosis (MS) gets its name from the buildup of scar tissue (sclerosis) in the brain and/or spinal cord. The scar tissue or plaques form when the protective and insulating myelin covering the nerves is destroyed, a process called demyelination. Without myelin, electrical signals transmitted throughout the brain and spinal cord are disrupted or halted. The brain then becomes unable to send and to receive messages.

MS is categorized as an autoimmune disease. Autoimmune diseases are characterized by the body being attacked by its own immune system. Researchers are unsure why this happens, but it results in loss of the myelin insulation that covers the nerves, making transmission of nervous impulses difficult or impossible. As a result, the main early symptoms of MS are numbness and tingling, fatigue, difficulty with muscle use and normal movements, loss of balance, and blurred vision. These symptoms can progress and lead to slurred speech, loss of coordination, and even paralysis.

Some recent research has explored a correlation between MS and toxic heavy metals in the body and some researchers believe that there is a link specifically between mercury, aluminum and other toxic compounds and MS. A hair analysis test or blood test should be performed to examine for the presence of heavy metals like mercury and other toxins as well as mineral imbalances. Different tests for heavy metals are also available through blood and urine by labs such as Genova Diagnostics and others. To find a physician familiar with these tests, you can contact the lab for a directory in your area (see Appendix D p. 357 #17 for information). Work with a qualified, holistic physician to test for the presence of these problems and for the correct course of action.

Mercury in vaccines, allergy and flu shots, contaminated fish, and even dental amalgams can leach into the body and wreak havoc. Aluminum present in antiperspirants can do the same. It blocks the nerve transmission to the sweat gland. The problem is, it can accumulate there and throughout the body and cause illnesses like MS or even breast cancer. I recommend that each person facing the condition of MS consider having their mercury amalgams removed by an experienced, knowledgeable holistic dentist. To gain further insight into how mercury dental amalgams may be causing illness, read *Radical Medicine* by Louisa Williams and *It's All in Your Head* by Hal A. Huggins. In Appendix D there is information on how to contact the Holistic Dental Association in order to find a qualified holistic dentist in your area. Also consider the connection between root canal procedures and MS. This has been the case for several of my patients over the years. I refer my readers concerned with this possible connection to read *Root Canal Cover-Up* by George E. Meinig to learn about the dangers of root canal procedures and the connection with MS.

In my experience, MS responds very well to diet. First and foremost, all wheat and conventional pasteurized dairy must be removed from the diet. There is emerging research that shows that in people with a leaky, inflamed intestinal lining, certain proteins in wheat called gliadins as well as proteins in milk can leak through the intestinal lining. When this happens, they enter the bloodstream and cause an immune reaction. This can lead to inflammation and degeneration in the brain and nervous system. An excellent book on this topic is *Gut and Psychology Syndrome* by Natasha Campbell-McBride, a London-based physician who has been working for many years on psychological and neurological disorders related to diet. She describes the GAPS diet, which is based on the Specific Carbohydrate Diet (SCD) developed by Elaine Gottschall and discussed in her book *Breaking the Vicious Cycle*, and how this can improve and even resolve difficult conditions like MS, Attention Deficit Disorder (ADD & ADHD) and even depression.

Ultimately, all preservatives, colorings, sweeteners etc. must be removed from the diet. It must be based on whole food vegetables, fruits, and proteins. In some cases, raw dairy products from grass-fed cows can be introduced slowly. Lactofermented vegetables are also important in the process of rebuilding the gastrointestinal tract by providing a rich source of probiotic bacteria.

The next part of my protocol for MS involves the use of flax seed oil. Flax seed oil contains fats which play an important role in the anti-inflammatory pathways of the body. Flax seed oil also helps with the utilization of calcium and other minerals crucial to nervous system function. Several tablespoons of high-quality flax seed oil, such as Udo's Oil, is a standard dosage.

With any condition of the body involving degeneration and inflammation, an acidic condition almost always prevails. Therefore, an alkaline-based, whole food diet must be maintained indefinitely. I refer you here to Section III of this book on pH balance for guidelines on how to correct the alkaline/acid balance.

Perhaps most important is the topic of fats in the diet, and specifically fat soluble vitamins like vitamin D. The myelin sheath that covers and insulates the nerves is composed of 70–85% lipids (lipids are composed of fats, fatty acids and cholesterol) known as galactocerebrosides and sphingomyelin. Since MS involves a deterioration of this fatty nerve covering, it is important to supply the body with the fats needed to repair the damage as well as to prevent the autoimmune aspect of the disease which results in the degeneration of the myelin sheath. Recent research from Johns Hopkins published in the Proceedings of the National Academy of Sciences found that vitamin D blocks the damage-causing immune cells from migrating to the central nervous system. In doing so, vitamin D is able to keep the immune T-cells away from the places in the body where they can do the most damage. Since vitamin D deficiency, and an overall "quality fats deficiency" is rampant in the SAD, it is no surprise that researchers are finding that fats and fat-soluble vitamins can be efficacious in treating MS.

I encourage the use of flax seed oil, coconut oil, raw organic dairy like cream and butter as well as fish in the diet of those struggling with MS in order to supply the much needed saturated fats, cholesterol and fat soluble vitamins. These are rich sources of much needed fats not only for the myelin production, but for good health in general.

SECTION XIII
DERMATOLOGICAL PROBLEMS

Dryness and Cracking of Skin on Hands and Feet

The first skin problem I would like to address is dry and cracking skin on the fingers and on the heels of the feet. This is caused by a lack of the fat soluble vitamins A and D and often the unsaturated fatty acids as well. The Standard American Diet (SAD) has become highly deficient in these factors. These fat soluble factors can all be tested for by using Genova Diagnostics Fat Soluble vitamin panel as well as the Fatty Acids panel. To add to the problem, most people do not spend enough time in the sunshine, which is vital for converting cholesterol in the skin to active vitamin D. Many people believe that the sun is dangerous and that sunscreen should be worn at all times during sun exposure. This phobia has furthered the vitamin D deficiency epidemic.

The commonly held belief that all sun exposure will lead to skin cancer is only true if the skin is burned frequently. Taking a little sun from time to time is not only safe, it is absolutely necessary for good health. I urge my patients to refrain from using conventional sunscreen, and to cover up and wear a hat if they are going to be in the sun for prolonged periods of time. If you must use sunscreen, do not put anything on your skin you wouldn't eat. Conventional sunscreens are loaded with toxic chemicals including titanium dioxide which find their way into the body through the skin's sweat glands and themselves cause cancers of the body and skin. For prolonged periods of time in the sun and to avoid burning, cover up and use natural sunscreens available at your local health food store. Better yet, visit the Environmental Working Group's website at ewg.org for their up-to-date list of the safest sunscreens.

Supplementation for dry and cracking skin is simple. Use a high quality fermented cod liver oil supplement which provides vitamins A and D in their natural, active forms. In our office we use Blue Ice™ brand fermented cod liver oil, but there are several other brands of cod liver oil that are of excellent quality, including Dr. Ron's brand. Refer to the Weston A. Price Shopper's Guide (available online from the Weston A. Price Foundation at www.westonaprice.org) for other brands. Dosage is based on the patient's individual needs and test results. A typical dosage is between three and six capsules per day or the equivalent of one teaspoon to one tablespoon for adults. For children the dosage varies by age and weight. See the information in Appendix A p. 320 for recommended dosages.

For topical relief, use either coconut oil or USF Ointment® made by Standard Process. This will moisturize and soothe the skin until the deficiency is corrected.

Fungus of Fingernails/Toenails

One of the best treatments for this condition involves the use of grapefruit seed extract (GSE) and tea tree oil. These items are available in most health food stores. The procedure first involves getting under the nails to clean out all the white, dead tissue. This can be done with a nail file or a cuticle instrument. Then take a toothpick and cotton and make a small q-tip. Dip the q-tip into the tea tree oil or GSE and place it under the nail getting as much as possible of the area coated. Next, take cold pressed unrefined castor oil on a q-tip and coat the entire nail bed. It is best if, when doing this, you lift the nail cuticle a little bit before applying the castor oil. The entire procedure should be done every night before going to bed. Continue until you see the new nail growing out. Reduce the procedure to once a week after you have killed the fungus. To get at the fungus internally as well, purchase a bottle of GSE and take it internally as directed on the label by putting the drops in water.

A second and very effective treatment for nail fungus is montmorillonite clay which is even edible and very helpful for gastrointestinal problems. But for nail fungus, the clay is placed on top of the nail around the entire nail bed. It can be molded around the nail like putty. Then wrap it up with some gauze or a large Band Aid and leave it. This should be repeated twice per day, once in the morning and once at night until the fungus is gone. It works very well, but be patient, it takes time, up to several weeks in some cases.

A side note: fungus of this type can indicate an internal dysbiosis and fungal infection. An astute physician will check this, make necessary adjustments to the patient's diet, and support the immune system. It is often necessary to use probiotics, Argentyn 23 silver hydrosol, and make dietary changes to address the internal environment. Refer to this book's section on Candidiasis p. 72 as well as *The Yeast Syndrome* by John Parks Trowbridge, MD or *The Yeast Connection* by William Crooks, MD for suggested dietary changes.

Eczema

According to the Mayo Clinic, eczema, also known as atopic dermatitis, is an itchy inflammation of the skin. It is typically a long-lasting, chronic condition that may be accompanied by asthma or hay fever. Though it may affect any area of skin, eczema typically appears on the arms and behind the knees. (Mayoclinic.com). There are many forms of dermatitis including contact dermatitis, cosmetic, plant, perfume, etc. Some forms can be avoided by not coming into contact with the offending agent, poison ivy for example.

Several key components involved in most cases of eczema are an imbalance in the pH of the body, food allergies, and a condition known as leaky gut. We spoke of pH in detail in the section regarding allergies. In many ways that is what we are dealing with here, an allergic skin reaction. Skin is the largest body organ. If your body is not eliminating poisons properly through the bowel and urine, it is forced to push it out of the body through the skin. Many researchers believe that it is this mechanism that is behind the cause of eczema. Others believe that the nutritional deficiencies caused by poor digestive function are at the heart of the breakdown in the integrity and health of the skin. Either way, we must look within for the cause and the solution. It is important to understand this concept and to realize why conventional medical treatment of eczema with anti-histamines, antibiotics, immunomodulators, and corticosteroid creams (usually hydrocortisone based), does not treat the cause of the problem, and can result in dangerous side effects.

Leaky gut is a term used when inflammation of the intestinal tract causes malabsorption of nutrients from food and creates the environment for bacteria, yeast, and undigested foods to enter into the bloodstream. In response, an immune system reaction is mounted against the foreign invader. This gets complicated since no two people are exactly alike. One person may have an overload of yeast in their system related to extensive antibiotic usage as the culprit while another case may be caused by poor diet. Some cases are combinations of both. The point is that diet and the digestive system must be examined first. I have treated many cases of eczema and dermatitis occurring in children as well as seniors. In most if not all of these cases, the cause was directly related to the digestive system. Some lacked digestive enzyme function; others had really poor dietary habits.

Regardless, when examining the patient with this condition, we invariably find that there are spinal subluxations in the thoracic spine as well as the C1 vertebra (also known as the Atlas for the way the skull sits upon it like a globe). A thorough physical examination of these patients will include an abdominal exam that usually reveals multiple sensitivities of the different digestive zones including the stomach and small intestines. Furthermore, we usually find gallbladder tenderness/involvement as well when we palpate the right lateral side.

Patients suffering with eczema need a diet that removes all of the common food allergens for a time. This will include pasteurized dairy of all kinds, grains of all kinds, soy, corn and nuts. Digestive enzymes (usually with HCL) must be given to aid in the complete breakdown of food. We must also assist the gallbladder in functioning more efficiently to produce adequate amounts of bile, to ensure proper fat breakdown, and also to stimulate peristalsis and the release of pancreatic enzymes. Many doctors do not know that a healthy functioning gallbladder will stimulate three healthy bowel movements a day, providing that the patient is eating three meals per day. Coffee enemas may be necessary at first to cleanse the bowel and to stimulate the gallbladder. In more difficult or severe cases, it may be important to flush the gallbladder repeatedly using the protocol given in Appendix A p. 333. Be sure to work with a qualified physician when treating this problem.

One product that can be used topically to temporarily soothe the skin and help it heal as we address the real cause from the inside is called Itch Calm Cream and is made by a company called Artemis (See Appendix D). For more information visit their website (www.herbalmedicine.co.nz/creams.html).

Dr. Angelo Rose; Dr. Christopher Amoruso

Urticaria/Hives

Urticaria, commonly known as hives, is an outbreak of swollen, pale red bumps or plaques (known as wheals) on the skin that appear suddenly. Hives can itch or burn and vary from the size of a penny to the size of a dish. Webmd.com states they are from some type of allergic reaction or unknown cause. In my experience, hives are the result of a fundamental problem with the pH balance of the body, resulting in immune system dysfunction with concomitant metabolic disturbances. They can even be trigered by stress. The pH disturbance involved with hives is that of an overly acidic condition in the body. This sets up an environment which aggravates the immune system and the tissues of the body. When a certain food is consumed which augments this overly acidic condition, the body responds with an allergic type reaction on the skin. I believe this is due to dilation of the small capillaries in the skin as the body attempts to eliminate acidic toxins that have accumulated. When the body's elimination pathways (liver, kidney, skin, etc.) are overwhelmed by a toxic diet/lifestyle, hives result.

Another mechanism involved in the appearance of hives is tissue calcium starvation. As mentioned in the sections on arthritis, when the body is overly acidic, calcium is forced from the bones, teeth, and muscles and is moved into the blood to buffer the acidity there. This is a necessary protective mechanism to maintain the strict control of our blood's pH range (7.36–7.40) Therefore, a patient with hives must be put on an alkaline-based diet for a few months in order to rectify this problem. The importance of pH balance and foods is covered in detail in the book *Alkalize or Die* by James Baroody. It offers a complete list of alkaline and acid foods as well as an in-depth discussion of the importance of pH and health.

Once diet is corrected and the pH balance of the body restored (a salivary pH of 6.8–7.0 is ideal) there are a few other considerations that will help resolve the hives. The patient must be given Calcium Lactate by Standard Process (a vegetable source form of calcium which is easy to assimilate) at a dose of 6–9 per day. Along with the calcium, he/she will also need flax seed oil at a dosage of one tablespoon per 100 pounds of body weight or Cataplex® F by Standard Process at a dosage of 6 per day. The vitamin F found in the flax seed oil helps the body utilize calcium without difficulty. Lastly, cod liver oil (one teaspoon for children, one tablespoon for adults) is also helpful for its vitamin D content. Vitamin D brings calcium into the blood from the intestinal tract, and vitamin F along with vitamin K takes it from the blood into the bone and muscle.

After several weeks on a more alkaline diet, digestion will improve, pH will normalize and so will immune function. We often give the patient Congaplex® from Standard Process to strengthen the immune system and aid in this process. With this type of condition, as with most others, a pre-existing digestive problem is at the root of the problem. Work with a physician who can help you identify your specific area(s) of concern.

Skin Cancer/Sun Tanning

Many people shun the sun for fear of skin cancer. Regularly I see patients' blood reports showing low vitamin D levels.

Important things to know if you are concerned about skin cancer: First, if you will be out in the sun during the hotter times of the day, be sensible, cover up and wear a hat. I recommend that most people get sunlight on their face and arms for at least an hour or two each day, especially in the morning hours and later in the afternoon. It is never acceptable to burn. Burning damages the skin and can lead to skin cancer. Furthermore, never use conventional sunscreens. They are loaded with chemicals that can be absorbed through the skin and have been shown to cause cancer. In fact, some recent studies suggest that up to 68% of people who use sunscreen get cancer of the skin. Use only natural sunscreens made from plant botanicals when you are going to be out in the sun for a long period of time. Zinc oxide can be used sparingly on the most vulnerable areas, but covering up and limiting exposure is the smartest and safest approach. A very good topical treatment for sunburn is an ointment or gel called Combudoron by Weleda (www.weleda.com).

Lastly, never use artificial tanning beds or spray-on tanners. They damage the skin and contain chemicals that can cause cancer and other problems. An important consideration with tanning is making sure that a person is also getting adequate calcium. A proper amount of calcium intake per day will ensure a good balance with vitamins A and D. It is best to start in the early spring and take a half hour of upper body sun per day when possible. If you continue this as the weather gets warmer, you can increase to one hour and then slowly more and more time can be spent safely in the sun. If you remember to take sunlight in slow, increasing intervals like this, you will be able to enjoy all of the wonderful health benefits that the sun has to offer. Getting proper sunlight in the summer protects from vitamin D deficiency later in the winter months. Adequate vitamin D will protect you from colds and the winter depression that so many people experience. If you absolutely cannot get enough sun in the summer months because of working indoors, then you must supplement with a high quality cod liver oil.

Psoriasis

John O. A. Pagano, DC writes in *Healing Psoriasis: The Natural Alternative*, p. 73, "The significance of an effective diet has been questioned for as long as the disease has been researched." He emphasizes: ". . . as early as 1932, the beneficial effects that diet has on psoriasis were clearly demonstrated by Jay F. Schamberg, MD, a former professor of dermatology at the University of Pennsylvania." (Ibid p. 73) To be more specific, in my experience this condition is caused by a disturbance in fat metabolism with a concomitant inability of the body to eliminate waste. The cure is then quite straightforward, as Pagano points out:

> Frequently, the culprit in psoriasis is improper elimination due to poor eating habits, which in most cases can be corrected. Both require discipline on the part of the patient. With regard to eating, the patient should select easily digestible and more absorbable types of foods. (Ibid p. 43)

Following such a protocol will naturally have to involve cleansing the liver and the kidneys, as these two organs are our body's major players in detoxification/elimination. A good tip for keeping your kidneys cleansed, as Pagano notes, is to drink "an adequate amount of pure water daily . . . six to eight glasses of water each day . . . and, if desired, add the juice of a few fresh limes or lemons."(Ibid p. 45) For cleansing the liver periodically, follow the Seven Day Liver and Gallbladder Flush as outlined in Andreas Moritz's book *The*

Amazing Liver and Gallbladder Flush. Using the herb milk thistle along with bitter herbs and foods to complement the cleansing process is highly advisable. Work with your holistic physician to accomplish this properly.

In assessing the psoriatic patient, start with IgG4 food allergy and stool testing (Genova Diagnostics) to determine any offensive foods and to assess the overall health of the gut. This includes a few very important markers that evaluate pancreatic and gallbladder function, hence the need for a lower/proper fat diet. In psoriasis there is always a sluggishness of the bile route, and bile is crucial for proper fat metabolism. A common indication of this is frequent belching, nausea, and even constipation; however, many patients may have only slight signs of one of these symptoms.

A temporary, low fat diet including only healthy fats is the best avenue of approach with this condition. Please see the specifics of what fats to avoid and which to accentuate as outlined in previous segments as well as in the "Guide to Knowing Your Fats" in Appendix C pp. 353-354. More important is a diet that helps maintain a proper acid/alkaline balance. Dr. Pagano stresses this point, stating:

> Nature demands that the body remain more on the alkaline side rather than on the acid side for the preservation of good health. The body becomes more resistant to all types of disease and physical ailments when engulfed in this internal chemical atmosphere. Arthritic joints are greatly relieved, colds and congestion are counteracted, skin problems diminish, and internal organs become less burdened. (Ibid p. 76)

In order to control psoriasis, as stated above, choose foods that will help to keep the body's pH alkaline. Do this by taking two alkaline foods to one acid food in your diet plan. Removal of all processed foods laden with artificial colors and preservatives is a must. This includes alcohol, refined sugars, pasteurized/homogenized dairy, and hydrogenated oils. Using lacto-fermented vegetables and beverages is an important factor in helping clear psoriasis. Read p.298-308 on the 4 Rs Protocol to understand the basic approach to cleansing the intestinal tract. *Real Food Fermentation* by Alex Lewin has recipes that will help you incorporate lacto-fermented foods into your diet.

Since it is crucial to keep the body's pH alkaline so it can heal, use the alkaline/acid chart provided as a guide and read the section in this book on pH balance. It may take several months to accomplish, so be patient. It will probably be necessary to begin a 4 Rs Protocol based on the results of a stool test and food allergy panel. Your holistic physician should be able to help you accomplish this and get you on the path to clear skin and vibrant health.

Most doctors give psoriasis patients topical cortisone creams or toxic drugs which help little if at all. When the creams and drugs are stopped, the patient is left to find that the condition has returned and was merely being masked. When an area of skin that is affected is chemically analyzed it shows that the cells have a higher than normal potassium content. This elevation of potassium is related to the chloride levels in the blood. Therefore one must not consume food and supplements with high levels of potassium.

Several vitamins and supplements helpful for this condition are:

1. A and F Betafood® (Standard Process) – helpful for the functioning of the gallbladder and liver. It is usually necessary to take 6 a day in divided doses.
2. Zypan® (Standard Process) – one to two tablets per meal to aid in digestion.
3. Dermatrophin PMG® (Standard Process) – to help regenerate the damaged skin; take 3-9 a day according to your physician's recommendations.
4. Udo's Perfected Oil Blend (Flax Seed Oil) – two tablespoons a day with food.
5. Blue Ice™ Fermented Cod Liver Oil – dosage varies depending on condition, age, etc. Typical dosage ranges from one teaspoon to one tablespoon a day.
6. Pure Radiance Vitamin C – dosage varies according to the person. Typical dosage ranges from one teaspoon twice a day to one tablespoon three times a day.

An important part of healing psoriasis is the chiropractic adjustment of the spine. The most important parts of the spine which relate to psoriasis are those which are intimately connected to the stomach, intestines, kidneys and liver. For this, we specifically adjust the 6th-9th thoracic vertebrae. We also concentrate on evaluating and adjusting the 3rd cervical, 9th thoracic and 4th lumbar "because these are the areas of the spine where lymph centers and their neural and circulatory connections are disturbed."(Ibid p. 136) Dr. Pagano reminds us of the wisdom of Hippocrates when he states, "Look well to the spine for the cause of disease."(Ibid p. 139)

Dr. Pagano's book *Healing Psoriasis* is full of helpful tips on how to deal with the itching and joint discomfort so common to psoriasis as well as a more in-depth description of the pathogenesis and successful treatment. He offers case studies with dramatic before and after pictures of patients who were cured by following this approach.

Acne

Acne is often associated with a hormone change during adolescence. These hormone changes can be aggravated by fluctuations in blood sugar and insulin levels, metabolic occurrences that are very common in the Standard American Diet today. The best approach for young people is to start reducing the harmful fats in the diet because these are responsible for hormone movement in the body. If there is an excess of processed/industrial fats in the diet this imbalance can occur. Instruction must be given in how to eat properly in order to establish a stable blood sugar.

Start by eliminating all of the detrimental fats and strictly limiting carbohydrates in the diet, especially refined carbohydrates. At the same time advise the patient on which specific foods to avoid and why. This includes all trans fats, hydrogenated oils, margarines, shortenings, vegetable oils, soybean oil, corn oil, safflower oil, cottonseed oil, and canola oil. Also temporarily eliminate foods that are too high in fat content. Some of the more common foods to avoid are pasteurized/homogenized dairy, cheese and cheese products, pork, conventional chicken and beef from Concentrated Animal Feeding Operations (CAFOs) that feed the animals GMO corn and soy laced with pesticides, chemicals, and hormones. Be aware that many of the convenience foods Americans eat are a hidden source of bad fats. Bagels, pizza, cookies, and even common snack foods like chips are all made with these offensive oils and refined sugars.

What the body needs for acne is good fats, and lots of them. Good fats such as unrefined walnut oil, expeller pressed flax seed oil, extra virgin coconut oil, raw organic pastured butter, wheat germ oil and extra virgin olive oil are healthier choices and not the fats that cause acne. Nor are the saturated fats found in animal products like eggs as long as they are raised on pasture and are organic.

For the most part, the diet should be kept simple. Fruit is best in the morning for breakfast while salads and a starch or two at lunch work best. If there exists an underlying yeast condition (properly known as candidiasis, or candidal enteritis), fruits may have to be restricted. Dinner should be two green vegetables and a small salad with salmon, organic and/or pastured chicken, turkey, lamb or veal. This is the most practical way of treating acne and other skin problems.

Vitamins crucial for the treatment of acne are as follows:

1. Cataplex® A (Standard Process vitamin A) – chew three to nine a day with Blue Ice™ Fermented Cod Liver Oil at a dosage of two to three teaspoons a day.
2. Cataplex® E (Standard Process vitamin E) – chew three to nine a day.
3. Catalyn® (Standard Process Multi Vitamin) – chew three to six a day.

We often recommend a gallbladder and liver flush once a month in order to facilitate the cleansing of the liver and better bile flow into the intestines. Not only does this improve digestive ability, it also helps to remove toxins. See the detailed instructions in Andreas Moritz's book *The Amazing Liver and Gallbladder Flush* and work with a knowledgeable holistic physician.

There are also cases of acne that occur in older people. Often more severe, it is known as acne vulgaris, and presents as large cysts and pustules. The same dietary procedure outlined above is pivotal in clearing this condition; however, the treatment is different.

First the skin must be cleaned and treated by using Swiss Kriss facial steam treatment. Second, using red potato and cucumber, make a poultice and place it over the skin in the affected areas. Make the poultice by grating either a cucumber or red potato using a hand grater. Place the gratings on a piece of cheesecloth and place that on the face for 45 minutes to an hour. One day use the cucumber and the next the red potato alternating until the skin has cleared. After the poultice treatment you can flush the face with witch hazel by wiping a cloth soaked in witch hazel over the affected area, dampening the skin and then patting the face dry. Finally, Standard Process makes an ointment called USF Ointment® which is excellent for this condition. A very thin coat of the ointment can be spread on the affected area up to twice a day.

One final topic related to this condition is the sun. Regular exposure to the sun is very important to the health of the skin and body. Get a good share of sun exposure during the summer months if you live in the northern hemisphere so you can build up your stores of vitamin D. People who live in climates closer to the equator are more likely to have adequate exposure to the sun. Over the past decade warnings regarding skin cancer have made some people sun shy. I believe this has been a grave mistake.

The most important reason for staying out of the sun is to prevent excessive burning. It is never good to get burned tanning. However, taking in sunshine a little at a time is very important to maintaining vitamin D levels and also for stimulating the pineal gland in the brain. The pineal gland secretes melatonin, influences aspects of sexual development, and coordinates circadian rhythms of the body. The best avenue of protection is to tan a little at a time each day. This gives the skin a chance to adjust to the sun exposure and will allow you to stay in the sun a little longer each day. If you must use sunscreen, use a sunscreen with all natural ingredients/botanicals. Consult the Weston A. Price Foundation's website for literature regarding safe sunscreens, or the Environmental Working Group's list at ewg.org.

Boils

To treat a boil, follow the protocol below. Between the treatments, keep the area around the boil coated with a high-quality castor oil, unrefined and cold-processed.

Boil Treatment

Items Needed: Octagon soap (supermarket), water, sugar.

Procedure

1. Using a knife, scrape a small portion of shavings of the Octagon soap off so that you have enough to cover the ulcer. Place the shavings into a dish or onto a small plate.
2. Take a small amount of water and sugar and add it to the soap shavings in order to make a paste the consistency of toothpaste.
3. Put the paste onto the boil and cover with a piece of gauze. Use medical tape to fasten the gauze in place and keep the boil covered.
4. Refresh the paste and gauze bandage once every day until the boil comes to a head. Once the boil has come to a head, contact the doctor who will need to lance it and drain it.

SECTION XIV
WOUND HEALING

Cuts, Scrapes, Open Wounds, Bed Sores

For wound healing, there are two important things to remember: first, if the patient has poor circulation, as is common with diabetes and peripheral vascular diseases, healing will be slow and difficult, especially in the extremities. Therefore it is very important that circulation in the patient be improved whenever possible/necessary. Second, the wound must be kept clean. Castor oil and chlorophyll ointment are valuable tools that can be used in this process as well as Argentyn 23 Silver Hydrosol. If circulation is poor, the wound will not heal, so consult with Section XI regarding circulation and diabetes for more information on how to rectify this situation. And at all times, the wound should be kept clean with a natural antibiotic like Argentyn 23.

Bed Sores

Bed sores are caused by poor circulation and constant pressure applied to an area of the body while lying in bed. Although most bed sores will heal once circulation is restored and the pressure removed (usually by getting the patient upright and ambulatory) they are still a significant and common problem afflicting the elderly. The best treatment I have seen is to use a pure chlorophyll salve and to keep the area free of pressure. A helpful way to handle this problem is to utilize an air mattress and to move the patient as often as possible.

If circulation is poor, one can use cayenne pepper internally in the form of capsules as, when taken with food, this will get the blood to the smallest blood vessels. Cayenne pepper is also helpful when applied directly to the wound to stop bleeding and hemorrhaging, although it can sting significantly. For improving the circulation one can also use grapeseed extract at two to three capsules a day combined with 50 mgs. of niacin (vitamin B3).

One of the best topical applications for open wounds is a form of silver hydrosol, Argentyn 23 First Aid Gel, made by the company Natural Immunogenics Corporation. This form of silver hydrosol is the purest and safest colloidal silver on the market and it will not cause argyria (an irreversible cosmetic discoloration of the skin that is caused by cheaper forms of colloidal silver that contain impurities and silver bound to proteins). Argentyn 23 reduces topical pain, calms skin inflammation, and promotes healing of the skin. Simply apply a liberal layer of the gel on the wound in order to allow for consistent, sustained delivery. Leave wet. Do not rub until dry. After absorption, repeat as often as needed to prolong its activity. This works well in combination with using Cold Pressed Castor Oil (made by the Heritage Company and also known by the name Palma Christi or "hand of Christ") spread about ¼ inch away from the opening of the wound around the perimeter (roughly one inch in width). Do not put the castor oil directly on the opening, just around the perimeter (See Appendix D for details on where to purchase high-quality castor oil).

Supplement directions for wound healing are as follows:
1. Pycnogenol (grapeseed extract) – two to three capsules twice a day for first 48–72 hours then decrease to two to three a day.

2. Butcher's broom (standardized herb) – two to three capsules a day.
3. Cayenne pepper – take two to three capsules a day with food.
4. Wobenzyme – take as directed on the label.
5. Vitamins A, C, E and zinc are crucial for wound healing. Green Pasture™ Fermented Cod Liver Oil is an excellent source of active Vitamin A (retinol) at a dose of 2–3 capsules a day. I use The Synergy Company brand Whole Food Vitamin C known as Pure Radiance Vitamin C at a dose of six to twelve capsules a day (or one to two tablespoons a day) until healing is well established. For Vitamin E, I use Standard Process Cataplex® E at a dose of 6 a day and Zinc Liver Chelate at a dose of 3 a day.
6. Organic Super B-Complex – by The Synergy Company at a dose of two a day.

Burns

It is important to remember that with any burn there is an immediate adrenal reaction. Some people that get severe burns and die, usually do not die of the burn but from the adrenal failure that follows. These types of burns are usually 2nd and 3rd degree, the most severe kinds. In this book we will focus on the treatment of a minor burn or a severe case of sunburn. The home remedy for these is as follows:

1. 1 lb. of corn starch to a tub of water, keep the person in the bathtub for at least 30 minutes. This soothes the burning and gives the skin a chance to balance the fluid lost during a burn.
2. 2 cups of organic apple cider vinegar in a tub of water. This will also soothe the skin and even take pain out of the sunburn.
3. Willard's Water is an excellent water to place on a cloth and put on any burn. You may also make a poultice and lay it on the burned area.
4. On very severe burns a salve of chlorophyll (Standard Process) will relieve a severe burn in 20 minutes or less.
5. For sunburns, use a salve called USF Ointment® made by Standard Process. It is excellent for burns as well.

6. Colloidal Silver Salve – Sovereign Silver First Aid Gel is available through doctors only. To contact the company for doctors who carry this product in your area, visit http://www.natural-immunogenics.com.
7. Wipe the patient down 3 or 4 times a day with 8 ounces of water containing three tablespoons of organic apple cider vinegar. This is also very good for sunburn.
8. Organic raw honey unfiltered and unheated – apply to a burn several times a day and the burn will not scar.

Bruising

When one is injured through blunt trauma or a fall of some kind, the area of contact is damaged without breaking open the skin. A discoloration is seen which indicates that small capillaries underneath the skin have ruptured and blood is leaking into the surrounding tissue. After the subdermal bleeding clots, a discoloration that appears purple in color forms. This can happen very easily in the elderly, those on warfarin or other blood thinning medications, and in patients with nutritional deficiencies of the vitamin C and vitamin P family.

Treatment for this condition is simple. Use moist heat and then a high quality, unrefined castor oil spread around the area of bruising. Castor oil is an emollient which is also effective at bringing oxygenated blood to the area of a wound. This enables the damaged cells to be taken away and processed by the liver and allows fresh, oxygenated blood to deliver the material necessary for healing. This application should be repeated a few times a day. However, in cases where a patient does not recall any trauma and remarks that they don't know where their bruises are coming from, the remedy is more involved. With these patients you must first discern whether or not they take a blood-thinning medication. If so, they will have to speak to their primary care doctor and have their clotting time checked (INR) to make sure that their medication does not have to be adjusted. Ideally, you work with them to get them off the medication. If they are not on blood thinners of any kind, their bruising indicates an entirely different problem. Patients who bruise easily are deficient in the vitamin C Complex including the P and K factors which are the bioflavonoids and rutin. The real vitamin C Complex contains the vitamin P factors and vitamin K which maintain vascular integrity. These are deficient in people who bruise easily or who have "pink toothbrush" syndrome (indicating that the gums bleed easily). Vitamin K promotes prothrombin to help with coagulation of blood and clotting. Like vitamin D, vitamin K is a fat soluble vitamin. Deficiencies in both are becoming more and more common. A recommended whole food source of Vitamin C Complex is Cataplex® C from Standard Process or The Synergy Company's Pure Radiance C combined with Blue Ice™ Fermented Cod Liver Oil.

Here is an interesting story involving bruising and castor oil. Many years ago a young friend of mine worked at a castor oil plant. He and another fellow got into a fight and both ended up with black eyes. On my advice, my friend applied castor oil around the area of his bruise daily, and in less than a week his bruising was gone. The other man's bruises, which did not receive the castor oil treatment, lasted twice as long.

When cells are ruptured as they are in a bruise, a chemical called biliverdin is released. Biliverdin is a green bile pigment, and is a product of heme catabolism (breakdown of our red blood cells). Heme is the protein portion of a red blood cell that carries iron and binds oxygen and is the pigment responsible for the greenish color sometimes seen in bruises (Boron W, Boulpaep E. Medical physiology: a cellular and molecular approach. United States: Elsevier Saunders; 2005. p. 984–6). Biliverdin is rapidly broken down into bilirubin which then gives the bruise its characteristic yellowish hue (Mosqueda L, Burnight K, Liao S. The life cycle of bruises in older adults. J Amer Geriatrics Soc. 2005 June 8;53(8):1339–43).

SECTION XV
PREGNANCY AND INFANT CARE

Pregnancy and Prenatal Nutrition

I am frequently asked "Can a chiropractor treat a pregnant woman safely?" The answer to this question is not only a resounding "yes," it is also, in my opinion, absolutely necessary, especially in today's modern, fast-paced/fast-food culture. Chiropractic is not only very important for a woman, it is essential in facilitating a comfortable and uncomplicated pregnancy.

Chiropractic adjustments help a pregnant mother maintain the pelvis in the proper, balanced structural position. Adjustments allow the woman's pelvis and spinal column to remain flexible and provide for an easy delivery. For over 50 years I have helped women during their pregnancy, and almost without exception, the pregnancies were smooth and easy.

Many women who have never had chiropractic care have trouble with the pelvis opening properly during childbearing. This prevents the baby from being able to get through the birth canal properly and will often result in a cesarean section being performed. To further complicate the problem, most doctors have resisted changing the way they deliver children. They place a woman on her back and can cause her to have back pain and pelvic problems for the rest of her life. In the past, midwives assisting in the birthing process would have told the doctors to use a birthing chair or to position the patient in the squatting position for delivery. This makes it easy for the pelvic canal to open by relaxing the pelvic musculature and ligaments, thus making it less painful for the mother.

Another common problem pregnant women encounter is improper positioning of the child in the womb or the birth canal. There are many times when the baby will move and the mother then becomes uncomfortable. Therefore it is important to teach the mother to get down on all fours and crawl around periodically. This positions the baby in an advantageous position with respect to gravity, enabling the baby to more easily move and reposition. I have used this positioning technique in my office to help gently maneuver the baby into a better position thus avoiding a breech birth.

Dr. Angelo Rose; Dr. Christopher Amoruso

This provides a perfect segue into the topic of ultrasound. Ultrasound is often used to check the positioning, sex, heartbeat, and other important factors of the baby's health and wellbeing during pregnancy. However, I believe that it is overused and may be dangerous to the health of the infant. Scientifically solid studies to discern what detrimental effects, if any, ultrasound has on the long-term health of the baby do not exist. Its correlation to children with developmental disorders, autism, attention deficit disorder, and learning disabilities has not been determined. An overview of the studies to date and the real facts about ultrasound, can be found in Chapter 3 of *Nourishing Traditions Book of Baby & Child Care*, by Sally Fallon Morell and Thomas S. Cowan, MD, and in Jim West's book *50 Human Studies In Utero Conducted in Modern China Indicate Extreme Risk for Prenatal Ultrasound*.

Furthermore, women are having multiple ultrasounds during their pregnancy, often with no clinical indication of the necessity for the test. Ultrasound technology has been applied in obstetrics since the late 1950s and early 1960s. It is offered to almost all expectant mothers, several times throughout the pregnancy. Parents just want a "picture" of their baby. Although I can understand the sentiment, I think, in most cases, that the risks outweigh the benefits.

Advanced techniques such as Doppler Ultrasounds and 3D/4D ultrasounds, are contributing to longer periods of exposure. Both prolonged exposure to ultrasound and increased frequency of use increase the risk of harm to the fetus. In addition, I have seen cases where a woman is told, after an ultrasound, that her baby is too large and she will need a cesarean, only to find out after the procedure that the baby was of normal weight and size. Ultrasound can lead to unnecessary cesarean procedures and undue stress on the mother and infant.

Transvaginal ultrasound, although providing a clearer, more detailed image, poses an even greater threat because it is performed by inserting a probe into the vagina. This carries with it a heightened risk of infection, not to mention the effects the ultrasound may have on the fetus, including creating a heating-up of the brain tissue. I would caution any mother to consider these risk factors and only use this type of ultrasound if the situation is of a medical emergency as, for example, if bleeding is occurring or if there are abnormal findings on physical examination such as growth, fibroids, etc.

I try to give my pregnant patients multi-faceted advice. This includes suggestions about nutrition and proper eating habits, exercise, and rest as well as other counseling specific to their needs. Obviously there should be no tobacco or alcohol use of any kind. Avoiding refined sugars, conventional wheat products, pasteurized/homogenized dairy products and soy are the most important dietary restrictions a pregnant woman can make. I stress the danger of soy to the health of the baby and the pregnant mother. Soy is known to be a goitrogen, or a food that can damage the thyroid gland. Furthermore, most soy in this country is genetically modified (GMO) making it unsafe for anyone to consume. And even if soy is organic, it still contains trypsin inhibitors, phytic acid and other anti-nutrients which can leach minerals from the woman's body, cause digestive disorders and create severe allergies. The Weston A. Price Foundation website, www.westonaprice.org gives information on the dangers of soy. They also have a regular section in their quarterly publication *Wise Traditions* entitled "Soy Alert" which keeps the public up to date on the latest information regarding soy. They alert readers to the hidden dangers of soy as well as other dangerous sources of soy ingredients like hydrolyzed soy protein, a hidden source of MSG according to Food Babe (Hari V, Hyman M. The food babe way. New York: Little, Brown and Co.; 2015. p. 54). The Weston A. Price Foundation even has a section on their website about raising healthy babies. Following these simple dietary and lifestyle guidelines will keep any woman healthy during her pregnancy and ensure a healthy baby.

Some women will want a doctor to give them an epidural (an injection to the spine to numb the pain associated with pregnancy). Then the doctor will use forceps to pull the baby out. This can be very dangerous for the baby. These procedures come with risks and repercussions. I advise any pregnant woman to consider avoiding them if at all possible. I also recommend working with a midwife and/or doula who is familiar in alternative pregnancy care. Consult *The Nourishing Traditions Book of Baby & Child Care* to learn critical information regarding pregnancy, both for pre-pregnancy preparation as well as during and after pregnancy.

Dr. Angelo Rose; Dr. Christopher Amoruso

Simple guidelines to follow during pregnancy:

1. Avoid routine IV stent
2. Use non-invasive Verinata's Test or Panorama Prenatal Test to screen for genetic problems like Down's Syndrome, Patau and Edward's Syndrome and more. See the websites http://www.panoramatest.com and http://www.verifitest.com.
3. Avoid ultrasound to hear the baby's heartbeat. Instead, have your midwife or doctor use a fetoscope at or after 20 weeks gestation.
4. Do not allow the vitamin K shot to be given to your baby. It has been linked to childhood leukemia, is synthetic, and unnec-essary. Instead, follow a nutritious diet like the Weston A. Price Foundation's diet, and include plenty of high-vitamin fermented cod liver oil and butter oil before, during and after your pregnancy.
5. Do not allow antibiotic eye ointment to be placed in your newborn baby's eyes. If need be, simply use a drop or two of your own breastmilk to prevent eye irritation/infection.
6. Absolutely no vaccines. If you are not sure or are afraid, before making a decision, read and study the facts. Your child deserves that much. Read the book *Vaccine Epidemic* and consult *The Nourishing Traditions Book of Baby & Child Care*. Vaccines are not as necessary or as safe as portrayed by media and regulatory agencies. However, ignorance is not an excuse for bliss. You must feed your child a nutritious whole food diet after breastfeeding and keep his/her immune system strong.
7. Demand that your midwife or doctor use *delayed cord clamping*. This ensures that the baby will receive the full amount of blood from the cord prior to life on his/her own. It is a fact that the cord will continue to pulsate and pump blood to your baby for up to 20 minutes after birth.
8. Leave the *vernix caseosa* intact and do not allow the staff to wipe it off. It protects the baby's skin and will flake off on its own after a few days.

In conclusion, I would like to say that for low risk pregnancies, homebirth is as safe or safer than hospital birth. Furthermore, medical interventions commonly used in hospital births such as epidurals, induction with synthetic oxytocin, and cesarean sections have risks and complications often not adequately communicated to pregnant women. *The Nourishing Traditions Book of Baby & Child Care* is an invaluable tool in sorting through these important topics and in the decision-making process.

Morning Sickness

Professional experience leads me to believe that morning sickness is a deficiency condition. It can be solved by correcting the diet (which varies with each patient's individual condition) and adding to the diet the supplements vitamin B6 and one zinc tablet per day. This has been effective in my work with most patients suffering from this malady. Foods rich in B6 like turnip greens, spinach, asparagus, and organic, grass-fed meats and fish are a great option. Lacto-fermented vegetables and fermented beverages like beet kvass and kombucha settle the stomach and eliminate morning sickness. *Real Food Fermentation* by Alex Lewin is a recipe book for those interested in making these superfoods easily at home.

I also recommend Sally Fallon and Thomas Cowan's book *The Nourishing Traditions Book of Baby and Child Care*. Chapter 3 p. 56 has recommendations for holistic treatment of morning sickness.

Prenatal Nutrition

This section deals with prenatal nutrition for healthy fetal development from conception to birth. My goal is to teach the expecting mother and father what needs to be done dietarily/nutritionally to ensure or maximize the health of the baby. Disturbingly, a large number of American mothers do not give prenatal nutrition sufficient thought. That should be a husband and wife's main concern. I know that *in vitro* fertilization has enabled otherwise childless couples to have children. In cases where diet could be an issue, it would be sensible to teach young mothers and fathers-to-be how to eat properly and take care of their health. I believe it would be more reasonable to try a more conservative approach, one that enriches the health of the family unit and increases the likelihood of having a healthy child naturally. I have seen many couples having difficulty conceiving, do so simply by making some basic changes to their diets and by taking some key supplements. Poor nutrition can be the cause of the problem. Attentiveness to one's body is critical and should be the first aproach.

As for *in vitro* fertilization, it has consequences. Children born from *in vitro* fertilization have a greater risk of autism, ADHD, and other degenerative conditions. A study done in 2010 and published by the American Society of Reproductive Medicine found that, when it came to risk factors for chronic diseases, they were up to 11 times more likely to be diagnosed with certain psychological disorders, such as clinical depression and attention deficit hyperactivity disorder (ADD/ADHD). In fact, it is growing more common that women who are not in good enough health, are conceiving through *in vitro* fertilization, thus forcing an unhealthy body to maintain a pregnancy. Good maternal nutrition during the pregnancy should be the parents' primary concern. I advise young parents who are unable to conceive to look in the mirror first and then work with a qualified holistic physician or nutritionist who can help address the situation and improve their own health first. Take at least six months to a year to prepare your body. Lose weight, work on learning traditional nutritional wisdom, and supplement appropriately. It is just common sense to do so and your child deserves it.

This is an appropriate point to discuss what women and men can do to improve their reproductive health prior to and during pregnancy. I will highlight some main points and direct the reader to further sources for more in-depth information. It is well known that most traditional cultures had pre-conception and pregnancy diets emphasizing nutrient dense foods high in specific nutrients amenable to a healthy pregnancy. Weston Price found this to be universally true throughout his travels and studies of traditional cultures. I offer below some of the more common areas of deficiency in the SAD with regard to prenatal nutrition and what can be done.

Embryonic and fetal development is dependent upon certain nutrients more than others, specifically fats and certain carbohydrates to fuel growth. (Masterjohn C. Vitamins for fetal development: conception to birth. Wise Traditions. Weston A. Price

Foundation. 2007 Winter;8(4):25.) "Amino acids form structural proteins and enzymes. Vitamins and minerals act as cofactors for those enzymes or as regulators of the entire process of growth." (Ibid) The most important point is stressed by Masterjohn when he states, "These nutrients are uniquely supplied by the mother's diet."(Ibid)

Weston Price found that all healthy traditional cultures had special pregnancy and preconception diets for mothers-to-be, and, in some cases, for fathers-to-be. In referencing *Nutrition and Physical Degeneration* from Weston A. Price, Masterjohn highlights the main foods prized by these traditional cultures for optimizing preconception/pregnancy nutrition, stating:

> All groups that had access to the sea used fish eggs; milk-drinking groups used high-quality dairy from the season when grass was green and rapidly growing. Some groups used other foods such as moose thyroids or spider crabs, and African groups whose water was low in iodine used the ashes of certain plant foods to supply this element. These foods were added against the backdrop of a diet rich in liver and other organ meats, bones, and skin, fats, seafood and the local plant foods. (Ibid p. 26)

Nutrients found in these traditional foods play an important role in the body's physiology for reproduction and development. I am not saying you have to eat spider crabs or moose thyroids to have a healthy pregnancy. There are other more palatable ways to obtain the critical nutrients found in these traditional foods. The take-home message here is to make sure your diet is supplying the vast array of these key nutrients, and if not, to supplement accordingly.

The first nutrient important to prenatal care is folate, or folic acid, as its synthetic form is known. Folate is necessary for proper replication of DNA during the cell division process as the fetus develops. Proper neural tube development is also dependent upon adequate folate which is best absorbed by the body from food and from whole-food supplements in its natural, methylated form 5-methyl-tetrahydrofolate. The best food sources of folate are organic calf's liver, legumes pre-soaked properly in an acidic medium, and organic green vegetables and leafy greens like spinach.

Second in importance for prenatal development is vitamin E, named tocopherol from the Greek word *tokos* for "offspring." Vitamin E is essential in constructing the human placenta, the transport system for nutrition from the mother to the growing fetus. The best sources of vitamin E are: palm oil; grass-fed animal fat; raw, organic nuts and seeds properly soaked and dried in a dehydrator prior to eating; fresh organic fruits and vegetables as well as freshly ground grains. Appendices C and D give sources of these life-giving traditional foods.

Vitamin A is also a critical nutrient possibly more important than vitamin E as it is "necessary for the differentiation and patterning of all of the cells, tissues and organs within the developing body."(Masterjohn C. Vitamins for fetal development. p. 26). Vitamin A is a crucial factor in proper kidney formation as well as in maintaining the cells which line the developing lungs. (Ibid) For this reason I recommend that patients planning to have a child take a high-vitamin fermented cod liver oil daily. Eating a few ounces of liver each week as well as raw organic milk, raw butter and pastured eggs ensures an adequate intake of this crucial vitamin. Pasteurized/homogenized dairy is not adequate, because the heating involved destroys heat labile nutrients like vitamin C, B12, folate and vitamin B5.

Some of my patients have been warned by their doctors that vitamin A is dangerous and can be toxic in doses of higher than 10,000 IUs per day. This information was based on a poorly designed study in 1995 using synthetic vitamin A. Masterjohn remarks, "There are several important flaws in this study . . . every other published study on this subject shows this amount of vitamin A to be safe." He emphasizes what I also believe to be true: the "[P]reponderance of the evidence clearly favors the view that 20,000–25,000 IUs of vitamin A during pregnancy is safe and may even reduce the risk of birth defects."(Ibid) Remember to get your vitamin A from a good quality, unprocessed cod liver oil such as Green Pasture™ Blue Ice™ Fermented Cod Liver Oil. Chapter I of *The Nourishing Traditions Book of Baby & Child Care*, by Fallon-Morell and Cowan explains how important vitamin A is in fetal development, for those looking for more detail.

Also crucial to prenatal nutrition is fat-soluble vitamin D, a common nutritional deficiency in the United States, due to lack of availability or the illegality of the sale, in most states, of wholesome, raw, pastured dairy products. This is combined with a culture that no longer values organ meats as part of the diet. Furthermore, fear of skin cancer, overuse of sunscreens, and having an indoor work place deprive people in northern climates of the benefits of the sun, a natural source of vitamin D. Vitamin D is necessary for lung and skeletal development of the fetus, and, as noted by Masterjohn, "protects the newborn from tetany, convulsions, and heart failure."(Ibid p. 28) I refer my readers to the Weston A. Price Foundation for more information on vitamin D and its important role in fetal development. Weston Price recommends taking 2,000 IUs per day of vitamin D from unprocessed cod liver oil, and small amounts from fish including shellfish, butter and lard (www.westonaprice.org).

Another important vitamin deficient in the American diet is vitamin K, found in leafy greens. "Although very little is known about vitamin K, it is understood that it is necessary for laying down calcium salts in bone tissue and to keep calcium out of the soft tissue where it does not belong."(Ibid p. 29) Vitamin K is believed to play a critical role in the formation of proper facial proportions and the fundamental development of the nervous system. It comes in two isomers, K_1 and K_2, both of which are severely lacking in the SAD. Vitamin K_2 is found in fermented foods as well as grass-fed animal fats, foods rarely consumed by many Americans. I recommend including them in a prenatal diet, and in any diet in general.

A nutrient many women are more familiar with as being crucial during the prenatal period as well as during growth and development of a healthy child is docosahexaenoic acid, better known as DHA. DHA is a component of fish oil and can also be made by the body from alpha-linolenic acid (found in flax, for example), unless the person has diabetes, in which case the enzyme delta-desaturase needed for the conversion does not function properly. Salynn Boyles on Web MD Health News points out that "babies whose diets include an abundance of essential fats seem to have an edge in terms of early development." The author further emphasizes that new research has shown that the same is true for infants born to mothers whose diets contain plenty of this essential fatty acid. "Although its role is not fully understood, it is well known that DHA is critical for the developing brain and nervous system, which accumulates large amounts of it during the first two years of life. In fact, in one recent study it was shown that children born to mothers with higher levels of DHA in their blood scored higher on attention tests as well as tests designed to measure visual acuity." (Colombo J, Kannass KN, Shaddy DJ, Kundurthi S, Maikranz JN, Anderson CJ, Blaga OM, Carlson SE. Maternal DHA and the development of attention in infancy and toddlerhood. Child development. 2004 July/August; 75(4):p. 1254-67.)

DHA is abundant in fatty fish like salmon, cod and tuna, although one must be careful not to purchase farm-raised fish whose levels of DHA are much lower. It is important to eat the skin of the fish as well to obtain this nutrient. Cod liver oil is also an excellent source of DHA and mandatory for any mother before, during and even after pregnancy. Chris Masterjohn notes, "A double-blind, placebo-controlled study showed that use of cod liver oil during pregnancy and lactation increased the child's IQ at the age of four years. The belief is that DHA is largely responsible for this fact" (Masterjohn C. Vitamins for fetal development. p. 30). A less well-known but equally critical nutrient in prenatal development is choline. "Choline has a direct role in brain development and is especially important for the formation of cholinergic neurons, which takes place from day 56 of pregnancy through three months postpartum. It also has a role in the formation of the connections between these neurons, called synapses, which occurs at a high rate through the fourth year of life." (Ibid p. 32) Pastured, organic eggs and liver, and raw, organic, grass-fed dairy are all excellent sources of choline.

Let me recommend some specific foods I believe all parents, especially mothers, should include in their diets prior to, during and after pregnancy. First and foremost is bone and vegetable broths. These broths (or stocks), fish, beef, chicken and vegetable, can be made according to the guidelines in *Nourishing Traditions* by Sally Fallon. Stocks, especially those made from the bones of chicken or beef, are rich in minerals as well as gelatin and amino acids crucial to the baby for building protein. "Folk wisdom worldwide values broth for its healing powers, and we have found confirmation of these traditional beliefs in hundreds of 19th and early 20th century studies on gelatin, and in thousands of modern investigations into glycine, cartilage, glucosamine, and other components found abundantly in broth." (Fallon-Morell S, Daniel KT. Nourishing broth: an old-fashioned remedy for the modern world. New York: Grand Central Life & Style Publ; 2014. p. 8)

Equally important to the prenatal diet for the mother are fats and the fat-soluble vitamins which come with them. We spoke earlier of Vitamins A, D, E, and K as well as DHA, but there are many more known and unknown that play a critical role in brain and nervous system development. These include fats in the form of organ meats, wild-caught fatty fish, pastured, organic eggs, raw organic dairy from pastured animals, and animal fats and skin.

Mothers should include green vegetables and leafy greens as well as some lacto-fermented foods like sauerkraut in the diet. This will help build probiotic flora which is handed down to the child in passing through the birth canal and even in breastfeeding. This is especially important for mothers who have a history of antiobiotic use, as this may result in yeast and other pathogens being passed on to the baby. I advise my patients to eat nuts, seeds, legumes and grains in moderation, only if they are properly soaked and dried, and in their raw, unprocessed form.

Lastly, parents-to-be need to forgo the refined sugars and grains, fast-foods, packaged foods, coffee, foods laden with artificial colors and sweeteners, sodas, and opt for a more traditional diet rich in fresh wholesome foods. What you eat is what feeds the child and fuels his or her development. Recent research finds evidence that the baby's future health is intimately intertwined with the health/nutrition of the parents at conception, and the health/nutrition of the mother during and after pregnancy. The fetus has no choice in the matter and is completely at the mercy of its parents.

Another area of confusion is prenatal supplementation. There is a differences between whole-food supplements and synthetic ones. Take calcium as an example. All calcium is not the same. Calcium carbonate, the most common form found in supplements, is chalk. Taking this form of calcium is the equivalent of chewing on rock. It takes the body over 20 chemical reactions to convert this form to the usable, ionized bicarbonate form the body needs. (All minerals must first be in an ionized or "charged" state to be usable by our body.) Calcium lactate is the form found in vegetables and takes only one reaction to become the usable bicarbonate form. There are many other forms of calcium, some better, some worse. The simple fact is that when you use whole food supplements, you eliminate the need to worry about whether your body can even use the vitamins you are consuming. Therefore, the best prenatal vitamins will be made of whole food ingredients free of soy, sugars, yeast, colorings, and additives and made with minimal processing.

I recommend using Standard Process Catalyn® chewable as a starting point for a good multivitamin. They also make a Folic Acid/B12 supplement and calcium lactate which are crucial for prenatal use. Add a high-vitamin cod liver oil like Green Pasture™ and you have a strong foundation for prenatal supplementation. What we recommend most women do prior to conceiving is to have a nutritional work-up including using the Genova Diagnostics Lab's testing to customize a complete nutritional program and eliminate as much guesswork as possible.

Monthly maintenance care for the pregnant mother should include routine chiropractic adjustments to maintain good structural position of the pelvis and spine. The adjustments are pivotal in maintaining the flexibility of the body including the pelvis thereby facilitating easier passage of the baby through the birth canal. The pelvis is composed of three bones: the ischium, pubis, and ilium. These three bones spread as the hormone relaxin is produced and released from the placenta, the chorion, and the deciduas, making flexibility of the birth canal possible and creating room for the baby's head and shoulders. Assuring proper positioning of the pelvis through proper chiropractic care is critical for a smooth, uncomplicated delivery.

For all prospective parents I recommend *The Nourishing Traditions Book of Baby & Child Care* by Fallon and Cowan, MD. On p. 15 the book includes an resource for prenatal nutrition, and a summary entitled "The Diet For Healthy Babies." It covers the highlights of a proper diet prior to and during pregnancy. For comprehensive prenatal information this book is essential. It is packed with relevant, concise and accurate information which meshes perfectly with my protocol for preparing women for childbirth.

Another guide on proper pre/postnatal diet and nutrition is *Real Food for Mother and Baby* by Nina Planck. I recommend it for any woman who is pregnant or considering pregnancy. The Weston A. Price Foundation also provides helpful information on pregnancy and child rearing on their website (www.westonaprice.org).

Infant Care/Raising a Healthy Child

The newborn needs special care including bathing, feeding and all of the love and attention possible. Parents, as primary care-givers who are responsible for their children, need to be educated as to the alternatives and options available for their child's health.

We begin with bathing. For the first 2–3 weeks, bathing is not really necessary since the baby's skin has a protective coating known as the *vernix caseosa* (a waxy substance which coats the infant's skin, acting as a moisturizer, helping preserve heat and protect the newborn's skin from the outside environment). Therefore, it is best to wait a week or two before bathing the child so as to allow this waxy coating to naturally slough off. Also, it may take up to three weeks or so for the baby's *umbilicus* to fall off; bathing can wait until that time. Prior to that point, all that is necessary is cleaning the baby's bottom using a warm, damp cloth with each diaper change. Bathing should be done in tepid water and a gentle soap made only from natural botanicals used to rinse the baby's head. Rinsing the baby's head well with a natural, botanical-based moisturizing soap will help to keep the baby's scalp moist. A good choice is Poya Baby Shampoo which is a gentle formulation that contains no harsh, synthetic chemicals or fragrances. It soothes baby's delicate scalp while gently cleansing the hair and nourishing the scalp. This mild shampoo will not cause tears, and uses natural, coconut-derived surfactants that lather without stripping the skin of its natural oils. You can also use a little homemade mayonnaise on the scalp one or two nights a week and then rinse it off in the morning. Mayonnaise is rich in lanolin which is excellent for the hair as well. (Easy recipe for mayonnaise found in *Nourishing Traditions*.)

Feeding infants has become an area of misinformation and controversy. In the past, mothers and fathers knew that babies were to be breastfed. This was the best and healthiest way of feeding a newborn. Synthetic infant formulas now crowd the shelves of food stores. The convenience and ease of using these products have consequences. Infants and toddlers are brought into my office with allergies, skin conditions, learning disorders, and developmental delays. Parents assuming the responsibility of having a child should make diet/nutrition before, during and after pregnancy a number one priority. This includes breastfeeding which helps develop a strong, healthy child and is best for the child. Fallon agrees, stating in *Nourishing Traditions*:

> Couples planning to have children should eat liberally of organic liver and other organ meats, fish eggs, and other seafood, eggs, and the best quality butter, cream and fermented milk products they can obtain for at least six months before conceptions. A daily cod liver oil supplement is also advised. Organic meats, vegetables, grains, and legumes should round out the diet, with a special emphasis on the leafy green vegetables rich in folic acid, which is necessary for the prevention of birth defects like spina bifida. (p. 598)

A baby also needs adequate calcium for the developing skeleton as does the mother in order to maintain her bone health during the pregnancy. Eating a diet rich in the aforementioned foods will ensure adequate calcium and maintain a proper body pH for both the child and the mother.

Breast milk is the best and only complete food for the infant. A purchased formula is not just as good and the child will not "grow just as well" as some doctors tell expectant mothers. Breastfed babies do much better with overall health and wellness as well as with better development of the immune system. One study carried out at Duke University and published in the journal *Current Nutrition & Food Science* found, "Human milk promotes the growth of "biofilms" of beneficial bacteria that line the intestinal tract of healthy babies, helping digestion and the development of the immune system and acting as a barrier to bad germs."(Zhang AQ, Ryan Lee SY, Truneh

M, Everett ML, Parker W. Human whey promotes sessile bacterial growth, whereas alternative sources of infant nutrition promote planktonic growth. Current Nutrition & Food Science. 2012 Aug; 8(3):168–76) Many more studies support the superiority of breast milk. Breastfeeding is common sense. It is nature's design.

If a woman is contemplating having a child she should do everything in her power to maintain good health and nutrition. In this way she will give her baby the best chance to develop with robust health. Put succinctly, this means proper diet, adequate rest, appropriate whole-food vitamin supplementation and exercise as well as staying clear of alcohol, drugs, and medications. As a doctor, I have seen all types of pregnancy problems: morning sickness, allergies, fatigue, sciatica and other back problems, and more commonly today, gestational diabetes. In all there was a common thread. The woman was not following a healthy lifestyle in one or more of the areas outlined above. When the parents follow the lifestyle addressed by the holistic physician, health and wellness is invariably restored.

Author Sally Fallon says:

> A good rule for pregnant women is two eggs, raw milk or bone broth, and cod liver oil daily, and liver once a week. Appropriate amounts of superfoods, such as high-vitamin butter oil, evening primrose, borage or black currant oil, bee pollen, mineral powder, wheat germ oil and acerola powder, will provide optimal amounts of nutrients for your unborn child. (Fallon, S. Nourishing Traditions. p. 598)

In this book Fallon shares recipes for beet kvass and kombucha which are useful for preventing morning sickness as are foods rich in vitamin B6 such as turnip greens, spinach, asparagus, organic grass-fed meats and fish. It should also be noted that the quality of a mother's milk will reflect the mother's diet and lifestyle habits. Eating sufficient quantities of organic, pastured animal products will ensure adequate levels of vitamins B12, A, and D as well as the minerals calcium and zinc. An excellent and simple rule of thumb for the expecting mother is to eat plenty of green vegetables and drink plenty of pure, clean water.

Breastfeeding is all that is necessary for a newborn child, and should be done every 3 to 4 hours and continued for roughly the first year of life. "Breastfeeding should ideally be continued for six months to a year. If mother's milk is not adequate or of good quality, or if the mother is unable to breastfeed for whatever reason, a homemade baby formula, rather than a commercial formula, can be used," says Fallon (Fallon S. Nourishing Traditions. p. 599). I recommend every woman read the section Feeding Babies in *Nourishing Traditions*. Further insights can be gained from *The Nourishing Traditions Book of Baby & Child Care* by Thomas S. Cowan, MD and Sally Fallon.

In preparing for breastfeeding it is helpful to "toughen" the nipple of each breast. This can be done by taking a dry wash cloth and grabbing the nipple firmly between the thumb and index finger. Then, firmly tug on the nipple on and off for a few minutes each morning and evening beginning in the 3rd month of pregnancy. The goal is to toughen the nipple, not to cause pain. Doing so will prepare it for the suckling of the baby and prevent it from cracking if the baby sucks too hard.

Caring for the nipple and breast after nursing should include using some natural vitamin E or castor oil spread around the nipple and areola of each breast. This will ensure proper circulation in the nipples and will keep the circulation in the breast moving well. Lastly, after you wash the breast just before nursing, it is a good habit to tug at the nipple for approximately 30 seconds to keep the nipples firm and make them easier for the baby to latch on to.

When nursing, it is best for the mother to lie down and relax while the baby is suckling. Thus both mother and baby are in a restful position. Though some women prefer to nurse in the seated position, I think this can be a mistake because it can lead the woman's breast to become engorged with milk (because of gravity pushing it down toward the nipple). This can force the milk to come out too fast and lead to the child spitting up. In the lying position, gravity is removed and the flow of milk is easier for the baby to handle.

A traumatizing situation for a new mother and father is when their infant runs a fever for the first time. Their instinctual panic may lead to rash decision-making including doctor's visits, antibiotics, Tylenol, baby aspirin, and other harmful medications. Never give a baby Tylenol. "There is evidence that increased acetaminophen use is a major cause of the epidemics of autism, ADHD, and asthma."

(Shaw W. Evidence that increased acetaminophen use in genetically vulnerable children appears to be a major cause of the epidemics of autism, attention deficit with hyperactivity, and asthma. Journal of Restorative Medicine. 2013 Oct; 2(1)14-29.) This was also found to be true in babies whose mothers took Tylenol during pregnancy. (Ibid) Natural methods of fever reduction have served my family and my patients very well. They are all based on helping the body deal with the problem at hand and allowing the body to reduce the fever on its own, not by treating the symptoms or forcing the body into submission. They are as follows:

1. Give the child a plain water enema. For infants under the age of 2, use 1 ½–2 ounces of water. Remember to place a small amount of Vaseline on the tip of the syringe. After administering the fluid into the rectum by squeezing the syringe, hold the infant's buttocks together for a few minutes, laying the baby on his/her right side. This should be repeated within a 5-minute period, and can be done 2 or 3 hours later as well. Do not worry if the water does not come out; if the temperature is high the body will absorb the fluid.

2. Wipe the baby down with tepid water – 8 ounces with one tablespoon of apple cider vinegar added to it. This is done to reduce body temperature and to replace through the skin some of the minerals lost during the high temperature.

3. Wrap the child in a towel soaked in cool tap water then a dry towel around the wet one. Let the baby stay wrapped like this from 10–12 minutes allowing the towel to absorb the body heat. This can be repeated 2 or 3 times according to how the body responds.

4. After you have tried A–C above, give the child sips of water with a pinch of Celtic brand unrefined sea salt added. Doing so replaces the electrolytes lost during the fever. A mouthful is adequate for infants under 12 months of age. You can use a teaspoon to administer the liquid.

If the temperature persists, any of the above can be repeated until the temperature abates and the baby returns to normal. In 98% of the cases in my experience, these simple home remedies are effective. There are some natural herbs and liquid preparations that can be given to any child without causing internal trouble or side effects. One can use homeopathic tissue cell salts numbers 4, 5, 6 and 12. They can be administered under the tongue or dissolved in a little water on a spoon. Dosages vary according to age but generally 2 under the tongue every few hours will suffice for infants running a fever. You can use primarily numbers 4 and 12 for basic fevers and use numbers 5 and 6 if the baby's tongue is covered with a white coating and if there is constipation. Another remedy that is helpful is Occillococcinum homeopathic remedy. It can be taken as directed on the label.

An important note: It is never safe to use an aspirin for children. *Do not make this mistake.* Some people will give their children Tylenol and other over-the-counter medications without even thinking of the consequences. But as the news reports on Tylenol earlier in 2012 showed, these medications are toxic to the liver and gastrointestinal system and can even cause permanent brain damage in children. A web search on Reye's syndrome and aspirin is very important for uninformed parents to learn these facts. As previously mentioned, Tylenol is equally dangerous.

A colicky baby can cause anxiety for new parents. A colicky baby is a malnourished baby. This may be the result of poor diet in the mother during pregnancy and breastfeeding as well as a result of commercial formula. Colic can be remedied quite simply by restoring the diet of the mother as outlined previously (if breastfeeding) OR by taking the baby off of the harmful commercial formulas and using homemade formulas as outlined in Nourishing Traditions. The protocol below is also helpful in dealing with the colicky baby.

Colicky Baby Protocol

1. If the mother is breastfeeding *she must avoid all of the following foods without exception:*
    - processed dairy of all types
    - grains (including wheat and whole wheat)
    - soy products of all types
    - gas-forming vegetables including beans
    - cabbage, kale, corn, onions
    - white and sweet potato; all raw vegetables

2. Tissue Cell Salt #4 (Ferrum Phosphate) – Give the baby two crushed tablets 3 times/day.
3. Tissue Cell Salt #5 (Magnesium Phospate) – Give two cell salts crushed every 30 minutes until bowel movements return and then slowly cut back the dosage until reaching a final dosage of two cell salts 3 times/day.
4. Use a Baby Fleet Enema (*containing sterile water only*) to administer a few ounces of water (2–3 ounces per enema) into the baby's rectum. If you cannot find the Baby Fleet water enema you may use an adult size and simply administer only a few ounces instead of the whole enema. Make sure to gently hold the baby's buttocks closed for a few minutes to allow movement of the water through the intestinal tract. This may be done easily in a sink basin or bathtub. Repeat this 2–3 times a day or as directed by the physician.

Another important area of infant care is allowing the baby access to fresh air. This may not always be possible for those living in industrial centers and cities. Whenever possible, it is important to put the baby in a carriage and take the child outside to get fresh air. I did this with all of my six children, even throughout the winter. My wife and I would always make sure the baby had a knit hat and gloves, and was bundled-up appropriately in the colder weather. But it never deterred us from putting the baby outside. This is because after being indoors all evening the child will need a good lung cleansing with access to the outdoors and fresh air. Putting the child outside will enable the baby to get more oxygen and sunlight. Obviously in the summer months you must take care to not leave the baby in the direct sun too long, but it is certainly important for making vitamin D that the baby has some sun exposure every day.

In spite of today's fast-paced culture, it is still important for there to be time for the mother and baby to rest and relax together. A simple walk around the block in the stroller or a visit to a local park for an hour or two may suffice. The importance of this time for mother and baby together cannot be overstated. Today we need to rebuild the family unit by learning to balance our lives and prioritize our choices. I realize that a mother needs a social life too, but this shouldn't mean running around with the baby in a car seat all day.

Wisely, some mothers choose to keep a more relaxed profile for the first few months after the birth of their child. This time together gives mother and child time to bond, free from distractions and stress thus keeping a quiet and relaxed environment as much as possible.

Furthermore, it gives the mother's body and immune system a chance to "recharge" and recover from the tremendously stressful event of childbirth. After 3 or 4 months, the baby has grown and the mother and child can begin to go out a little more.

Let me cover a few more suggestions in caring for a newborn. First of all, it is very important to keep a hat on the baby's head and socks on the baby's feet. The baby's head and feet must always be kept warm. Since the head is the main area through which a baby will lose heat, it is crucial to keep the head warm to protect the baby's developing immune system. Obviously if you live in a warmer climate like Florida, this will not be necessary at all times. However, in most northern climates, this is a crucial point to remember. A simple rule of thumb is this: never under-dress a child, you can always take things off if necessary.

What should a woman do if she cannot breastfeed? First, it is very important to understand a few things about commercial baby formulas. Author and nutrition pioneer Sally Fallon makes the point that "commercial infant formulas are highly fabricated concoctions composed of milk or soy powders produced with high-temperature processes that overdenature proteins and add many carcinogens (cancer-causing compounds)." (Fallon S, Enig MG. Nourishing Traditions: the cookbook that challenges politically correct nutrition and the diet dictocrats. Washington DC: New Trends Publishing Inc; 2001. p. 99) These denatured proteins and compounds weaken the immune system, create allergies, and can lead to mineral deficiencies. Moreover, many formulas have added simple sugars like fructose without the full complement of cofactors and enzymes, many of which have yet to be identified. Furthermore, the vitamins and minerals added to these formulas do not come from whole food sources. Rather they are synthetic, made in a laboratory and do not contain the many unidentified compounds yet to be discovered in breast milk. Processed, pasteurized milk and most soy products are leading allergy-causing foods, and thus are not appropriate for daily consumption, especially by an infant. So a woman facing this decision is best served by learning to make her own formula using the recipes in *Nourishing Traditions*.

Another area of concern for new mothers is the danger of soy-based formulas. Soy has several characteristics that make it dangerous to give to anyone as a food, let alone an infant. To begin with, most of the soy produced and used in formulas is genetically modified (GMO), and toxic for the human body. Genetic modification uses viral and bacterial DNA injected into the DNA of the seed of a given plant to produce a desired characteristic not previously present in nature. In the case of soy and corn, companies like Monsanto have developed these technologies to enable the crops to be sprayed with pesticides and not be harmed. Monsanto's Round-Up Ready technology gives them a virtual monopoly on the chemical sprays used to combat weeds while allowing them the patent rights on the crops which are being sprayed. The consumer is left to ingest these pesticides which are difficult to wash off and contain the foreign proteins created by the genetic modification process. For an enlightening journey through the dark world of Monsanto and similar companies, and the dangers inherent in genetically modified foods, read *Seeds of Deception*, by Jeffrey M. Smith and *The World According to Monsanto* by Marie-Monique Robin.

Soy contains mineral blocking phytic acid which deprives the baby of the ability to absorb minerals via the intestinal tract. Potentially more dangerous are the estrogen-mimicking compounds found in soy. Estimates vary, but experts believe that feeding a baby soy-based formula is equivalent to giving a birth control pill a day to the infant! This can have devastating effects on the child's hormonal development.

Fortunately there are products available that closely resemble mother's milk and which do not carry the dangers of commercial soy and milk-based formulas. The best option for a woman seeking alternatives to breastfeeding is a homemade formula made from wholesome, organic, unprocessed nutrients. Sally Fallon notes, "Whenever possible this formula should be based on raw organic milk, from grass-fed cows certified free of tuberculosis and brucellosis. Ideally, the milk should come from Jersey or Guernsey cows, rather than Holsteins, so that it has a high butterfat content."

She goes on to note that "Properly produced raw milk does not pose a danger to your baby, in spite of what numerous public health propagandists may assert."(Fallon S, Enig MG. Nourishing Traditions. p. 599.) She includes in the book several recipes for making natural, wholesome formulas and where to find the ingredients. Another option is the meat-based formula she provides, which is best suited for children who may be allergic to milk. Consult her book for details.

Another important need for the baby during the transition off of breast milk includes the introduction of solid foods. A crucial supplement for all babies is egg yolk. The eggs should be organic and from pastured chickens allowed to roam freely and never given antibiotics or soy and corn-based feeds. I recommend supplementing an egg yolk per day beginning at about the sixth month mark. Egg yolks are loaded with B-vitamin factors including inositol and choline as well as crucial fats that are an integral part of the developing brain. You may also give the baby small amounts of finely ground or grated raw, organic liver added to the egg yolk with a pinch of sea salt, as Fallon notes. (Ibid p. 600)

The biggest dietary mistake mothers make with the developing infant is to begin feeding them cereal grains, especially Cheerios and crackers. Many medical doctors tell new mothers that it is smart to introduce cereal and blended foods after the age of six months. This is when trouble starts with constipation, allergies, intestinal problems including irritable bowel, gas and colic. These are the warning signs of a malnourished baby. For the first six months to a year, the baby really only needs what the breast milk of a nutritionally healthy mother can provide. As for fruit juices, their overuse with young toddlers is a comon mistake. It is unwise to give the baby fruit juice, especially apple juice, which provides only simple carbohydrates, and will often spoil an infant's appetite for more nutritious foods (Fallon, p. 601). Fruit juices are often sweetened with high fructose corn syrup and are pasteurized, further diminishing enzymes and other nutritional value.

After one year it is time to introduce regular food into the diet. This coincides with the beginning of the appearance of the first teeth which occurs around the eighth-month stage and terminating with the molars at approximately 32 months. Mother Nature is wise, timing the development of the teeth with the proper time to introduce more solid foods. Fresh, preferably organic, ripe fruits in the mornings such as apples, pears, plums and bananas are excellent choices. I also recommend organic pastured eggs and egg yolks. Some people like to use whole, unprocessed cereals like millet, amaranth, steel-cut oatmeal, and even barley. These are acceptable as long as they are soaked properly and then cooked. Begin this after the first birthday since earlier than this the baby's digestive system cannot produce sufficient amylase to properly digest the starch in grains. A baby's earliest solid foods should be animal-based foods because the baby's digestive system is more adapted to supply enzymes to digest fats and proteins rather than carbohydrates.

For lunches it is wise to give steamed, half-cooked, blended/pureed green and yellow vegetables flavored with some raw, organic butter and a pinch of sea salt. Sweet potato, carrots, turnips, and pre-soaked beans are also a good choice.

Organic pastured meat, chicken, turkey, liver, lamb, or fish should be given for dinner with two non-starchy vegetables. This balance helps keep the baby alkaline, and an alkaline baby will be a strong and healthy baby. Test your baby's saliva first thing in the morning using litmus paper which can be ordered online or purchased in most reputable health food stores; it should register 6.6–7.0.

Fevers in the Infant and Young Child

This is a general condition with many unique and specific causes. In children, it can be caused by teething, constipation, sinus problems, ear infection and so on. Chiropractors take the natural approach, not to simply suppress the fever, but to help it along. Fever serves a very important function for the immune system and the body. In order to increase the speed and efficacy of the chemical reactions our immune system needs to fight off infection and process waste, body temperature must rise. The thyroid gland plays a role in this process, raising the body temperature and assisting the immune system. The fever isn't really a culprit; it is a side effect of the accumulating waste and infection the body is dealing with.

Fever Caused By Teething

Teething is a time of great growth and development for a child. Tissue is growing and changing at a rapid pace, especially in the mouth. This growth and development necessitates an elevation in body temperature to facilitate the immune system in helping remove old, damaged tissue while aiding in the building of new tissue, specifically the teeth. Here is what you can do:

1. Make the child some barley cereal. Purchase pre-soaked or sprouted barley or soak it yourself. Barley has a calming effect on the body because it gives the body the essential minerals needed in the production of teeth. You may also use the barley water that results as you cook the cereal. Soak the barley overnight in an acid medium first. See the directions in Appendix C p. 344-46. Give it to the child in a bottle throughout the day, little by little.

2. Learn to use a plain water enema – 2 ounce syringe given 2–3 times per day. This will replace some of the water that the body has lost due to the fever. (Baby fleet enemas can be purchased in most pharmacies.) High fever can also cause electrolyte loss and these electrolytes must be replaced. You can do this by giving a pinch of Celtic sea salt (available in health food stores and in Whole Foods) in 8 ounces of water. Have the child take mouthfuls every 5 minutes or so until they have consumed all 8 ounces.

3. Make bone broths. Follow the directions on pages 116–125 in *Nourishing Traditions* for making your own stocks. Give small amounts of this mineral rich broth to the baby throughout the day. It is one of the most nourishing foods you can feed a child and is extremely rich in minerals. These minerals are crucial for the growing skeleton, to replace electrolytes, and are tremendously important for the immune system.

4. Where vomiting accompanies the fever, add approximately 1 tbsp of raw honey (see Appendix D #22) to the enema by dissolving the honey in the water prior to administering the enema as described above in #2. This is the best way to replace the electrolytes that have been lost through the fever, vomiting and any diarrhea.

5. If there is an infection somewhere in the body, you must first give the child good, unprocessed cod liver oil (see Appendix D p. 355

#4). You can do this in younger children by administering drops directly on the tongue with a dropper or straw. Give the equivalent of ½ teaspoon up to 2 times per day for children up to the age of four. A full teaspoon can be used 1–2 times per day for children over four. A natural vitamin C Complex like Standard Process Cataplex® C is helpful as well. It can be chewed or crushed and given with the child's food. I recommend one per meal for children under four and two per meal for children over four. The Synergy Company makes a whole food vitamin C in powdered form which is easily mixed in water and has a delightful taste. See Appendix D.

6. To further reduce the fever, wrap the child in a cool, wet towel and then, around the wet towel, wrap a dry towel to draw the heat out from the body. Do this for up to 10 minutes, repeating if necessary.

7. Calcium (preferably calcium lactate from Standard Process) can be crushed into a powder and given to the child with water. Crush two tablets of Standard Process calcium lactate tablets and mix with water. This can be repeated up to 3 times per day. It will cause the body to become more alkaline and assist in detoxifying the body. Calcium is also crucial to the immune system in cases of fever.

8. Another helpful procedure is to wipe the child's body down with a solution of 2 tablespoons organic apple cider vinegar, preferably raw, in a quart of water (see Appendix D p. 358 #27). This will help replace the electrolytes lost through the fever and can be done 2 or 3 times a day if necessary. When a child has diarrhea, vomiting, or a high temperature he/she is losing important electrolytes along with the water. This can become a very serious problem, so it is best to act as quickly and as intelligently as possible to help the body.

Children's Anti-Fever Protocol

Items Needed
A hot water bottle with enema attachment for *children 8 or older*:

1. Administer the enema to your child according to the physician's directions (see Appendix A p. 321-22 for instructions). Ask for a complete set of directions from your physician if you have never administered an enema before. This protocol can be repeated twice to three times a day during the fever without worry. Please consult with your holistic physician if you have any questions.

2a. For children under the age of five: take 6 tablets of Calcium Lactate and 3 tablets of Cataplex® F and grind or crush them in a seed or coffee grinder. Add the contents to homemade apple sauce or other food and allow the child to eat it.

2b. For children over five who are able to swallow small pills, give the supplements described in 2a above as pills. The pills can be taken with a small amount of water or with food.

3. Congaplex® Chewable for children and regular Congaplex® for children above the age of ten. Give children under the age of ten 2 Congaplex® Chewable tablets every hour while they are awake for the first 48 hours, reducing to 4–6 per day thereafter until the fever is relieved. For children over the age of ten, repeat the same procedure using regular Congaplex® Capsules.

To Vaccinate or Not to Vaccinate?

The decision not to vaccinate my children was an easy one for me. I say this, both from the standpoint of a father, and as that of a physician. It was important that my wife and I shared a unified front on this decision. We decided that injecting foreign bacterial/viral material, material containing mercury, aluminum, and other toxins directly into our child's bloodstream was not a smart decision, especially when a baby's immune system is just beginning to develop. I did not let fear goad me into doing something dangerous and hazardous to my children's health, or the health of my patients' children, if I could help it. I intended to raise my children according to nature's laws, laws I believed in and knew would protect my children without the need for vaccination.

The debate regarding vaccinations has been hotly contested since its inception. Superficially, it may seem that vaccinations are common sense. Few realize the scarcity of research on the safety of vaccines, or that vaccine efficacy has never been proven. Also people do not realize the corruption that has been the foundation of vaccination mandates. Louise K. Habakus and Mary Holland in their book on the vaccine epidemic write:

> Many advisers on governmental advisory committees have deep professional and financial stakes in vaccination policy.

> Truly public participation in such committees is extremely limited. Voting members frequently have conflicts of interest, including stocks, patents, grants and honoraria from industry. Public health officials often benefit from a lucrative "revolving door" that may convert their public service into a private sector sinecure. Congressional interventions, including the 1986 National Childhood Vaccine Injury Act, have severely restricted the capacity for redress from a vaccine-induced injury. The net result is that public health decisions regarding vaccination policy may not be as truly democratic as they appear. (Habakus LK, Holland M. Vaccine epidemic: how corporate greed, biased science, and coercive government threaten our human rights, our health, and our children. New York: Skyhorse Publishing; 2010. p. 21–22)

Whether we accept the efficacy of vaccines or not, many state vaccination mandates are for diseases from which American children typically do not die. Habakus and Holland note, "Some diseases, such as chickenpox and rotavirus, have never caused a significant number of deaths in children."(Ibid p. 23) They continue, "young children are required to receive vaccines for diseases that do not routinely afflict them."(Ibid p. 23) For example, why mandate vaccination for hepatitis B or human papilloma virus when these diseases are spread primarily through sexual contact or intravenous drug use? Shouldn't a parent's right to decide what is injected into their child's body, especially in instances like this, be preserved?

> By age eighteen, children in the United States receive seventy doses of sixteen vaccines. Infants, whose immune systems are undeveloped, are exposed to more than thirty three doses of over one dozen vaccines by fifteen months of age, including hepatitis B, diphtheria, tetanus, pertussis, polio, rubella, measles, mumps, chickenpox, pneumococcal infections, haemophilus influenza type B, and influenza. Moreover, infants are being vaccinated not only against childhood diseases, but also against diseases to which they are unlikely to be exposed for the express purpose of protecting adults. For example, why are newborn infants

on the day of birth being vaccinated against hepatitis B, a disease contracted by having unprotected sex or sharing needles? Why are two-month-old infants vaccinated against tetanus, which is extremely rare and occurs primarily in older populations, is effectively treatable after exposure, and is uncontagious? (Habakus LK. Vaccine epidemic. p. 79)

Vaccines, much like the pseudo-science used to propagate the diet-heart hypothesis, are a big money-making business. If you do the research (parents owe it to their children to be informed) you will see the facts for yourself. In Chapter 8 of *Vaccine Epidemic* this exact point is emphasized by Robert Johnston, PhD:

> If vaccines have greatly improved the health of America's children, then it is fair to ask why the United States' ranking among world nations in infant mortality has plummeted from twelfth in 1960 to twenty-ninth in 1990, down to forty-sixth in 2010. The U.S. Center for Disease Control and Prevention (CDC) acknowledges, "The U.S. infant mortality rate is higher than those in most other developed countries, and the gap between the U.S. infant mortality rate and the rates for the countries with the lowest infant mortality appears to be widening.... The United States lags behind nearly every developed country and even poor countries such as Cuba, whose healthcare expenditure is $230 per capita, whereas the United States' is $6,096 per capita. (Ibid p. 79)

Johnston continues:

> U.S. medicine is dominated by corporate interests — physicians, academic institutions, and government agencies whose financial interests are intertwined with drug and vaccine manufacturers. Physicians, professional associations, medical institutions, and government agencies are collaborating partners in the business of medicine.... Thus individuals and communities are viewed as the means by which to increase profits. Neither individuals nor the citizenry are well served when the integrity of medicine is debased, its scientific method is tainted, and its humanitarian and moral principles are violated with impunity. (Ibid p. 80)

Consider the theory of vaccination. The justification for it relies completely on the work of Edward Jenner from the last part of the 18th century and on Louis Pasteur's mid-19th century Germ Theory. See Section V, thesegment in this book on the Germ Theory and the treatment of the common cold.

Commenting on the theory of vaccination, Annemarie Colbin, PhD in *Food and Healing* writes:

> Modern vaccination theory is, at its core, a hybrid of Jenner's and Pasteur's models. It claims that microorganisms cause disease, and the way to avoid a particular disease is to introduce the disease artificially so that the body can set up defenses in the event that the "real" disease shows up later. A healthy immune system creates antibodies in the blood to specific diseases, and these antibodies depend on what we have been exposed to in the environment since birth. Vaccines introduce the microorganisms, either live or inactivated, to provoke the body's production of antibodies to that disease. Vaccination theory posits that a vaccine offers "protection against an infectious disease by inducing a mild attack of the disease beforehand." The theory also assumes that the body will react to the introduction of the disease by setting up a defense mechanism, or immunity, to that same disease only; the theory ignores or mimimizes other reactions.
>
> Proponents of the vaccination schedule also argue that aggressive vaccination is necessary to maintain "herd immunity." This theory, according to the Centers for Disease Control and Prevention (CDC) and the World Health Organization (WHO), holds that if a high percentage, between eighty-five and ninety-six percent, of the population is immunized, they will protect the unimmunized.
>
> This theory ignores many crucial facts: In many outbreaks, a significant portion of those contracting the disease have been vaccinated; for certain vaccines, recipients may shed the virus following the vaccination, risking the spread of disease; and vaccination does not prevent individuals from being carriers of a disease although they may remain asymptomatic. (Ibid p. 193-94)

There are multiple problems with this theory. First, and foremost, there have been *no peer-reviewed, randomized, double-blind, placebo-controlled scientific studies carried out to prove that vaccination even works, nor are there any studies comparing vaccinated and non-vaccinated populations.* This is due in part to ethical issues involving using children in human studies. Perhaps a larger problem comes from the financial gains that would be jeapordized if the truth came out.

> The late pediatrician/author Dr. Robert Mendelsohn was adamantly opposed to mass vaccination. He noted that while we attribute the end of polio epidemics in the 1940s and 1950s to vaccination programs, polio ended simultaneously in Europe where people did not use the vaccine extensively. Diseases are known to be cyclical, and some, such as bubonic plague, and scarlet fever, have disappeared without any vaccinations whatsoever. This fact weakens the claims about vaccines' effectiveness in preventing epidemics. (Ibid p. 196)

Improved hygiene, better quality in the food supply, and even modern plumbing and waste removal may be the most responsible components in reducing infectious diseases. Proving this simple point with regard to childbed fever, Dr. Ignaz Semmelweis discovered that mortality rates were reduced ten-fold when doctors (often coming from dissection labs or autopsy rooms) washed their hands with a chlorine solution between patients. His hand-washing suggestion in the hospital was initially met with scorn and rejection, so much so that he lost his position, only later to be vindicated and proven correct. In another example, Dr. Thomas McKeown, states in his book *The Modern Rise of Population* that "vaccinations were introduced **after** (my emphasis) infectious diseases, such as whooping cough and measles, had declined by about ninety percent." He points out that "of much higher impact was the increase in the available food supply leading to improved nutrition," as well as "the purification of water, efficient sewage disposal, and improved food hygiene, particularly the pasteurization of milk, the item in the diet most likely to spread disease."(Ibid p. 195-97) This demonstrates a pattern found in the medical field. Arthur Schopenhauer, famous

German philosopher, lamented that "All truth passes through three stages. First, it is ridiculed. Second, it is violently opposed. Third, it is accepted as being self-evident."

Pediatrician and author Mendelsohn also stated "there is no convincing scientific evidence that mass inoculation eliminated any disease" calling immunizations "a medical time bomb" and urging parents to "reject all vaccinations for their children." He also believed vaccines to be at the heart of the rise in autoimmune diseases in the United States in this century. (Ibid p. 99) If you do the research, you will find a long list of brilliant doctors, researchers, authors and others who feel the same way. Professor Richard DeLong, a retired microbiologist has been warning the medical community since the 1960s of the dangers of live or attenuated viral vaccines. These vaccines, he warned, can cause mutations, chromosomal aberrations, birth defects, cancer, and new diseases. (Ibid p.199)

Plan ahead before having children. Review the literature. Read *Vaccine Epidemic*. Get to know the facts about vaccinations before you make a decision based on ignorance, fear and haste. *Fear of the Invisible* by investigative reporter Janine Roberts is a wonderful book to help new parents make informed decisions. I have listed further resources in the back of this book. Do not believe everything the media says, especially when fear is being used to drive people to action. Vaccines are not effective and safe as we have been led to believe. The parent should determine what is allowed into the child's body. I was able to do this for my entire family as well as for friends and patients who listened and trusted me. We used traditional, unprocessed foods, sound nutrition, good hygiene practices and plenty of love. You owe it to yourself and, most importantly, to your child. For a list of individual state laws and requirements for opting out, see Appendix D p. 356 #9. Ignorance is not an excuse. If you choose not to vaccinate, you must also shun the SAD and opt for a traditional diet of unprocessed foods.

Dealing with Picky Eaters

For over a half-century I have counseled patients on how to deal with children who are picky eaters. Most picky eaters have been created by their parents. For many, it begins the day the decision is made whether or not to breast-feed. Research published in *Pediatrics* in April of 2004 found that "early introduction to different flavors may alter food preferences later in life. Breast milk exposes infants early on to different flavors through a mother's varied diet. This is now believed to encourage a wider palate later in life."(Mennella JA, Griffin CE, Beauchamp GK. Flavor programming during infancy. Pediatrics. 2004 April; 113(4):840-845.) Remember, whatever you eat, your baby eats too. If your baby is commercial formula-fed then his or her nutritional health is already off to a bad start. So whatever you do, start with breastfeeding. If you are having trouble breastfeeding, try some of the suggestions in *Nourishing Traditions*. Pump and freeze your breast milk if you have to. And if you absolutely cannot breast feed, then use the homemade formula recipes recommended in *Nourishing Traditions*.

For toddlers, sitting down to meals together as a family is very important. In our home, we sat down to meals together as a family as much as possible. This encouraged the family to bond and to share food. This is especially important for toddlers, as laying a foundation of different flavors and textures begins before they develop the control to choose for themselves. Jen Albritton, CN writes in *Wise Traditions*,Vol 7, No 3, p. 59, "A study reported in the Archives of Family Medicine found that kids who regularly sit down with their families for an evening meal make wiser food choices, eat more vegetables, and get more nutrients than those who do not." Some parents feed their young children large amounts of sweets (whether from fruits, juices, cereals, or formulas loaded with sugar). When youngsters are given whatever is "convenient" or "easy," it sabotages their taste buds and sets them up to be picky eaters. In Albritton's article "Taking the Icky Out of Picky Eaters." *Wise Traditions*, Vol. 7, No.3 Fall 2006, she gives the reader excellent suggestions on how to deal with picky eaters. The book is available from the Weston A. Price website at www.westonaprice.org .

My children were fortunate enough to have access to a garden in their yard. I included them in my garden work, from planting seeds, to weeding, and harvesting. This way they established an intimate relationship with the food put on the table, where it comes from, and the work it takes to provide it for our family. Gardening makes food fun and teaches children where real nourishing food comes from. Even planting a few potted herbs or tomatoes on the balcony or window sill can serve as a starting point for nourishing your children and establishing better eating habits.

Children need variety. They especially need fats and protein from wholesome, homemade foods to fuel the growth of their young brains. Cook your meals at home as much as possible. A simple wholesome, traditional dinner is a start. How you prepare makes all the difference. Stock your refrigerator and cabinets with wholesome foods and snacks so that you are prepared when your children are looking for food. Also remember that you are the boss. Establish ground rules without being too forceful. Reward your child when appropriate, but be firm and you will build a foundation of health and structure for a lifetime.

SECTION XVI
ATTENTION DISORDERS:
ATTENTION DEFICIT DISORDER (ADD) ATTENTION DEFICIT HYPERACTIVITY DISORDER (ADHD) OPPOSITIONAL DEFIANT DISORDER (ODD)

ADD/ ADHD/ ODD

I want to discuss these three topics together. I think they are close cousins caused by the same problems: poor gut health, food allergies, overuse of antibiotics and vaccines and poor eating habits — specifically too much sugar. My approach is centered on what is now known as a 4 Rs approach explained in detail at the end of this section. It is important to work with a physician well-versed in the 4 Rs approach so that he/she can individualize it to your specific needs. Better yet, find a physician familiar with the GAPS Diet developed by Dr. Natasha Campbell-McBride.

Over the years many pioneers like Dr. Royal Lee, Dr. Weston A. Price, Dr. John Pagano, Elaine Gottschall, William Dufty, Natasha Campbell-McBride, Sally Fallon-Morrell, Mary Enig, and many more have contributed pieces to a larger puzzle that has become the 4 Rs approach. No one person can take credit for it. And when it is applied judiciously and correctly, there is no greater healing mechanism.

To diagnose these disorders, the first place we look as chiropractors is the spine. Subluxations tell us a lot about the body because the spine is a relay station from all regions of the body up to the brain (afferent) and from the brain back out to the body (efferent). Therefore, the spine can be used as a wonderful diagnostic tool to identify what areas of digestion and even what specific glands are involved. So first and foremost, a spinal evaluation is performed to isolate subluxations and identify structural imbalances. X-rays may be needed in some cases involving scoliosis, injury, etc. From there, the information can be correlated with the information from the history and from nutritional and functional testing.

Without exception children with ODD, ADD, and ADHD must first have very specific functional testing done to identify the condition of the gastrointestinal lining (inflammation, parasites, predominant and pathogenic bacteria and yeast), digestive function, food allergies like gluten sensitivity, pH and more. As with previous tests we use Genova Diagnostics Labs stool analysis or CDSA (Complete Digestive Stool Analysis). From there we can custom design a plan of attack that may require natural antibiotics, anti-fungals, digestive enzymes and other gut-healing nutrients. See below for our 4 Rs approach including the various supplements we typically use. If food allergies are suspected we will order an IgG and/or IgE food allergy panel known as the Allergix panel (again by Genova Diagnostics Labs). This will eliminate guesswork and make custom tailoring the diet much easier for both the clinician and the parents.

The first test we typically order is known as the GI Effects Stool Profile. This test uses advanced microbial DNA analysis to improve the accuracy of what was once an unreliable test. Anaerobic bacteria comprise over 95% of the bacteria in the gut and are difficult to detect with old culture methods. Furthermore, using DNA analysis, the specimen taken is placed in a fixative tube that stops microbial growth and offers a highly accurate snapshot of the microbial balance in the gut. This gives us a very important look at the environment of the gastrointestinal tract and enables us to make crucial decisions as to our protocol.

Typically we see what is termed dysbiosis, or literally "abnormal life." Dysbiosis occurs as a result of poor diet, increasing use of cesarean sections, as well as the overuse of antibiotics and other drugs on children at a very early age. The term dysbiosis was originally introduced in the early 1900s by Russian-born biologist Dr. Elie Metchnikoff to describe an imbalance of the bacteria in the gut. Metchnikoff was famously known to say, "Death begins in the gut!" In 1908, Metchnikoff was awarded the Nobel Prize for his work on friendly bacterial flora (E Lipsky. Leaky gut syndrome: what to do about a health threat that can cause arthritis, allergies and a host of other illnesses. New York:McGraw Hill; 1998, p.18). He introduced the idea that fermented milk products could prove beneficial to the gut, inhibiting bacterial infection. Metchnikoff believed that the root of most illness came from intestinal bacteria decomposing protein in the bowel. Lactic acid producing bacteria were believed to stunt the production of the pathogenic bacteria.

Antibiotic usage for ear infections, colds, etc. comes with dire long-term consequences of which the public is often unaware. These antibiotics destroy all of the beneficial bacteria responsible for protecting the intestinal lining and maintaining its integrity. As a result, the intestine is exposed to toxins produced by these pathogenic bacteria. If there is enough damage to the intestinal lining over time, the toxins can get into the bloodstream and wreak havoc. The stool analysis allows us to see more clearly what type of environment is present in the gut, and what steps we may need to take to move the patient back to health.

A second important test for ADD/ADHD and ODD patients is the Fatty Acid Profile. Today's Standard American Diet is overwhelmingly imbalanced in the area of fatty acids. Specifically, it allows children and adults to consume far too many processed vegetable oils high in omega-6 (Ω-6) fats and far too low in omega-3 (Ω-3) fats. Although both types of fats are needed by the body, it is the imbalance that makes controlling inflammation and cell signaling difficult. Many researchers feel that it is this variable which differs so greatly from our Paleolithic ancestors and is responsible for many of the degenerative and cognitive diseases of our time.

In their book *Perfect Health Diet*, (pp. 59, 75), Paul and Shou-Ching Jaminet note that Ω-6 polyunsaturated fats are healthful in modest amounts — at the levels contained in meat, fish and eggs — but become toxic in excess. The authors point out that clinical trials have repeatedly shown that reducing the Ω-6 to Ω-3 ratio relieves depression, improves mood disorders, decreases anger and anxiety, reduces aggression, and can improve cognitive functioning. Although ranges vary, it is generally held that our Paleolithic ancestors had a ratio of between 1:1 and 2:1 Ω-6 to Ω-3. Shockingly, the SAD today provides the average person with a ratio of between 10:1 and 20:1 depending on the research you look at.

When we combine this with a mentality that foolishly shuns healthy saturated fats and cholesterol from sources like raw pastured butter, coconut oil, and pastured animal products, while consuming excessive amounts of refined carbohydrates and sugars, we have a recipe for cognitive dysfunction. Even though EPA and DHA (Ω-3 fish oils) get most of the press today, saturated fats are an important part of the equation as well. As Fallon points out, saturated fatty acids are crucial for proper utilization of essential fatty acids, enhance the immune system and constitute at least 50% of the cell membranes (Fallon S, Enig MG. Nourishing Traditions. p. 11). These are three of the most important benefits of saturated fats regarding ADD/ADHD and ODD. Without saturated fats, our cells cannot maintain their form, function, or their structural integrity. Interestingly, in early 2015 the FDA acknowledged that it is not saturated fats but the trans fats found in industrial vegetable oils that are linked to disease.

Cholesterol and saturated fats are so crucial to our body's natural functioning that if we do not consume them in our diet, they can be made by the body from sugar (Erasmus U. Fats that heal, fats that kill: the complete guide to fats, oils, cholesterol and human weight. Burnaby BC Canada: Alive Book Publishing; 1998. p. 35). For the most part, consumable cholesterol comes from animals and animal products where saturated fats are also found. Cholesterol has been conclusively shown to be vital to the functioning of the brain. As pointed out by Enig and Fallon, cholesterol is needed for proper function of serotonin receptors in the brain, and low cholesterol levels are associated with aggressive and violent behavior. Is it any wonder that one of the common, major side effects of statin drugs, which lower cholesterol, is cognitive impairment?

More importantly, mother's milk is especially rich in cholesterol and contains a special enzyme that helps the baby utilize this nutrient. Babies and children need cholesterol-rich foods throughout their growing years to ensure proper development of the brain and nervous system (Wise Traditions. Heart Disease Issue. p. 24). Fallon adds emphasis to this, stating "Mother's milk provides a higher proportion of cholesterol than almost any other food. It also contains over 50% of its calories as fat, much of it saturated fat. Both cholesterol and saturated fat are essential for growth in babies and children, especially the development of the brain (Fallon S, Enig MG. Nourishing Traditions. p. 6).

If the infant is denied breastfeeding and given an infant formula depleted in crucial nutrients, is it any wonder that we have an ADD/ADHD, ODD epidemic? We should be looking at how we are raising and feeding our children before readily giving them Ritalin, lithium, Wellbutrin and other toxic drugs.

Research shows that fat may be the most crucial nutrient with regard to brain function. Chris Masterjohn points out deficiency consequences in *Meat, Organs, Bones and Skin: Nutrition for Mental Health*.

> There are a number of potential deficiencies and imbalances that could develop on a diet devoid of nutrient-dense animal foods: some people may become deficient in cholesterol if they do not make enough of their own; plant goitrogens, some of which require vitamin B12 and sulfur amino acids for their detoxification, could contribute to thyroid problems; deficiencies of vitamin B6, long-chain omega-6 and omega-3 fatty acids, zinc and fat-soluble vitamins A, D, and K_2 could also develop. This article, however, will focus on the role of vitamin B12, sulfur amino acids, and glycine in supporting and regulating a process known as methylation, which is critical for mental health. (Masterjohn C. Meat, organs, bones and skin: Nutrition for mental health. Wise Traditions. WAPF. 2013 Spring;14(1):40.)

Both organic acid testing (to identify B6 deficiency) and the fatty acid test are crucial parts of evaluating these points and the patient for specific imbalances. This type of testing enables more specific corrections in diet and supplements, and gives a better understanding of the diet plan for the patient.

Methylation, or adding a methyl group (one carbon atom, three hydrogens) to another compound, is an important process in how the body regulates compounds such as creatine and the neurotransmitter dopamine. Dopamine is critical for mental stability as well as focus and attention. Information presented on ADHD from WebMD states:

> Recent studies show that the brain chemical, dopamine, may play a role in ADHD. Dopamine is an important chemical that carries signals between nerves in the brain. It is linked to many functions, including movement, sleep, mood, attention, and learning. Another dopamine study involving adults with ADHD showed that adults with ADHD had a sluggish dopamine system. The study helped explain why

stimulant ADHD medications such as Ritalin and Adderall are beneficial. Stimulant ADHD medications increase dopamine by strengthening the weak dopamine signals in the brain. That counters the decreased brain dopamine activity in adults with ADHD.

Masterjohn points out the effects of controlling methylation with regard to dopamine, stating, "methylation regulates the balance between mental stability and mental flexibility: too much methylation will favor too much flexibility, not enough methylation will favor too much stability, and the level of methylation that is just right will provide the appropriate balance between the two." "Thus," he notes, "our goal is not to increase methylation or decrease methylation, but to provide our brains with the raw materials they need to regulate the process properly." How does this translate to our diets? Quite simply, it points the arrow in the direction of including nutrient-dense animal foods. But not just the meat we are used to eating. We must, as Masterjohn goes on to point out, include glycine-rich skin and bones (in the form of bone broth) in the diet.

Interestingly, the majority of studies performed looking at the relationship between vegetarianism and mental disorders found that "vegetarians are more likely to suffer from mental disorders at least in part because nutrient-dense animal foods are required for optimal mental health."(Ibid p. 53-54) In considering today's children, we see that their diets are overloaded with sugar. This excess serves to deplete vital minerals and vitamins like zinc, magnesium, vitamin B6 and many others.

An important point to note is that neither a vegetarian diet nor omnivorous diet is necessarily suitable when dealing with mental illnesses. However, if the diet is geared more toward vegans, there is a greater likelihood for mental illness. "People who exclude all animal products from their diets thus likely consume three to five times less methionine than those who eat a diet rich in animal products, leading to a dramatic decrease in the raw materials needed for methylation." (Masterjohn C. Meat, organs, bones and skin: nutrition for mental health. Wise Traditions. WAPF. 2013 Spring; 14(1):40.)

Saturated fats and cholesterol are crucial to healthy brain function. So is reducing the amount of sugar in the diets of children and adults. Clinical research has proven that destructive, aggressive and restless behavior is significantly correlated with the amount of sugar that is consumed, according to Jen Allbritton in "Zapping Sugar Cravings" (Wise Traditions. 2010 Winter;11(4)53). When you combine excessive sugar with a lack of healthy fat/overabundance of unhealthy fat in the SAD, you have a recipe for behavioral disorders. Allbritton emphasizes that, "The main reason for this is the fact that refined carbohydrates, which include sugar and its cousin white flour, cause hypoglycemia [**as a reaction to the initial surge in blood sugar** — my emphasis], or low blood sugar. Because glucose (blood sugar) is the primary fuel for the brain, when blood levels are too low, the brain is affected first."(Ibid pp. 53-54) She explains the process in more detail:

> The chain of events goes something like this: a soda drink or other sugary food is consumed and blood sugar rapidly goes up, the body releases insulin in response, and the sudden increase in insulin causes a drop in blood glucose. This yo-yo scenario stresses the body, causing a fight-or-flight response, which involves a rapid increase in adrenaline. Both the low blood sugar and surge of adrenaline exacerbate aggressive behavior and contribute to hyperactivity, anxiety and attention difficulties. (Ibid p. 54)

Also, overconsumption of sugar causes a loss of the alkaline ash minerals calcium and magnesium whose functions are to calm the nervous system and maintain proper blood pH.

In conclusion, depending on the situation and the specific needs of the patient, allergy testing may be necessary to identify food sensitivities so common in patients with leaky gut and digestive dysfunction. We use the Allergix IgG4 and IgE food testing through Genova Diagnostics Labs. The IgG4 test can reveal food reactions due to intestinal permeability (leaky gut) issues. Because they are distinct from IgE-mediated allergies, we describe them as "food sensitivities." IgG4 antibodies are associated with delayed hypersensitivity reactions. Symptoms may not appear until hours or even days after ingesting the offending foods. Though these are the most common food reactions, they are the most difficult type to detect. These profiles allow us to design appropriate diets that exclude the offending foods.

The following is our basic dietary framework for treating ADD/ADHD and ODD. Not everyone is the same. In some patients, yeast (candidiasis caused by candida albicans) may be the central player that needs to be addressed. In others, food sensitivities or fatty acid imbalances may require specific dietary changes and supplementation with cod liver oil or even flax seed oil. Still in others, vitamin B6 may be a crucial nutrient needed supplementally. If other nutrient/metabolic imbalances are suspected, we may order an Organic Acids test as well. Regardless, we begin with our 4 Rs approach as outlined below and make specific adaptations for the individual patient as needed.

The 4 Rs Cleansing Protocol (Dysbiosis)

This cleansing protocol is broken into three distinct phases, each several weeks long; the duration of each phase, ultimately determined by the physician, will vary based on the individual patient, severity of the case and compliance of the patient. Phase one, weeks 1–6, is an initial dietary cleansing in which all digestively difficult and harmful foods are removed from the diet. This phase removes all animal products and overly starchy foods to take the burden off of the digestive system and therefore the immune system as well. It is mostly a liquid diet to allow the body to "rest" digestively, further allowing the body to devote its energy toward cleansing the intestines, liver and other organ systems. Much of the diet will be in a liquefied form, i.e. shakes and soups to further aid in simplifying the digestive process. The key ingredient in this phase is bone stock made from beef, chicken, fish or vegetables. These stocks are very nutritious, easy to digest, and healing to the inflamed digestive tract.

Several supplements are used to promote ease of digestion and elimination of harmful microbes such as yeast and pathogenic/opportunistic bacteria. A broad spectrum digestive enzyme is used to facilitate complete breakdown of all foods. Also, depending on the patient's specific needs and in some cases test results, a natural antibiotic and/or antifungal is used to treat the dysbiosis.

Phase two, weeks 7–12, reintroduces organic, preferably pastured animal protein in the form of wild-caught fish, chicken and eggs. Since each patient is an individual, the time frames vary. The important point to remember is what each phase is designed to do. You must work with a qualified practitioner who can assess your individual needs and progress, and to determine timing. As previously noted, the best animal products are those from healthy, pastured animals raised without the use of antibiotics or hormones and fed their natural diet. To promote better digestion and to facilitate the cleansing process, this second phase involves the use of supplements, the most important of which is the probiotic. It helps restore the natural balance of healthy gut flora which protects the intestinal tract and immune system. Furthermore, herbs such as okra pepsin and edible clay (montmorillonite/bentonite clay) are used to give the intestinal lining a "scrubbing" and promote better contact of the intestinal villi with the food and therefore more complete digestion. Lastly, the use of colonics and/or enemas is encouraged to further facilitate the cleansing of the intestines.

Phase three, weeks 13–19 and beyond, consists of providing further nourishment to the body to promote a rebuilding including prebiotics and probiotics. The diet is broadened to include a wider variety of healthy traditional food choices including lacto-fermented foods such as raw yogurts, kefir, kombucha, and others.

Treatment Using the 4 Rs Program for Intestinal Health

The 4 Rs program is not a new concept and has been around for decades in holistic therapy circles. It is a framework which, when applied on an individual basis, can be very effective at restoring the health and function of the gastrointestinal lining and therefore the health of the patient. I have used it successfully to treat all types of conditions ranging from chronic fatigue syndrome, IBS, and even "incurable" autoimmune illnesses. I have used it to successfully treat my own mother who, for multiple reasons was stricken with polymyalgia rheumatica. At 75 years old, she had degenerated from completely healthy to the point where she could not walk without a cane, could no longer drive her car and suffered with terrible muscle pains in her arms and legs that limited her ability to move in a normal way. As a result she began to wither away, going from 120 pounds down to 95 pounds within a few short weeks. After extensive medical testing (including bloodwork and CT scans) she was told by a medical physician and long-time friend that there was no cure and she would have to take prednisone to treat her illness. Within 3 months of implementing the 4 Rs approach, and with some simple nutritional testing mentioned earlier, she was back to her healthy self.

The 4 Rs program is generally defined by the following:

Remove offending foods, medications and gluten (if sensitive) and reduce poor quality fats, refined carbohydrates, sugars and industrially fermented foods (if yeast is present). Consider antimicrobial, antifungal and/or antiparasitic therapies in the case of opportunistic/pathogenic bacterial, yeast, and/or parasitic overgrowth.

Replace what is needed for normal digestion and absorption such as betaine HCL, pancreatic enzymes, herbs that aid in digestion such as bitters, deglycyrrhizinated licorice and marshmallow root, dietary fiber, and water.

Reinoculate with favorable microbes (probiotics such as Lactobacillus spp., Bifidobacter spp., and Saccharomyces boulardii). To enhance the growth of the favorable bacteria, supplement with prebiotics such as inulin, xylooligosachharides, larch arabinogalactans, beta glucan, and fiber. Eventually introduce lacto-fermented foods and beverages to aid in the restoration of the normal, healthy bacterial flora through better food choices rather than supplements.

Repair mucosal lining by giving support to healthy intestinal mucosal cells, goblet cells, and to the immune system. Consider L-glutamine, essential fatty acids, zinc, pantothenic acid and vitamin C.

Weeks 1–6: Dietary Simplification/Rest Phase

Supplements

1. Digestive Enzyme – Use either Multizyme® (Standard Process) or digestive enzyme containing betaine HCL (*to be determined*

by the physician) at a dosage of one per meal. This will facilitate the proper breakdown of your food. ***Continue this supplement during and after the cleanse.***

2. Gastrofiber® (Standard Process) – Take three capsules 3 times a day with any of your meals throughout the day. *Once finished with 2 bottles, most patients may discontinue.*

3. GI-Microb-X™ (Designs For Health) – This will help to eliminate pathogenic bacteria and parasites. Take two capsules 3 times a day on an empty stomach. *This product will be continued until the physician determines that it is appropriate to stop.*

4. Candicid Forte (Ortho Molecular) or Candidase (Enzymedica) – take two capsules, 3 times a day on an empty stomach. This is a specific product to treat yeast (Candida) overgrowth. *Necessity will be determined by the physician based on test results.*

Breakfast Choices

1. **Fruit** (low sugar only – see vegetable/fruit list) – including stewed prunes or apricots; baked apple or pear; mixed berries; papaya; Asian pear; grapefruit; lemon. Fruits may be spread throughout the morning and should not be mixed. Leave 45 minutes minimum between fruits. If you eat any other food first, you must wait 2–3 hours to eat the fruit.

2. **Eggs** (preferably pastured, organic, found at Whole Foods or through a local CSA) – you may eat the eggs soft-cooked or lightly scrambled using butter or ghee *or* you may make a green vegetable omelet (see vegetable list).

3. **Vegetarian Shake** (Rice-based-hypoallergenic–Standard Process) (SP Complete® Dairy Free/InflammaCore – OrthoMolecular) – many delicious shake recipes may be made using low-sugar fruits and flax seed oil. You may also use PaleoMeal Dairy Free by Designs for Health or Ultra Meal by Metagenics. Ask medical professional for sources and where to purchase. *You CANNOT use SP Complete® if you have a known milk allergy or have tested positive for an IgG4 reaction to casein or milk. In this case you MUST use the Dairy Free version known as SP Complete® DF or InflammaCore shake which are rice based. Also,* see shake recipe list provided by our office.

Lunch Choices:

1. Mixed Green Vegetable Salad with Homemade Dressing – using extra virgin, cold-pressed olive oil, lemon juice, fresh cracked pepper, Barlean's or Udo's Flax Oil and Celtic sea salt as a dressing. Add fresh spinach, avocado, peppers, cucumber, etc to your liking according to the vegetable list provided.

2. Cucumber Salad – puree or mash avocado; remove seeds from cucumber and mix; chop up some red onion; add some fresh lemon juice to taste; fresh oregano; olive oil and organic unpasteurized apple cider vinegar *(Do not use vinegar if you are diagnosed with yeast/candida by the physician)*. You may also add cherry tomato if you desire. Unpasteurized apple cider vinegar can be purchased at Whole Foods (Bragg's Apple Cider Vinegar) or at the following website: www.healthalertstore.com.

3. Lentils or Brown Rice Stir Fry – Lentils and rice (basmati, wild, or brown) must be soaked overnight in warm water to improve digestibility (see directions in *Nourishing Traditions*). It can be done simply by adding 2 tbsp of lemon juice per cup. Use one serving (1/4 cup rice *or* ½ cup lentils) Soak overnight and then drain off water. Add fresh water and cook as per directions on box/bag. Use organic raw pastured butter or ghee from Udder Milk Creamery and add steamed or sautéed vegetables of your liking. You must add at least one green vegetable.

4. Blended Green Vegetable Soup – using zucchini, escarole, cauliflower, kale, broccoli, asparagus, brussel sprouts, broccoli rabe, and other vegetables from the lower-starch list provided in Appendix G p. 367. (No potatoes, rice, or beans). You are encouraged to make your own homemade broth preparing the soup as given in the directions from the *Nourishing Traditions* cookbook by Sally Fallon. *If you do not want to make your own broth, I recommend using Pacific Organic Chicken or Vegetable Broth* **or** *Nature's Promise bonebroths which are free of MSG. Also, use herbs like oregano, garlic, and others as long as they are fresh and not too spicy or hot. For information about using other vegetables, ask the physician.*

Dinner Choices:

1. SP Complete® Shake/InflammaCore Shake – refer to the shake list in Appendix C p. 346 and following.

Nutritional Shake Recipes

Whey protein (cow) based options:

Tips: Adding a half or quarter of a ripe avocado to your shake will make it smooth and thicker in texture rather than watery.

Use Nutiva or Native Forest brand Coconut Cream/Water or Milk available at Whole Foods and in health food stores.

Rice/Hemp Protein in the form of Warrior Food Extreme, LifeCore, or Inflammacore (by OrthoMolecular) may be substituted for the whey protein in any of the shakes for those seeking hypoallergenic protein (Dairy Allergy) or as directed by the physician. They come in a variety of flavors.

For the dairy-sensitive, substitute coconut milk/water *or* you may use your own homemade almond milk in any shake above. (See the book *Nourishing Traditions* for recipe.)

For a more complete meal replacement shake, use either PaleoMeal protein from Designs for Health in place of Whey Cool *or* K-Pax Fuel of Life Protein Blend by OrthoMolecular.

For those with more serious gastrointestinal issues, food allergies, etc. Warrior Food, Inflammacore (OrthoMolecular) are the best choices for the protein source for the shakes above.

GT's Kombucha is available at Whole Foods or Fairway Markets.

Experiment with recipes by adding Flax Seed Oil (Udo's or Barlean's), Pure Radiance Vitamin C, Raw Honey, Calcifood® Powder, etc.

2. Vegetable Soup as above or any of the aforementioned salads from lunch suggestions – with ¼ cup of rice (basmati, wild or brown) *or* ½ cup lentils. Use butter, preferably pastured, raw butter from Uddermilk.com. Pastured butter is also available at Whole Foods, though it is not as good because it is pasteurized.

In this phase, patients are encouraged to drink homemade bone broths like a tea, having several cups throughout the day. This will promote faster healing of the digestive tract.

Weeks 7-12: Gastrointestinal/Liver Cleansing Phase

Supplements

1. Probiotic 225 – a special high-potency probiotic product made by OrthoMolecular specifically for treating dysbiosis. There are 15 packets. Take one a day mixed in water. When the box is finished, transition to Ortho Biotic at a dose of one capsule/day.
2. Digestive Enzyme – continue as in Phase One
3. Cholacol® II (Standard Process) – Take two tablets, 3 times a day with a glass of water just prior to each meal. *When finished with the bottle, you may discontinue.*
4. Okra Pepsin (Standard Process) – Take two capsules, 3 times a day each meal. *When finished with the bottle, you may discontinue.*
5. GastroMend-HP (Designs For Health) – Take two capsules, 2 times a day on an empty stomach 10–15 minutes before you eat. *When finished with the bottle, you may discontinue.*

Dietary Changes

This phase reintroduces animal proteins in the form of organic, preferably pastured chicken and wild-caught fish. Bake, broil, steam, grill or sauté as you like. The animal proteins you are adding must be consumed with two green vegetables from the list *or* one green vegetable and a small salad. In more severe cases of gastrointestinal inflammation, salads may be restricted due to difficulty of digestion. Use the dressing suggested in Lunch Choices #1 for the salad. Feel free to use garlic, oregano, parsley and other natural herbs and spices to flavor. *All foods should be cooked in ghee, organic raw butter or coconut oil or lard/tallow.*

Colonic Cleansing

What is an enema/colonic, and what is its purpose regarding the general headache? An enema, or colonic, is a procedure by which sterilized water or other fluid is gently circulated through the intestinal tract and allowed to "wash" out the contents. It is very important to understand one main facet of our digestive tract. It is estimated that over 65%–75% of our body's total immune system is located throughout the intestinal tract. Every inch of our digestive tract is covered with specialized immune cells specifically to protect the barrier between the outside world (the lumen of the intestine) and what is truly the inside of our body (the bloodstream and cells of the organs and tissues themselves). Therefore, regarding detoxification of the body as a whole, it is logical to start in the intestinal tract which is the main barrier protecting us from toxins waiting to enter into our bloodstream and wreak havoc. These toxins come not only from the foods we eat (i.e., preservatives, colorings, fillers, flavoring agents like MSG, trans fats and other man-made additives) and the air we breathe, but also from some of the bacteria that inhabit our intestine. Harmful bacteria not kept under the control of the immune system release toxins (often byproducts of their own metabolism) that are harmful to our body.

Understanding the importance of the intimate interrelationship between our intestinal/digestive tract and our immune system is very important. Because of this relationship we use the enema/colonic as a tool to support both functions. In doing so, we use an enema/colonic to facilitate better elimination of waste through a "washing" of the intestinal contents and therefore removing some of the toxic burden facing the immune system.

The kit for performing an enema can be purchased at most good drug stores or pharmacies as well as from www.enemakit.com. The kit is made up of a hot water bottle (usually a rubber bag with a screw-in plug at the top), a small rubber hose with a tip, and a douche attachment. You simply fill the bag with 12–16 ozs. of sterilized water for an adult; boil the water, cover it and let it cool to room temperature or use organic coffee (the same is done for the coffee; it is brewed and then covered and allowed to cool to at least a luke-warm or room temperature). Using coffee may sound strange but coffee has an excellent detoxification effect when used in this manner. Furthermore, coffee introduces an acidic medium to the digestive tract, making it inhospitable to many of the pathogenic bacteria that are responsible for causing disease. The procedure is in Appendix A p. 321-22.

This procedure should be repeated once every evening for approximately one week. If the condition is severe, then it must be done twice per day for one week. Consult with your alternative physician if you are unsure. An important concept here is the establishment of normal, regular, cyclical bowel movements. Our bodies are not meant to hold onto waste, especially in the intestinal tract. Three bowel movements per day is ideal considering that we normally eat three times per day. Furthermore, bowel movements are supposed to be more buoyant in nature. If they are not, this is an indication that you are not digesting your food properly and/or are not getting the adequate nutrition from your food. The dietary recommendations discussed earlier in this book and here provide the framework necessary for accomplishing this goal.

Once the enema protocol is completed, a strict focus on dietary changes must be made. The diet should temporarily be changed to a higher carbohydrate type consisting of whole foods. Breakfast should be ripe fruits spread out throughout the morning. A different type may be eaten every 45 minutes to an hour, but do not mix fruit types at any one time. Lunch should consist of a starch meal including either a sweet potato, brown or wild rice, or lentils combined with two green vegetables (all legumes, beans, grains, nuts and seeds should be soaked to remove antinutrients and enable proper digestion; see Appendix C for soaking instructions). Dinner is to include a small salad of mixed greens. Make your own dressing from olive oil, flax seed oil, unpasteurized organic apple cider vinegar, fresh lemon, celtic sea salt, mashed avocado (optional) and fresh cracked pepper. With the salad have two steamed or lightly sautéed green vegetables and a small 6–8 oz. piece of protein (either fish, chicken, turkey, or lamb). Nuts may be taken as a snack but they must be soaked first and then dried in an oven on low temperature or in a dehydrator (see Appendix C for soaking instructions). Nuts must be organic and purchased in sealed packages not from open bins.

Weeks 13 and Beyond: Intestinal Rebuilding and Maintenance Principles:

This phase requires the use of naturally fermented/lactofermented foods such as yogurt, kefir, sauerkraut and kvass. For guidance use the book *Nourishing Traditions* by Fallon available at Amazon.com. Your regimen during this week is to continue with the diet as in Phase II. However, you must make use of the following foods, all of which can be ordered from Uddermilk.com (go to their website and become a member; they deliver directly to you) or from Westonaprice.org. For more information, consult with the physician.

1. Raw organic pastured yogurt – This may be eaten for breakfast with mixed berries or plain. You may also use this as the base for shakes and smoothies.

2. Raw organic pastured milk/kefir – This is an excellent adjunct for making delicious shakes.

3. Sauerkraut and other lacto-fermented vegetables – all recipes are found in the book *Nourishing Traditions* and are quite simple to make. *Include at least one lacto-fermented vegetable a day.* Many of these foods can be purchased from local farms or CSAs (Community Supported Agriculture). To find availability, contact the Weston A. Price Foundation to reach a representative in your area (See Appendix D for information on the Weston A. Price Foundation).

Supplements

1. ProSynbiotic (Standard Process) – can be purchased from the doctor or at Vitamin Shoppe and other health food stores. Take one a day on an empty stomach for the first week and then increase slowly up to four each day until the bottle is finished. Take a maintenance dose of one a day.
2. Digestive Enzyme – Take as recommended in weeks 1–6.
3. Blue Ice™ Fermented Cod Liver Oil (can be purchased at several websites. Ask physician for sources) – Take at a dosage of four a day in divided doses with food.
4. Catalyn® (Standard Process' MultiVitamin) – three a day taken one per meal.
5. Congaplex® (Standard Process) – Take two capsules every 2-3 waking hours for the entire week. Then decrease to three a day.

Dietary Changes

In this phase, nuts, seeds, whole grains like steel cut oatmeal, and beans may be introduced *as long as they are soaked*. Directions can be found in Appendix C and in *Nourishing Traditions*. Soaking makes foods much more digestible by freeing the nutrients for absorption by the body. Some people may not be able to digest some nuts and beans despite proper soaking. Always listen to your body and consult with the physician should any symptoms such as gas, bloating, or itchy throat occur.

Resources

1. Nourishing Traditions, by Sally Fallon – both a cookbook and an educational tool teaching the basics on traditional foods. Its excellent resources guide in the back helps locate needed products.

2. Ghee – Pure Indian Foods Ghee can be ordered online at pureindianfoods.com. This brand has great taste, quality and is made from grass-fed organic dairy.

3. www.realmilk.com – a Weston A. Price Foundation website that helps one locate raw milk and other dairy products in one's own area.

4. www.westonaprice.org – This website excellently promotes truth in nutrition and diet information and is a resource for all patients.

5. The Gut and Psychology Syndrome by Natasha Campbell-McBride, including the GAPS Guide Book, explains the connection between the health of our digestive system and illness, especially illnesses like ADD/ADHD and depression.

I cannot conclude the discussion of ADD/ADHD/ and ODD without emphasizing the work of Dr. Natasha Campbell-McBride. Her book Gut and Psychology Syndrome: Natural Treatment for Autism, ADD, ADHD, Depression, Dyslexia, Dyspraxia and Schizophrenia is helpful for anyone hoping to gain insight into a truly effective approach for these illnesses. It is a must for any adult suffering with one of these conditions or for a parent with a child with one of these related conditions. The author explains the gut-brain connection including food sensitivities and allergies. I highly recommend this book as well as the GAPS Guide Book that can be purchased with it.

SECTION XVII
HOLISTIC TREATMENT OF CANCER

Natural Treatment of Cancer

It has been my experience that most people who are ill are in a state of acidosis and have been that way for many years. By this I mean that their cells are bathing in a fluid that is chemically imbalanced (pH too low/too acidic) and therefore irritating. This prevents the cells from functioning properly. Consider the example of a pool: when the water is clean and properly balanced, you can swim in the pool and enjoy it; when it's not, algae grow and the water becomes unsafe to swim in. In the case of the cells, this leads to immune system compromise; the cells are no longer able to get nutrients in and wastes out. Essentially, the body becomes inundated with its own waste, and is unable to remove it. Add to this a diet overloaded with processed foods including refined sugars, in which cancers thrive, and hydrogenated oils, as well as artificial sweeteners, colorings, and pesticides. These plus inadequate rest, stress, pollution and pharmaceutical medications are a recipe for cancer. This view of the causes of cancer differs from the medical model of the Germ Theory, which blames bacteria and viruses as the causes of disease.

The word "cancer" strikes fear into the hearts and minds of those with the misfortune of crossing its path. Yet many doctors around the world, often unrecognized and frequently maligned by the medical profession, have gotten excellent results and even cured cancer holistically. They have operated outside of the accepted medical dogma of drugs, surgery and radiation. They have dared to think outside the box.

I became interested in a natural cancer treatment one day when I picked up a book *The Cancer Cure* by Max Gerson, MD. He used juice therapy, coffee enemas, wheat grass juice, diet and supplementation to treat cancer. His ideas were so in line with what I had learned as a chiropractor that I began to take a great interest in the work of doctors having success with a similar natural approach. This was in the 1950's when few people understood what cancer was and even fewer knew what a chiropractor or nutritionist was. Dr.

Max Gerson was soon the victim of a vicious smear campaign and ostracized from his own medical profession.

One of the many other doctors in the cancer field that I studied was Dr. William Donald Kelley, a dentist from Texas. In 1962, Kelley, then a practicing dentist, developed a disease involving body pains, weight loss, and depression. His doctor diagnosed pancreatic cancer, gave him only months to live, telling him that no treatment was available. Kelley then used diet and alternative medical methods as proposed by Dr. Gerson to treat his cancer. He went on to formulate his own cancer cure, adapted from Gerson therapy. The treatment included using pancreatic enzymes, an individualized diet of vitamins, minerals, and other nutrients, and detoxification, including the use of coffee enemas. Kelley also added prayer and osteopathic manipulations to his treatment regime.

Intrigued by his story, I called Dr. Kelley and asked him if I could visit him to talk about his method of treating cancer, explaining to him my interest as a physician. He was very cordial and invited me down to see him. When I arrived he had me sit in his dental chair and we began talking about his methods. I noticed that he was very nervous and cautious. When I asked him why he seemed uneasy, he remarked to me that the FDA was investigating him and that he had to be very careful because they had threatened him. I later realized that he had seated me in his dental chair to give the appearance to any spying eyes that he was merely treating me as a dental patient. His life's work and his livelihood were at stake, and I could see how important this was to him. By the time I was ready to leave, Dr. Kelley and I had developed a plan to use blood samples from my patients to study cancer. He asked me to take samples of blood from my patients' fingers so that he could show me how to identify which patients were prone to cancer.

When I came back to New Jersey I began to pipette blood into little glass tubes of some of the more sick patients that I had in my office. I labeled them by number, using no names, so as to maintain anonymity. I later took all of the blood samples back to Dr. Kelley and we examined them under a microscope. He showed me which characteristics were likely signs of a patient being prone to cancer. This may sound hard for many of my readers to believe, but it is true. Dr. Kelley eventually went on to treat many patients with his protocol, and was even able to help cure some patients of their cancer. His book called *One Answer to Cancer* documented his experiences as well as his methods for treating cancer. However, after many years of being harassed by the government, put through expensive lawsuits and ostracized by the medical community, Dr. Kelley died in 2005 of a heart attack. He was able to successfully cure himself of pancreatic cancer, the most deadly cancer known, yet never given the opportunity to share his methods openly with the medical community.

Nicholas Gonzalez MD, author of several books on the natural treatment of cancer including *The Trophoblast and the Origins of Cancer*, spent time with Dr. Kelley studying his methods. He refined the Kelley method and developed his own version of this natural treatment, using enemas and enzyme therapy. A randomized phase III clinical trial for the possible treatment of pancreatic cancer with the Gonzalez Regimen was funded by a $1.4 million grant from the National Center for Complementary and Alternative Medicine, and co-sponsored by the National Cancer Institute, awarded in 1999 to Columbia University's Rosenthal Center for Alternative Medicine. Dr. Gonzalez was not allowed to control the study and his protocols were altered and manipulated in order to doom the research to failure and "prove" his treatment worthless. Dr. Gonzalez wrote about this manipulation and the corruption within the National Cancer Institute, Academia, and the National Institutes of Health in his book entitled *What Went Wrong: The Truth Behind the Clinical Trial of the Enzyme Treatment for Cancer*. The story is one of conviction, persistence and dedication in the face of opposition by the medical field.

Sometimes the simplest things are overlooked by the smartest people. So I urge you to keep an open mind. Do not be afraid to go against the grain; make your own judgement after reading this and other recommended books and investigating the topic for yourself.

Those in the cancer research field know that cancer cells do not develop in an oxygen-rich environment. If healthy cells cannot get enough oxygen, they become toxic, unable to eliminate their own cellular waste. And it is this toxicity that signals the beginning of the disease process. When a cell cannot get rid of its own waste, it begins to malfunction and eventually behaves abnormally, as cancer cells do.

For a long time, the medical profession has asserted that chemotherapy, radiation and surgery are the only acceptable ways of treating cancer. Perhaps this began with the acceptance of Pasteur's Germ Theory in the latter part of the 19th century. But it was certainly promoted by industrialists like Andrew Carnegie and John D. Rockefeller, men who influenced the way medical education in this country would be structured. Detailed information on this topic is available for those who wish to search it out, but is beyond the scope of this book.

Cancer as defined by Thomas Cowan, MD is "the situation that occurs when a certain type of cell out of the many different types of cells in our body — such as blood cells, pancreatic cells, brain cells, liver cells, connective tissue cells — decides to grow in an uncontrolled way, in an excessive way, and at the expense of all the other types of cells in the body."(Cowan T. A holistic approach to cancer. Wise Traditions. Weston A. Price Foundation. 2009;10(4):24.) This leads to the next question: What triggers this uncontrolled cell growth?"

Cowan likens cancer to civilization. As people abandoned the hunter-gatherer way of life, agriculture began. This defines a civilization. Grains became a diet staple. People relied heavily on the resources of the specific area they inhabited. As civilization grew, the resources of the area were exhausted, the soil depleted, and elements of that specific community died. The Dust Bowl occurred in the 1930s because of over-farming of grains leading to erosion of top-soil. One species grows until it eventually exhausts and kills the landbase or the people themselves. This is not unlike cancer. "As the Tigris and Euphrates Delta became the desert of Iraq solely through organic agriculture and some over-grazing," says Cowan, "so does cancer follow hand-in-hand with the consumption of a primarily grain-based diet." (Ibid p. 26)

At this point you may be saying, "What does this have to do with cancer?" Everything, actually. For much of our history on this planet, human diet was that of hunter-gatherer, not grain-based agriculture. When you compare our digestive tract to that of a gorilla and that of a dog, the point becomes clear. Our digestive tract is not nearly as long as a gorilla's, which is designed for a vegetarian-based diet of mostly carbohydrates (gorillas do eat insects) which must be fermented with the help of bacteria in order to digest. Yet our intestinal tract is not nearly as short as a wolf's or dog's which is designed for meat as they are carnivores. "The human anatomy is precisely designed for a hunter-gatherer diet of about 70 percent animal food, predominantly fat (as much as they could tolerate and digest) including organ meats and bones (usually in the form of broth), but not so much protein-something like two to four ounces of protein, two to three times a day was what people ate."(Ibid p.27)

If you are not familiar with the Thrive Movement, read about it and visit their website at www.thrivemovement.com:

> The current healthcare system took root around the turn of the century when the AMA, Rockefeller Foundation, and Carnegie Foundation forged a partnership. They put their money into drug-based research and made that the main focus of "healthcare." Since then, the Rockefellers and other prominent banking elite have been able to control and profit enormously from the drug industry. The AMA – which is the largest association of physicians in the U.S. – enforces the drug-treatment paradigm by heavily lobbying Congress and publishing one of the most influential journals, JAMA, which is largely funded by pharmaceutical advertisers. It is also engaged in suppressing alternative health treatments, such as the Royal Rife cancer cure.

Timeline of Suppression of Alternative Cancer Cures

Here follows a timeline taken from the Thrive Movement's website detailing the suppression of alternative cancer cures and the Rockefeller Foundation's role in shaping the healthcare industry:

1901 – Rockefeller Institute for Medical Research opens
Based in New York, this became one of the most "richly endowed" research centers. By the year 1928, John D. Rockefeller had given it $65 million in endowment funds. The Institute later became Rockefeller University.

1910 – Flexner Report published, establishes new standards for medical education

This highly influential report, sponsored by the Rockefeller and Carnegie Foundations, evaluated medical schools and restructured American medical education. It set up a new standard so that schools could be accredited only if they showed an emphasis on drug-based research and treatment. Homeopathy and other alternative approaches to medicine were no longer recognized. Abraham Flexner, author of the report, was on the staff of the Carnegie Foundation for the Advancement of Teaching. In 1910, 161 medical schools existed. By 1919, there were only 81 left.

1913 – Rockefeller Foundation establishes the International Health Commission

This laid the foundation for how health and science research and development were to be conducted. Many of today's health institutions such as the UN's World Health Organization, the U.S. Government's National Science Foundation, and the National Institute of Health, were modeled on this commission's practices, policies, and research processes.

1918 – Public health becomes Rockefeller Foundation's top priority

"The Foundation identifies public health education as one of its principal areas of interest, and builds and endows the first school of public health at Johns Hopkins University." (http://www.rockefeller100.org/exhibits/show/education/medical-education/public-health-at-johns-hopkins)

1921 – Rockefeller Foundation contributes $357 million to medical schools around the world

This funding spreads the drug-based approach to the most prominent schools around the world.

1922 – Dr. Royal Raymond Rife begins cancer research

In the 1920s, Dr. Rife – a brilliant bacteriologist and former student of John Hopkins University – began researching and developing an alternative cancer cure.

1924 – Morris Fishbein becomes primary editor of JAMA

The Journal of the American Medical Association, JAMA, is one of the most influential medical journals in the world. As head of JAMA, Morris Fishbein became one of most powerful, prominent men in medicine at the time. He transformed the industry into a money-making machine and used negative campaigns to squash competitors. He was one of the key figures to suppress Dr. Royal Rife's cancer cure.

1924 – Harry Hoxsey founds first cancer clinic in Taylorville, Illinois

Harry Hoxsey offers a natural herbal formula to cure cancer that thousands claim to have worked. This is the first of 17 clinics to eventually open.

1926 – JAMA publishes first tirade against Hoxsey

The article scares doctors and researchers from being associated with Hoxsey.

1927 – John D. Rockefeller Jr. gives the first of his annual $60,000 contributions to Memorial (Sloan-Kettering) Cancer Center

1932 – Dr. Rife develops cancer cure

Dr. Rife developed a machine that could neutralize disease-causing micro-organisms, including cancer cells, with the use of frequencies.

1932 – Director of Rockefeller Institute, Dr. Thomas Rivers, denies success of Rife cancer treatment

In 1932, Dr. Arthur Kendall, director of Medical Research at Northwestern University, spoke before the Association of American Physicians at Johns Hopkins University about the preliminary successes with Rife's methods and treatments of cancer. Dr. Thomas Rivers, virologist and bacteriologist, Director of the Rockefeller Institute (a primary source of funding for medical research) and Dr. Hans Zinsser called Kendall a liar to his face in front of the assembled crowd.

1934 – Rife's treatment cures 16 terminally ill cancer patients

In 1934 at the Scripps Institute in La Jolla, Southern California, Rife conducted clinical trials on 16 terminally ill cancer patients, and successfully cured all of them. A team of medical specialists — including Dr. Milbank Johnson, Chairman of the Special Medical Research Committee of USC; George Fischer of the NY Children's Hospital; and Dr. Wayland Morrison, the chief medical officer of the Santa Fe Railway — confirmed the findings.

1938 – The AMA indicts Rife for fraudulent medical practices

1939 – Philip Hoyland files suit against Royal Rife's Company, the Beam Ray Corporation

Philip Hoyland admitted to accepting a $10,000 bribe from Hahn Realty Group (AMA Agents) to sue the Beam Ray Corporation.

1939 – New Memorial Sloan-Kettering Cancer Center opens – John D. Rockefeller donated the land and provided $3 million of funding

1940s – Rife's work is destroyed and findings continue to be suppressed

1949 – Hoxsey Sues JAMA and editors for libel and slander – Hoxsey Wins

1949 – Morris Fishbein is ousted from AMA

1956 – FDA issues public warning about Hoxsey cancer treatment

1960 – Hoxsey Method banned in U.S. by the FDA

1960 – Laurance Rockefeller serves as Chairman of Memorial Sloan-Kettering Cancer Center in New York from 1960-1982

This center is one of the most influential cancer centers in the world. During WWII it performed some of the first experiments applying chemical warfare weapons to the "treatment of cancer," which evolved into chemotherapy.

1963 – Bio-Medical (Hoxsey) Center opens in Tijuana, Mexico

It continues to operate and claims an 80% success rate.

1971 – President Nixon declares a "War on Cancer"

Signs $1.6 billion law to fund the "War on Cancer."

1977 – Sloan-Kettering rejects laetrile (derived from apricot kernels) as effective cancer treatment

This is despite positive results from Sloan-Kettering's own famous researcher, Kanematsu Suguira. In November of 1977 Dr. Ralph Moss, Assistant Director of public affairs at Sloan-Kettering, held a press-conference about the success and potential of laetrile, despite the Center's desire to cover it up. Dr. Moss was fired the next day for "failing to carry out the most basic job responsibilities."

1991 – Rockefeller Foundation helps start Children's Vaccine Initiative

The Foundation joins with the United Nations Development Program, UNICEF, WHO and the World Bank to form the Children's Vaccine Initiative (CVI).

2010 – More than half a million Americans die of cancer

Study the timeline carefully. We are not winning the war on cancer. In fact, if you look at the government database, www.cancer.gov, you can see the numbers for yourself. The statistics are not improving despite all of the early detection screenings, tests, new drugs, gene therapy, etc. The only thing that is happening is that the pharmaceutical companies and big businesses are getting richer, and our health is declining. Unfortunately, propaganda and lobbying prevent the average American from finding out the truth about cancer. Further complicating the matter is that data are often cherry-picked to suit the benefits of the company or group funding the research. Therefore, the only way in which we can know for ourselves what is really going on is to read the studies ourselves and evaluate the data/quality/etc., or have a reliable resource we can trust to do it for us. Either way, when you look at the numbers, you see clearly that we are not winning the war on cancer.

The New York Times published an article in 2009 by its American science writer, Gina Bari Kolata, which pointed out that the cancer death rate, when adjusted for the size and age of the population, has decreased by only 5 percent since 1950. Kolata argued that there has been very little overall progress in the war on cancer.

With regard to cancer treatment, I would like to recommend "Cancer is Serious Business", a DVD series produced by Stanislaw

Burzynski, MD. It documents Dr. Burzynski's innovative method for curing cancer using proteins taken from the patient's own urine. The content includes the FDA and other agencies' attempts to destroy Dr. Burzynski's practice by closing down his clinic, confiscating his files, bringing him to grand jury trial five times, each time failing to convict him and making attempts to steal his treatment and patent it for themselves. Thousands of his patients, all cured by his treatment, marched in Washington on his behalf. Proof is presented and interviews shown with many cancer patients who were given no hope for survival by mainstream medicine, but who were cured by Dr. Burzynski's treatment.

Cancer is a disease and its treatment has become a business. Many sufferers are gullible and ill-informed about the dangers of chemotherapy, radiation and surgery as well as the truth about the efficacy of these therapies in curing cancer. Manipulated statistics and false information add to the confusion.

Cancer has to be treated like any other symptom. We do not treat the cancer, we treat the causes in the patient. This involves examining, through appropriate testing, the digestive system for malfunction, the pH of the body and nutrient deficiencies. Before making a decision on what to do if you have cancer, start by working with a qualified holistic practitioner to design a plan that is appropriate for your individual case to strengthen your immune system and improve your overall health. This plan should involve dietary changes, pH correction, supplementation, detoxification, chiropractic care, stress reduction, and more. Addressing these areas can only help improve your odds of survival and cure, no matter what treatment you decide on. I also suggest looking into the Burzynski clinic and visiting their website at http://www.burzynskiclinic.com and also watching the above mentioned DVDs at http://www.burzynskimovie.com.

Below is a list of books and resources to help you on your journey of healing. Keep an open mind and pursue the truth for yourself. The patient's needs must be the first consideration. Here are some important resources and places to start:

1. Nicholas Gonzalez MD – author of several books including *One Man Alone: An Investigation of Nutrition, Cancer, and William Donald*

Kelley. Dr. Gonzalez practiced in Manhattan and had a website at http://www.dr-gonzalez.com. Unfortunately, Dr. Gonzalez died on July 21, 2015 under mysterious circumstances.

2. Stanislaw R. Burzynski MD, PhD – internationally recognized physician and biochemist-researcher who pioneered the development and use of biologically active peptides in diagnosing, preventing and treating cancer. In 1967 he graduated with an MD, first in his class from the Medical Academy in Lublin, Poland. The following year he earned his PhD in Biochemistry as one of the youngest candidates in Poland ever to hold both an MD and PhD. Anyone seeking to learn more about cancer should watch his DVDs (available from his website or on the internet) and consider visiting his clinic. His website is http://www.burzynskiclinic.com.

3. Ralph W. Moss, MD, PhD – Dr. Moss has gained credibility by writing eight books, including his most recent work, *Cancer Therapy: The Independent Consumer's Guide to Non-Toxic Treatment*. He also wrote *The Cancer Industry*, a documented research work telling of the enormous financial and political corruption in the "cancer establishment." He indicates that the motivating forces in cancer research and treatment are often power and money, and not the cure of the patient. He also writes The Cancer Chronicles, a newsletter reporting on new cancer treatments and preventive measures.

4. Max Gerson – a German-born American physician who developed the Gerson Therapy, an alternative dietary therapy used to cure cancer and most chronic, degenerative diseases. Gerson described his approach in the book *A Cancer Therapy: Results of 50 Cases*.

5. Weston A. Price Foundation – A wealth of overall health information, research, articles and nutritional advice based on traditional wisdom and the research of Dr. Weston A. Price.

6. Joseph M. Mercola, DO – For information on alternative cancer treatments visit his website at fwww.mercola.com.

7. *Beating Cancer with Nutrition*, by Patrick Quillin, PhD, RD, CNS – Much of the information Quillin provides is excellent, although there are some areas of his work I disagree with. (For example, he classifies oils from soybean, corn and safflower as "fair", whereas I classify them as "dangerous" and recommend avoiding them altogether.)

SECTION XVIII

APPENDIX A
Important Protocols for Natural Healing

General Recommendations for Cod Liver Oil Supplementation

These dosages are for high-vitamin fermented cod liver oil:

Children age 3 to 6 months: ¼ to ½ teaspoon or 1.25 to 2.5 mL, providing up to 4650 IU vitamin A and 975 IU vitamin D.

Children age one to 12 years: ½ to ¾ teaspoon or 2.5 mL to 3.75 mL, providing up to 6975 IU vitamin A and 1462 IU vitamin D.

Children over 12 years and adults: one teaspoon or 10 capsules, providing 9500 iu vitamin A and 1950 IU vitamin D.

Pregnant and nursing women: two teaspoons or 20 capsules, providing 19,000 iu vitamin A and 3900 IU vitamin D.

Hot Toddy Drink

Items needed: fresh lemon, whiskey and raw honey.

Procedure:

Step 1. Warm an 8 oz glass of hot water as for making tea.

Step 2. Add one tbsp of fresh-squeezed lemon juice.

Step 3. Add one tbsp of whiskey and one tsp of raw honey.

Note: *Drink slowly as you would a cup of warm tea. Repeat this several times throughout the day as directed by the physician.*

Parsley Tea

Items needed: one medium size bunch of fresh, preferably organic parsley, medium saucepan.

Procedure:

Place the bunch of parsley into a small saucepan filled with approximately one quart of boiling water. Reduce heat to low and simmer for 15–20 minutes. Then strain the liquid and allow to sit covered for a few minutes. Drink this tea several times per day.

Allergy Remedy/pH Drink

Mix ½ teaspoon of raw honey (preferably made from local honey in your area) and 2 teaspoons of raw, organic apple cider vinegar in 8 ounces of purified/filtered water. Drink this three times per day.

Enema Directions/Procedure

The kit for performing an enema can be purchased at most good drug stores or pharmacies as well as from www.enemakit.com. The kit is made up of a hot water bottle (usually a rubber bag with a screw-in plug at the top), a small rubber hose with a tip, and a douche attachment. You simply fill the bag with 12-16 ozs. of sterilized water for an adult; boil the water, cover it and let it cool to room temperature, or use organic coffee (the same is done for the coffee; it is brewed and then covered and allowed to cool to at least a luke-warm or room temperature). Using coffee may sound strange but coffee has an excellent detoxification effect when used in this manner. Furthermore, coffee introduces an acidic medium to the digestive tract, making it inhospitable to many of the pathogenic bacteria that are responsible for causing disease.

Procedure

1. Sterilize the 12–16 ounces of water or coffee and *allow to cool to a luke-warm or room temperature*. Fill the bag with the water or coffee.

2. Remove all air from the bag by using your hand to press the bag gently against your chest while screwing in the plug at the end.

3. Hang the bag upside down from either a shower door or closet using a hanger and the loop provided at the end of the bag. Open the valve at the end of the hose and allow some liquid to empty from the end of the tube into the sink or tub in order to allow all air out of the bag. Do this until some liquid exits the end of the hose.

4. Place a towel or mat on the floor and get onto your hands and knees with your chest to the floor and your buttock pointed up. Lubricate the tip of the enema tube with a small amount of Vaseline and insert into your rectum.

5. Open the valve at the end of the hose and allow the fluid to enter into the intestine (this should only take about 20–30 seconds). You can remove the hose as soon as the bag is empty.

6. Stay in this position, with your chest to the floor for approximately 3–5 minutes massaging your abdomen in a circular pattern from your left to right (counterclockwise if you were looking at yourself from the front).

7. Then, after the 3–5 minutes is up, lay on your right side and repeat massaging the abdomen. After another 3–5 minutes, switch to your left side and again massage your abdomen. If possible, it is best to try and hold the liquid in for 10 minutes or as long as you can. After this is completed, you may rise and sit on the toilet and release the fluid.

Note: For children under the age of 5, use a Fleet Enema or syringe according to the directions in Section XVI on infant care. For children over the age of 5, the procedure above may be followed using 6 ounces of coffee or sterile water.

Sore Throat Protocol

Requirements: One of the following: 3% hydrogen peroxide; Argentyn 23 Silver Hydrosol; pineapple juice; and slippery elm lozenges.

1. Mix 2 oz. of hydrogen peroxide and 2 oz. of distilled or purified water. Tilting your head back carefully (so as to enable the liquid further back into the back of the throat), gargle with a sip of the mixture and after approximately 30 seconds spit it out. Sip again and repeat until all of the mixture is gone. Repeat several times per day.
2. Using Argentyn 23 Silver Hydrosol Spray/Liquid, gargle with it several times per day as described in #1 above

    or

3. Using 2–3 oz. of pineapple juice, mix with 2 ounces of distilled water and gargle as explained in #1 above and repeat several times during the day.
4. In combination with all three protocols, suck on several slippery elm lozenges throughout the day as this will help to coat the throat and soothe it.

Dr. Angelo Rose; Dr. Christopher Amoruso

Laryngitis Protocol

Items needed: One large onion, cloth towel, raw sugar, saran wrap.

Procedure:

1. Cut large onion in five pieces. Lay the onion pieces on a cloth and wrap around the neck area in the front of the throat for one hour. Repeat a second time at bedtime.
2. To take internally:
Take a small onion and chop fine. Place in a glass. Sprinkle two teaspoons raw sugar on it and cover with saran wrap. The mixture will turn into a syrup. Take one tablespoon immediately, one at mid-day and one again before bed.

Fever Reduction Protocol

Items needed – Hot water bottle with enema attachment for children 8 years old and up (can be purchased in any reputable pharmacy); Fleet enema with sterilized water for children under the age of 8; Cataplex® F, Calcium Lactate and Congaplex® – all vitamins made by Standard Process.

1. Administer enema to your child as per the physician's directions. Refer to the enema protocol on the previous page for a complete set of directions if you have never administered an enema before. This can be repeated twice to three times a day during the fever without worry. Please consult the physician if you have any questions.

2a. For children under the age of 5 – take six tablets of Calcium Lactate and three tablets of Cataplex® F and grind or crush them in a seed or coffee grinder. Add contents to applesauce or other food and allow child to eat it.

2b. For children over the age of 5 who are able to swallow small pills, use the same dosages as described above in 2a. The child may use a small amount of water to take the pills which can be taken together with food.

3. Congaplex® Chewable for children and regular Congaplex® for adults. Take two capsules every hour for the first 48 hours as soon as signs of a cold or fever start. Then decrease to four to six a day.

Congestion of the Chest and Bronchitis
Mustard Plaster Protocol

Ingredients needed:
1. One heaping tbsp of Coleman's dry mustard powder (purchase in supermarket) 2. Three heaping tbsp of flour 3. White vinegar.

Procedure:
Step 1. Place mustard powder and flour into a cup.
Step 2. Add white vinegar into the cup, adding it slowly and mixing until the consistency is that of pancake batter.
Step 3. Place the ingredients onto a piece of cloth 5 inches wide X 10 inches long, covering only one half of the cloth.
Step 4. Fold the unused portion of the cloth over the other half containing the mixture.
Step 5. Place directly on bare chest for approximately 30 minutes. This may be repeated two times each day for three days. It can also be placed on the back in between the shoulder blades.

Caution: *This mustard plaster may become very hot. Remove it if the patient cannot tolerate the heat. The patient may place some USF Ointment® (Standard Process) or raw honey on the area of skin if it becomes irritated.*

Relief of Chest Colds and Congestion
Castor Oil Compress Instructions

Items needed: castor oil; one medium sized towel; saran wrap

Procedure:
Step 1. Warm several ounces of castor oil in a pan. Be careful not to overheat the oil. It should only be warmed to approximately body temperature.
Step 2. Dip the towel into the warmed castor oil and place the towel over the chest.
Step 3. Cover the towel with a piece of Saran wrap.
Step 4. Place a second cloth on the chest covering the saran wrap.
Step 5. Place hot water bottle over chest and leave for at least 30-40 minutes. Repeat several times a day until relief is established.

Note: *if any irritation develops, use USF Ointment® (Standard Process) or raw honey spread over the affected area.*

Protocol for Colds and Flu
Do the following *at the first signs/symptoms* of a cold:

Vitamin Protocol

1. Congaplex® (Standard Process) – 2 capsules every waking hour for up to 4 days. Then decrease to a dosage of 4 capsules daily.
2. Immuplex® (Standard Process) – 3 capsules 3 times daily until cold is resolved. Take maintenance dosage of 3 capsules daily.
3. Thymex® (Standard Process) – 5 tablets 4 times daily until the cold is resolved.
4. Blue Ice™ Fermented Cod Liver Oil – Take 4–5 capsules daily until the cold is resolved. Then take 3 capsules daily as a maintenance dose during the winter months. The liquid form is preferred. Give two teaspoons daily; for children under eight, give one teaspoon daily.

Alkalizing Drink
Mix one tablespoon of Braggs Organic Apple Cider Vinegar or any other organic, unpasteurized apple cider vinegar (order from www.healthalertstore.com) in hot water and add 1 teaspoon of raw, unheated, unfiltered honey. Drink this up to three times per day.

Dietary Instructions

1. Eat *only* fresh green vegetables and/or salad with either fish, chicken, or turkey (broil, bake, boil, steam or sauté). Make soups using the vegetables with either fish or chicken.
2. Fresh fruit is permissible as long as it is ripe and in season. It must be eaten separately from any other food.
3. Drink only water (away from meals), unsweetened herbal teas or fresh squeezed juices.

Children's Cold and Flu
Do the following *at the first signs/symptoms of a cold:*

Vitamin Protocol

1. *If under 8 years of age, take* Congaplex® Chewable (Standard Process) – 2 chewable tablets every waking hour for up to four days. Then decrease to a dosage of 4 tablets daily.

If older than 8 years, take regular Congaplex® at a dose of twocapsules every hour for 48–72 hours, then decrease to 4–6 per day until 100% cured or otherwise instructed.

2. Immuplex® (Standard Process) – one capsule three times daily until cold is resolved. Then take maintenance dosage of two capsules daily.
3. Thymex® (Standard Process) – two tablets 4 times daily until the cold is resolved.
4. Blue Ice™ Fermented Cod Liver Oil – Take 4–5 capsules daily until cold is resolved. Then take 3 capsules daily as a maintenance dose during the winter months.
5. Dr. Schulze's Children's Echinacea Drops – 60 drops (1.5 ml) in two ounces of water or unsweetened juice 2 to 4 times daily.

Ear Drum Inflammation Protocol

Items needed: Tissue Cell Salt #4 (Ferrum Phosphate); Tissue Cell Salt #12 (Silica); castor oil; olive oil; dried oregano (herb)

Directions:

Part 1. Castor oil is to be spread in a light coating around the back and front of the ear. This is to be done repeatedly for a few days.

Part 2. Oregano tea – take one heaping teaspoon of oregano and place into water that is boiling. Remove from the stove immediately after adding the oregano. Cover, letting steep (approximately 3–5 minutes). Allow to cool to tepid temperature so that it will not burn you. While lying on your side with the involved ear facing upward, place oregano tea into ear until ear is approximately half full. Place a piece of cotton in the ear and stay in that position for approximately 15 minutes. Repeat twice a day.

Part 3. Olive oil – At bedtime: place two drops of olive oil into the involved ear while in a side-lying position (with involved ear up). Place cotton in the ear and go to sleep. In the morning you may remove the cotton. Upon waking, place a new piece of cotton in the ear to keep it warm.

Part 4. Tissue Cell Salts – four tablets of each cell salt mentioned above three times per day under the tongue, waiting 5 minutes in between each cell salt. Taken until condition has resolved.

Basic Baby Diet (1 Year and Up)

Breakfast Choices

1. Fresh fruit – melon, apple, pear, grapefruit or berries. Give only one fruit type at a time. The fruit may be mashed, pureed, or blended using a small amount of water to make chewing and assimilation easier.
2. Eggs – Scramble or soft cook the egg and use alternating days with the fruit. If some bread is needed, put butter on the bread. *Do not use margarine.* Use only sourdough or sprouted bread.

Lunch Choices

1. Soft cook (steam) green vegetables – use endive, broccoli rabe, broccoli, dandelion, zucchini, string beans, etc. Puree or add water into a blender and make into a soup consistency. Add homemade bone broth and blend.
2. Steamed carrots – puree as described above.
3. Sweet potato – cook and mash finely. Add one or two green vegetables from above list and a liberal amount of butter for taste.

Dinner Choices

1. Use one of the following meats – lamb, chicken, liver, turkey. Mash the meat or chop it up very fine. Add any of the green vegetables from the list above. Use only organic/pastured meats when possible.

Important

1. The baby *should* be fed goat's milk (fresh only) from the health food store or locate fresh raw milk using www.realmilk.com's milk finder. Mix half with water and give the child a few ounces between meals.
2. *Do not use soy* for the baby. It is too difficult to digest and will cause problems for the baby including damage to the brain.
3. The baby must be given plenty of *water*. Give small amounts *before* and *between* meals. Never feed the baby water with the meal.
4. Supplement the baby's milk with the following: homemade almond milk or banana milk. You can make almond milk by taking a handful of almonds (they must be the type in the shell that you open yourself and have pre-soaked) and adding them into a blender with 8 oz. of water. Blend well and give to the baby. To make banana

milk, use a ripe banana (has brown spots) and make the milk in the same manner, blending with 8 ounces of water.

5. Try to limit the wheat products (white flour) you give the child including: cookies, crackers, breads and other flour products as these products will act as an irritant to your child's nervous system.

Supplements

1. Kyo-Dophilus (children's acidophilus). Give one tablet two times per day.
2. Tissue Cell Salt #2 – Calcarea phosphorica. Give two in the a.m. and two in the p.m.
3. Tissue Cell Salt #4 – Ferrum phosphate. Give two tablets in the a.m. and two in p.m.
4. Tissue Cell Salt #12 – Silica. Give two tablets in the a.m. and two in the p.m.
5. Catalyn® Chewable – multivitamin made by Standard Process. Grind up one tablet and add to food once a per day.
6. Calcium – powdered calcium lactate, citrate, or MCHC. Give three times a week as directed by the physician.

Progest E

Directions: Apply three drops of Progest E oil on the tip of your finger and rub into the gums of your mouth before going to bed. Do this every night for three weeks and then stop for one week. You are to apply the oil for the three weeks that you do not have your period. When bleeding begins, you are to stop using the oil until the bleeding stops (this is the one week period mentioned above). If your period should come prior to the 21 days of using the Progest E, stop for 1 week, then begin again, 3 weeks on, 1 week off.

Note: *Keep the oil refrigerated.*

Nail Fungus Protocol

Items needed:

1. Calcium Bentonite Clay (available at health food stores or on-line. One brand of Bentonite clay I have found effective is Aztec Secret Indian Healing Clay
2. Castor Oil (Heritage Brand sold at Whole Foods and health stores)
3. Nail clippers and cuticle device.

Procedure:

1. Clip the nail itself back as far as possible. This may be painful at first, but it is necessary in order for the treatment to be effective. Keep the nail trimmed back in this manner as far as necessary due to growth of the nail.
2. Push the cuticle back at least twice per day and keep the nail bed coated with castor oil twice per day.
3. Cover the nail front to back with the clay and wrap it in a bandage using gauze or a large square bandaid. Repeat this twice per day.

Note: It may take up to a few weeks for the fungus to be removed completely. Be patient and be diligent about the directions above. *Medications for this type of problem can be dangerous.*

Plantar Wart Protocol
Plantar warts are caused by the human papilloma virus (HPV). In order to resolve a plantar wart, you must understand that this condition is almost uniformly an internal problem. As such, it is important not only to treat the physical wart on the sole of the foot, but to also treat the internal environment of the body, enabling the immune system to eradicate the virus at its source. This must be done by making certain dietary adjustments as well as through the use of effective antiviral supplements. Therefore, the entire process will take several weeks (anywhere from 2-6 weeks) to complete.

Procedure for caring for the plantar warts:
You will be using either salicylic acid (commonly found over the counter in pharmacies as wart remover, or you may use Neutrogena's Clear Pore Oil Controlling Astringent, Salicylic Acid Gel Peel). The higher the percentage of salicylic acid in the product, the better. The most effective product in my opinion is Dr. Scholl Clear Away Wart Remover. Rite Aid also has a wart remover with 40% salicylic acid. If you cannot find these products, you may also use Tea Tree Oil. It must be applied over the area of the wart after the doctor removes the root. The most important thing is to apply the salicylic acid daily, changing the bandage twice per day. Since the surface will appear calloused, it is a good idea to file away the dead skin each time you change the bandage and apply the acid.

Dietary Considerations:

1. Eliminate all sources of refined sugar as this not only weakens the immune system, but promotes the acidic condition viruses thrive in. This includes sugar sweetened drinks; any products containing high fructose corn syrup (everything from candy/soda to dressings and sauces); white flour (bagels, bread, crackers, etc.; and white table sugar.
2. Limit the consumption of alcohol.
3. Try to emphasize the use of whole foods including fresh vegetables, fruits and salads.

Herbal/Supplement Support

1. Congaplex® – made by Standard Process, this is like a multi-vitamin for the immune system. It is to be taken at a dose of two capsules every 2 hours you are awake for the first three days. Thereafter it is to be taken at a dose of six a day (two per meal).
2. Coconut oil/Lauricidin – a very powerful anti-viral fat known as lauric acid is found in coconut. This may be purchased at Whole Foods, Fairway Markets, Trader Joe's or any health food store. The dosage is 2–3 tablespoons per day. It may be taken off the spoon directly as it is delicious *or* you may add it to hot water and drink like a tea. You may also cook with coconut oil as its heat stable properties make it great for sautéing. There is also a concentrated lauric acid extract from coconut called Lauricidin which can be purchased online. Take it according to the directions provided.
3. Blue Ice™ Fermented Cod Liver Oil – rich in Vitamins A, D, K and essential omega fats, this supports the immune system and is invaluable for this condition. Take at a dose of one tablespoon per day OR four capsules per day with food. Purchase from our office *or* order online. Other acceptable brands include Doctor Ron's (877-472-8701) and Radiant Life (888–593-8333).

Varicose Vein Treatment

Items needed: dry white wine, organic apple cider vinegar, mineral water. Do all three procedures.

Procedure 1
1. Mix two teaspoons of dry white wine into 8 ounces of mineral water (make sure you use mineral water from the supermarket/health food store, NOT any other type.)
2. Drink down once every day on an empty stomach.

Procedure 2
1. Take two teaspoons of organic apple cider vinegar, two teaspoons of dry white wine and add them to 8 ounces of mineral water.
2. Using a cloth soaked in the mixture, wipe down the legs and allow to air dry. Repeat two times every day.

Procedure 3
Blend together and drink 2–3 times per day:
Three ounces of unsweetened, concentrated black cherry juice.
Juice of 2–3 lemons (whole); limes may also be used.
Two tablespoons of aloe vera (scoop directly out of the aloe leaf).
Supplements: Collinsonia root – six per day (Standard Process); Cyruta® Plus – six per day (Standard Process).

Plantar Fasciitis Soaking

Items needed: Epsom salt; warm water; bucket or basin

Procedure:
1. Using a bucket or a small basin, filled with tepid/warm water, add one-half cup of Epsom salt and mix into the water.
2. Soak the foot before bed for at least 20 minutes. Repeat every night until relief is established.

Skin Eruption/Rash Treatment

Items needed: witch hazel, cucumber, gauze.

Procedure:
1. Wet a square piece of gauze with witch hazel until it is soaked. Lay it over the area of irritation for approximately 30 minutes. Repeat this every 2 or 3 hours.
2. Grate a cucumber up finely. Place gratings between two pieces of gauze. Place gauze over the area of irritation for approximately 45 minutes. Repeat two times per day initially for two or three days.

When there is excessive inflammation, procedure #2 can also be done with red potato grated as described above.

Supplements Support
1. Wheat germ oil capsules – take three a day; one with each meal.
2. Vitamin B6 – Must be in the form P-5-P (pyridoxyl-5-phosphate)- 50 mg taken twice a day with food.
3. Zinc – preferably in the form of gluconate or picolinate – take 50 mg on an empty stomach once every day.

Shingles Protocol
1. Undiluted Pure Witch Hazel – wipe down the area of the lesions 2-3 times per day. Do not dry the area off.
2. Organic Super B-Complex (B100) – 2 a day with food.
3. Lauricidin – go to www.lauricidin.com – use a 1/4 scoop 1x a day for 2–3 days, then up to ½ a scoop 1x a day, then up to 3/4 a scoop 1 x a day, continue to use until you can get up to 1 scoop 3x's a day
4. Miracle Mineral Supplement (MMS Drops) – Using the Chlorine dioxide bottle and the Citric Acid bottle from Ocean's labs, do the following:
   A. Mix one drop of each and wait 2–3 minutes. You will notice a color change to yellow and even a smell of chlorine as the two ingredients react. Then add a few ounces of water to the mixture.
   B. Drink the solution down. Do this once in the evening and once in the morning. Repeat this for a few days, then increase to two drops of each and repeat as in step one above.
   C. Work your way up slowly to ten drops of each mixed, increasing by one drop every few days. Once you have reached 10 drops of each you can decrease back to a maintenance dose of 3 drops of each per day.
5. Argentyn 23 Silver Hydrosol – See directions under Argentyn Information based on age and body weight.
6. Congaplex® – take two capsules every two hours while awake for the first 48 hours. Then decrease to four per day thereafter.

Dr. Angelo Rose; Dr. Christopher Amoruso

Swollen Joint Protocol
Items needed: kosher salt; organic apple cider vinegar; bucket or basin

Procedure:
1. Using a bucket or basin filled with cold water, add the following:
   4 ounces of organic apple cider vinegar
   4 tbsp of kosher salt
2. Soak body part that is swollen for 30 minutes.
3. Repeat as directed by physician.

Five-Day Liver and Gallbladder Flush
Directions: Start each of five consecutive mornings with the breakfast cocktail described below.

Step 1 Breakfast Cocktail
4 tbsp of extra virgin, cold-pressed olive oil
2 medium-sized cloves of fresh garlic
Juice of one fresh-squeezed lemon
Blend the above ingredients thoroughly in a blender and drink down.

Some patients may report slight to moderate nausea and rarely a mild abdominal discomfort when taking the breakfast cocktail. This nausea and discomfort will slowly disappear within an hour.

Step 2 Herb Tea
30 minutes to an hour after drinking the cocktail follow it with two cups of herbal tea. The following teas are ideal and should be chosen from: roasted dandelion root, ginger root, burdock root, red clover flower, yellow dock root, comfrey leaf, peppermint, milk thistle or any combination of the above. Celestial Seasonings makes an excellent tea for this program called Detox A.M. It contains milk thistle, dandelion and red clover. Numi Organic Tea, Rishi and Traditional Medicinals brands are also excellent choices

Step 3 Brunch
Eat a fresh fruit meal with or slightly after drinking the herbal teas. Eat only one kind of fruit during this meal. The fruit should be fresh, organic, in season, thoroughly cleaned, without added sweeteners. Suggested fruits include the following: pineapple, papaya, melon, grapefruit, nectarine, mango, banana and apple.

Step 4 Lunch and Dinner

While performing this cleansing, eat only fresh vegetables and sprouts that are half-cooked and/or raw. The best vegetables to eat are asparagus • beets • beet greens • bok choy • broccoli • Brussels sprouts • cabbage • carrots • cauliflower • celery • collard greens • cucumber • dandelion • eggplant • endive • garlic • kale • lettuce (butter, romaine, leaf) • mustard greens • okra • onions • parsley • peppers (red, green or yellow) • radish • spinach • squash • tomatoes • turnip greens • zucchini.

Eat any of the above vegetables either in a salad or steamed, or wok them in water. Eat no more than five kinds of vegetables at any one time. For salad dressings use a mixture of extra virgin olive oil, lemon juice and/or vinegar with your favorite herbs added. Eat as much as you like.

Avoid these foods:

All meats, sea foods, conventional processed (pasteurized/homogenized) dairy products, refined and processed foods (meaning all foods that come in cans, boxes or packages). Also avoid all sweeteners such as table sugar, brown sugar and honey. Avoid nuts and nut butters including peanuts. No bakery made products such as pastries, cakes, pies or white breads.

Beverages

Drink as much fluid as you desire. Drink ONLY WATER, HERB TEAS, or freshly made fruit juice and your breakfast cocktail. Try to drink at least six 8 oz. glasses of fluid each day.

Note: *This flushing of the liver and gallbladder stimulates and cleanses these organs as no other method does. For the next few days, lumps of green matter may appear in the stools. They will be irregular in shape and gelatinous in texture, varying in size from grape seed to cherry pits. If there seems to be a large number of these in the stool, then this "flush" should be repeated in two weeks.*

For a more simplified version of the cleanse, do the following:

For two days, stay on a fruit and vegetable diet only, including homemade bone broths and lacto-fermented vegetables when possible. You may eat soaked lentils and brown rice in moderation as well. Then, on the evening of the 2nd day, prepare 2 oz. of extra virgin, first cold-pressed olive oil and 2 oz. of freshly squeezed lemon juice. Mix them together well just before bedtime and drink down quickly. Lie immediately on your right side with your right knee up toward your chest and place a hot water bottle on your right lower rib cage on the side of your body. Stay in that position for 15 minutes without moving or talking. Then go to sleep. Do not get up and walk around. Repeat this procedure two nights in a row.

The following morning you may have a loose bowel movement. When you finish going to the bathroom you may notice small green or brownish green balls floating on the surface of the water. They are gallstones and can range from the size of a pea to as big as a grape. Some people will even notice white colored stones that sink to the bottom of the toilet. These are calcified gallstones. This is an excellent procedure to follow 3–4 times per year for detoxification. I recommend my patients do it with the changes in season as a good way to cleanse and prevent future problems.

For specifics on the 7 day liver and gallbladder flush please refer to the book, *The Amazing Liver and Gallbladder Flush* by Andreas Moritz.

Protocol for Prostate
Vitamin Protocol

1. Prostate PMG® – one with each meal. From Standard Process.
2. Vitamin E – chew one with each meal.
3. Vitamin D – two a day.
4. Selenium – 200 mgs one a day
5. Udo's Oil or any good flax seed oil including Barleen's brand – two tablets a day
6. Zinc Gluconate 50 mgs – two a day for first week then one a day. – Udo's oil and zinc gluconate can be purchased from a health food store.

Home treatment

Massage the Achilles tendon on both feet for two minutes every night before bed time.

Herbs
Pau d'arco, suma, golden seal – alternate all three as a tea
Green tea diuretic – oat straw, uva ursi, gravel root

For treatment of cancer of the prostate – the natural approach
Shark cartilege, MGN3 -Lane Labs, Pectin, Pygeum, Saw Palmetto – European studies have shown these are effective regarding cancer.

Dietary Instructions
Breakfast – Whole grain cereal: brown rice, millet, oats, oat bran
Nuts and seeds: almonds (from shell only) walnuts, sunflower seeds, pumpkin seeds and pumpkin seed oil, macadamia nuts, brazil nuts
Lunch – Cruciferous vegetables; broccoli, Brussels sprouts, cabbage, carrots, pumpkin, yams, squash
Any combination salad, oil and lemon juice or apple cider vinegar for dressing. *No meat with lunch.*
Dinner – Fish, organic pastured chicken, lamb or turkey with two green non-starchy vegetables, lacto-fermented vegetables and/or a salad.
Fruits – Apples, cantaloupe, all berries, cherries, grapes, plums (these can be also eaten for breakfast or can be used as snacks. Wait 45 minutes before having a different type of fruit. Do not mix different fruits at one meal.
Legumes – Chickpeas, red beans, lentils, fava beans (very good), kidney beans, black beans, etc.

Note: *Combining beans with brown rice creates a complete protein. However, never put beans and rice with meat. Consuming protein with starch causes gas as well as bowel trouble. It is a poor food combination.*

Prostate Procedure:
Lie on the edge of the bed with legs hanging off. Place the soles of your feet together as best you can. Raise your legs together in a circular motion from the floor up towards the body and out — to a holding position for 10 seconds. Do this 10 times every night before going to bed.

EXERCISE FOR PROSTATE

1. Soles together

2. Legs are bowed

3. Bring legs up in circular motion

4. Keeping soles together at all times, hold the extended 45 degree angle position for 10 seconds.

5. Then come down slowly and hold soles together until you get 6 inches from the floor and hold this position for 10 seconds. Do this exercise 10 times each night.

©T. Eppridge 2016

APPENDIX B
Important Patient Self-Tests

Adrenal Stress Assessment and Support Protocol

To access the Stress Assess Questionnaire and the three phases of adrenal support, at the request of Standard Process, please visit their website at the following links:

Adrenal stress assess survey link:
https://www.standardprocess.com/Products/Literature/Standard-Process-Stress-Assess-Questionnaire

Three phases of adrenal support link:
https://www.standardprocess.com/Body-Systems/Adrenal-Health-Managing-Patients-Stress-and-Energy#.V5E04Wf6uM8
Work with a qualified holistic practitioner familiar with Standard Process products to address your specific needs.

Thyroid Self-Assessment/AxillaryTemperature/Broda Barne's Basal Body Temperature Thyroid Test

Part I. Basal Body Temperature Record (Patient Instructions)

Patient Name_____

Date_____/_____/20_____

D.O.B._____/_____/_____

The purpose of this procedure is to obtain information about your thyroid gland's function. Please keep a 5 day record of your axillary (armpit) temperature, along with your associated symptoms, if any, below. The following procedure should be carefully adhered to:

1. The night before the procedure shake a glass/mercury thermometer down to below 96.0 and leave it near the bedside in a glass where it can easily be reached *without getting out of bed*. Basal body temperature should ideally reflect a "sleeping state" of bed rest for at least three hours. Have a clock or watch available for timing purposes.

2. For women: If scheduling allows, it is ideal for a woman to record her axillary temperature during the menstrual cycle (temperature

should be taken during the first 3 to 5 days of menstrual flow). Otherwise, any 5 days may be used.

3. When you awaken, *do not get up or move around a lot.* The ther-mometer should be placed in the armpit against the skin for 10 minutes. Press your arm against your body to hold the thermometer in place firmly. Be sure not to roll over on that side to prevent the possibility of breaking the thermometer.

4. Record your temperature to the nearest tenth of a degree (for example 97.8). Log these temperatures in the spaces provided below and bring them with you to your next doctor's visit.

Normal Axillary Temperature: (97.8°F to 98.2°F) **Normal Oral Temperature:** (98.2°F to 98.6°F)

Day #1____/____/20_____

Notable Symptoms_____

Day #2____/____/20_____

Notable Symptoms_____

Day #3____/____/20_____

Notable Symptoms_____

Day #4____/____/20_____

Notable Symptoms_____

Day #5____/____/20_____

Notable Symptoms_____

How many blankets do you use?_____

Do you have a sore throat, cold or other infection?_____

Do you have a chronic sinus problem and or post-nasal drip?____

Part II. Thyroid Self-Assessment

Thyroid Survey from Dr. Richard Shames, author of *Thyroid Power.* Used with permission. I encourage all of my readers concerned with the state of their thyroid function to read Dr. Shames' books

The following is a list of symptoms, conditions, and signs that could be indicators of low thyroid function. Take this self-assessment to see if there is a likelihood that you are suffering with a low functioning thyroid. *Simply mark/circle any of the symptoms in the four categories below that you feel apply to you. Then, add up your score as described on page 342 (scoring your self-assessment).*

1. Additional Symptoms
Do you have:

Significant fatigue, lethargy, sluggishness, or history of low thyroid at an earlier age
Hoarseness for no particular reason
Chronic recurrent infection(s)
Decreased sweating with mild exercise
Depression, to the point of being a bothersome problem
A tendency to be slow to heat up, even in a sauna
Constipation despite adequate fiber and liquids in diet
Brittle nails that crack or peel easily
High cholesterol despite good diet
Frequent headaches (especially migraine)
Irregular menses, pms, ovarian cysts, endometriosis
Unusually low sex drive
Red face with exercise
Accelerated worsening of eyesight or hearing
Palpitations or uncomfortably noticeable heartbeat
Difficulty in drawing a full breath, for no apparent reason
Mood swings, especially anxiety, panic or phobia
Gum problems
Mild choking sensation or difficulty swallowing
Excessive menopause symptoms, not well relieved with estrogen
Major weight gain
Aches and pains of limbs, unrelated to exertion
Skin problems of adult acne, eczema, or severe dry skin
Vague and mildly annoying chest discomfort, unrelated to exercise
Feeling off balance
Infertility
Annoying burning or tingling sensations that come and go
The experience of being colder than other people around you
Difficulty maintaining standard weight with a sensible food intake
Problems with memory, focus, or concentration

More than normal amounts of hair come out in the brush or shower
Difficulty maintaining stamina throughout the day

2. Related Conditions
Have you ever had any of these autoimmune disorders:

Diabetes, rheumatoid arthritis, lupus, sarcoidosis, scleroderma, Sjogren's syndrome, biliary cirrhosis, myasthenia gravis, multiple sclerosis, Crohn's disease, ulcerative colitis, thrombocytopenia (decreased blood platelets)
Prematurely gray hair
Anemia, especially the B_{12} deficiency type
Dyslexia
Persistent visual changes
Rapid cycle bipolar disorder (manic-depressive illness)
Raynaud's syndrome (white or blue discoloration of fingers or toes when cold)
Mitral valve prolapse
Carpal tunnel syndrome
Persistent tendinitis or bursitis
Atrial fibrillation
Alopecia (losing hair, especially in discrete patches)
Calcium deficiency
Attention deficit disorder (ADD)
Vitiligo (persistent large white patches on skin)
Neck injury, such as whiplash or blunt trauma

3. Family History
Have any of your blood relatives ever had:

High or low thyroid, or thyroid goiter
Prematurely gray hair
Complete or partial left-handedness
Diabetes
Rheumatoid arthritis
Lupus
Sarcoidosis
Scleroderma
Sjogren's syndrome
Biliary cirrhosis

Myasthenia gravis
Multiple sclerosis
Crohn's disease
Ulcerative colitis
Thrombocytopenia (decreased blood platelets)

4. Physical Signs
Have you or your doctor observed any of the following:

Low basal temperature in early morning (average of less than 97.6 degrees over 7 days)
Slow movements, slow speech, slow reaction time
Muscle weakness
Thick tongue (seemingly too big for mouth)
Swelling of feet
Swelling of eyelids or bags under eyes
Decreased color of lips or yellowing of skin
Swelling at base of neck (enlarged thyroid gland)
Asymmetry, lumpiness, or other irregularity of thyroid gland
Swelling of face
Excess ear wax
Dry mouth and/or dry eyes
Noticeably cool skin
Excessively dry or excessively coarse skin
Especially low blood pressure
Decreased ankle reflexes or normal reflexes with slow recovery phase
Noticeably slow pulse rate without having exercised regularly
Loss of outer one-third of eyebrows

Scoring Your Self Assessment

For Category I: Additional Symptoms
Give yourself 5 points for significant fatigue, and one point for each additional "yes" answer.

For Category 2: Related Conditions
Give yourself 5 points for autoimmune illness, and one point for each additional "yes" answer.

For Category 3: Family History
Give yourself 5 points for blood relatives ever having a thyroid problem, and 1 point for each additional "yes" answer.

For Category 4: Physical Signs
Give yourself 5 points for low basal temperature, and 1 point for each additional "yes" answer.

Interpreting Your Point Score

Add up your grand total of points from all four categories above.
5 Points = only mildly indicative low thyroid
Possible action: follow conservative suggestions (see your physician)
10 points = somewhat suspicious for low thyroid
Possible Action: obtain TSH level as first screening test
15 points = very suspicious for low thyroid
Possible Action: obtain additional tests, if TSH is normal
20 points = likely to be low thyroid
Possible Action: obtain all possible blood testing to help confirm a diagnosis
25 points = very likely to be low thyroid
Possible Action: obtain a trial of thyroid medicine, regardless of blood test results.

Our Suggested Panel of Thyroid Tests: the minimum amount of testing we think is needed before you can be told, "It doesn't look like low thyroid is causing your symptoms."

1. TSH
2. Basal Temperature Test
3. T-4 Panel (Total T-4, T-3 Uptake, Free Thyroxine Index)
4. T-3 Total
5. Thyroid Peroxidase (microsomal) Antibody

The Zypan Test (Taken from Bruce West's *Encyclopedia of Pragmatic Medicine p. 108–109*).
Purpose: To determine whether or not you have low stomach acid (hypochlorhydria). May also be useful in determining the presence of severe gastritis/stomach ulcers.

Requirements: Zypan® (Made by Standard Process)

Instructions: Start by taking one Zypan® tablet with meals. If indigestion lessens or if no noticeable discomfort occurs, begin taking 2 tablets of Zypan® per meal, and observe any symptoms. Again, if improvement is noted, or no symptoms of indigestion occur, increase to 3 tablets per meal. At this point, if improvement continues, it can safely be assumed that you are suffering from low stomach acid and need to take a digestive enzyme with betaine hydrochloride (like Zypan®) regularly until your stomach function is restored. Work with a qualified practitioner when evaluating stomach function and when performing the Zypan Test.

The Iodine Test

Purchase a small dropper bottle of liquid iodine solution at your local health food store. Then, first thing in the morning, apply a few drops to the skin of your upper arm, just on the inside of your bicep muscle. Make sure that you apply the drops slowly and cover a square area roughly 1 inch by 1 inch. Allow the iodine to dry so that it leaves a dry, stained area of your skin. Then get dressed and go about your day. Periodically take note of the stain on your skin, checking to see if it has disappeared. The stain should last roughly 24 hours before completely disappearing. Time how long it takes and report it back to your holistic physician. Anything less than 12 hours could indicate a need for iodine supplementation.

APPENDIX C
Recipes and Miscellaneous Information

Soaking instructions

The instructions for soaking, taken from *Nourishing Traditions* by Sally Fallon Morell, are used with her permission graciously given.

Instructions for Soaking Nuts

Pecans, almonds and walnuts – Soak in pot of warm water with 2 teaspoons of sea salt (must be Celtic sea salt) per pound of nuts (1 pound is approximately 4 cups). Soak for a minimum of 7 hours up to a maximum of 24 hours. Strain water off and dry in oven on warm (no more than 150 degrees) 12-24 hours or overnight, checking the nuts until they are crispy and dry.

Cashews – Soak for no more than 6 hours with 1 tablespoon of sea salt per pound of nuts. Strain water off and dry in oven on 200 degrees (no more than 220 degrees) overnight, checking for crispness and dryness of nuts to taste.

Purchase only raw, preferably organic nuts in sealed packages, not in open bins. Use unrefined sea salt, Celtic, Redmond, or Himalayan brands which can be purchased at Whole Foods or Trader Joe's.

Instructions for Soaking Oatmeal

Items needed:

1. McCann's Steel Cut Irish Oats. These come in an aluminum can and are found in most health food stores, Whole Foods, Trader Joe's and some supermarkets. Do not buy the instant version.
2. Whey liquid. It can be ordered from Uddermilk.com or you can use fresh lemon juice or Bragg's Apple Cider Vinegar.

Process:

1. First, spread 1 cup of oatmeal on a baking sheet. Place in the oven at 350° and allow oats to brown lightly. This should take about 10 minutes.

2. Remove oats from the oven and place in a food processor or grinder and grind down to a medium grind.

3. Place the oatmeal in a saucepan and add 1½ cups of fresh filtered *warm* water and 4 tablespoons of whey liquid. For the whey you may substitute lemon juice or Bragg's apple cider vinegar.

4. Allow the oats to soak in a warm place for a minimum of 8 hours, preferably overnight or longer.

5. Pour off the water when ready to cook. Add 1½ cups of fresh water and bring to a boil. Then reduce heat and cover slightly, cooking on a low heat for 10 minutes or until oatmeal reaches desired consistency.

Instructions for Soaking Beans, Rice and Legumes

Items needed:
1. Whole grain unpolished/unprocessed rice or dried beans.
2. Whey liquid (order at uddermilk.com) or fresh lemon juice or Bragg's Apple Cider Vinegar.

Process:
1. Cover rice or beans with warm, clean filtered water.
2. Add 1 tablespoon of whey or use lemon juice or apple cider vinegar.
3. Allow to soak overnight for a minimum of 8 hours. The longer the soak, the better.
4. Strain off the water when you are ready to cook. Take the amount of rice or beans you are going to cook and add fresh water accordingly. Bring to a boil and then reduce to a simmer allowing to cook the rest of the way on low heat. The remaining rice or beans may be left to soak longer or can be strained and stored in the refrigerator. (Sally Fallon Morell. *Nourishing Traditions.* New Trends Publishing newtrendspublishing.com.)

Nutritional Shake Recipes:

Whey Protein (cow-based options):
High Protein/Fat Shakes

1. **Chocolate-Almond Blast**
   1 scoop Whey Cool Chocolate Protein Powder
   1 tablespoon raw organic almond butter (may substitute cashew butter)
   1 tablespoon Udo's Perfected Oil Blend Flax Oil/Barlean's Flaxseed Oil
   1 raw organic pastured egg (Uddermilk or Whole Foods)
   6 ounces of full fat goat's or cow's milk (Uddermilk))
   Chopped ice as desired; blend

2. **Vanilla-Peanut Butter Crunch**
   1 scoop Whey Cool Vanilla Protein Powder
   1 tablespoon organic crunchy peanut butter
   1 tablespoon Udo's Perfected Oil Blend Flax Oil/Barlean's Flaxseed Oil
   1 raw organic pastured egg (Uddermilk or Whole Foods)

6 ounces of full fat goat's or cow's milk (Uddermilk)
Chopped ice as desired; blend

3. **Creamy Chocolate Dream**
   1 heaping tablespoon of raw heavy cream (Uddermilk)
   1 Scoop Whey Cool Chocolate Protein Powder
   1 tablespoon Udo's Perfected Oil Blend Flax Oil/Barlean's Flaxseed Oil
   1 raw organic pastured egg (Uddermilk or Whole Foods)
   6 ounces of full fat goat's or cow's milk (Uddermilk)
   Chopped ice as desired; blend

4. **Very Berry Blast**
   1 scoop Whey Cool Vanilla Protein Powder
   ½ cup of blueberries, strawberries or other berry of your choice
   1 tablespoon Udo's Perfected Oil Blend Flax Oil/Barlean's Flaxseed Oil
   1 raw organic pastured egg (Uddermilk or Whole Foods)
   6 ounces of full fat goat's or cow's milk (Uddermilk)
   Chopped ice as desired; blend

5. **Killer Almond Kefir Shake**
   4 ounces of raw kefir (Uddermilk)
   2-3 ounces of water *or* raw goat's or cow's milk (Uddermilk)
   1 tablespoon raw organic almond butter
   1 tablespoon Udo's Perfected Oil Blend Flax Oil/Barlean's Flaxseed Oil
   Chopped ice as desired; blend
   Berries may be substituted for almond butter if desired.

6. **Chocolate-Almond Espresso Boost**
   1 scoop Whey Cool Chocolate Protein Powder
   1 tablespoon raw organic almond butter (substitute cashew butter if preferred)
   1 tablespoon Udo's Perfected Oil Blend Flax Oil/Barlean's Flaxseed Oil
   1 raw organic pastured egg (Uddermilk or Whole Foods)
   6 ounces of full fat goat's or cow's milk (Uddermilk)
   1 shot decaffeinated espresso (2 ounces)
   Chopped ice as desired; blend

Probiotic/Fermented Shakes

1. **Original Kombucha Krush**
   4-6 ounces of GT's original flavored Kombucha
   1 tablespoon raw plain or vanilla yogurt (Uddermilk)
   1 scoop Vanilla Whey Cool
   ¼ - ½ cup of berries of your choice
   Chopped ice as desired; blend

2. **Mango Kombucha Madness**
   4-6 ounces of GT's Kombucha Synergy Mystic Mango
   1 tablespoon raw plain or vanilla yogurt or heavy cream (Uddermilk-optional)
   1 scoop Vanilla Whey Cool
   1 raw organic pastured egg
   Chopped ice as desired; blend

3. **Cranberry Kombucha Cream**
   4-6 ounces of GT's Kombucha Synergy Cosmic Cranberry
   1 tablespoon raw plain or vanilla yogurt or heavy cream (Uddermilk-optional)
   1 scoop Vanilla Whey Cool
   1 raw organic pastured egg
   Chopped ice as desired; blend

4. **Passionberry Kombucha Punch**
   4-6 ounces of GT's Kombucha Synergy Passionberry Bliss
   1 tablespoon raw plain or vanilla yogurt or heavy cream (Uddermilk-optional)
   1 scoop Vanilla Whey Cool
   1 raw organic pastured egg
   Chopped ice as desired; blend

5. **Strawberry Kombucha Creamsicle**
   4-6 ounces of GT's Kombucha Synergy Strawberry Serenity
   1 tablespoon raw plain or vanilla yogurt or heavy cream (Uddermilk-optional)
   1 scoop Vanilla Whey Cool
   1 raw organic pastured egg
   Chopped ice as desired; blend

Moderate/Higher Carbohydrate Shakes

1. **Chocolate Banana Nut Crunch**
   1 scoop Whey Cool Chocolate Protein Powder
   ½ of a ripe banana (use only when the skin has brown spots)
   1 tablespoon of organic crunchy peanut butter *or* almond butter
   1 tablespoon of raw honey (The Synergy Company's Healing Manuka Honey)
   6-8 ounces of raw goat's or cow's milk (Uddermilk)

2. **Vanilla Orange Cream Delight**
   1 scoop Whey Cool Vanilla Protein Powder
   ½ piece of a ripe banana (use only when the skin has brown spots)
   2-3 ounces fresh juice of Orange
   1 teaspoon of raw honey (Synergy Company's Healing Manuka Honey)
   6-8 ounces of raw goat's or cow's milk (Uddermilk)

3. **Orange Berry Blast**
   2-3 ounces fresh-squeezed orange juice
   ¼ - ½ cup of fresh (or frozen) berries of your choice
   6-9 ounces of water *or* raw milk (goat's or cow's)
   1 scoop Whey Cool Vanilla
   1 teaspoon Manuka Healing Honey

Specialty Shakes

1. **The Bone Builder**
   8 ounces of raw cow's milk (goat's optional) from Uddermilk
   1 Scoop chocolate or vanilla Whey Cool
   1 tablespoon of Calcifood® Powder from Standard Process
   1 tablespoon of Flax Seed Oil (Udo's Oil or Barlean's)
   1 tablespoon of Green Pasture™ Cod Liver Oil

2. **The Immune-O-Booster**
   6-8 ounces of raw cow's milk (goat's optional) from Uddermilk
   1 scoop chocolate or vanilla Whey Cool
   1 teaspoon Pure Radiance vitamin C powder
   1 teaspoon Pure Synergy Green Food
   1 teaspoon Green Pasture™ Cod Liver Oil

3. **The Killer Cleanser**
   2-3 ounces of fresh lemon juice (lime may be used as well)
   1-2 ounces of undistilled aloe vera juice
   6 ounces raw goat's milk or kefir (Uddermilk)
   1 scoop K-Pax Fuel of Life Protein
   1 teaspoon Pure Synergy Green Food
   1 teaspoon Green Pasture™ Cod Liver Oil

Whey Protein Tips *(cow-based options):*

Add a half or quarter of a ripe avocado to your shake to make it smooth and thicker in texture rather than watery!

Use Nutiva or Native Forest brand Coconut Cream/Water or Milk. Available at Whole Foods or in health food stores.

For the dairy-sensitive, substitute coconut milk/water *or* use your own homemade almond milk (see the book *Nourishing Traditions* for recipe) in any shake above.

For patients with more serious gastrointestinal issues, food allergies, etc., Warrior Food, Inflammacore (OrthoMolecular) are the best choices for your protein source for the shakes above.

Rice/Hemp Protein in the form of Warrior Food Extreme, LifeCore, or InflammaCORE (by OrthoMolecular) may be substituted for the Whey Protein in any of the shakes above for those seeking hypoallergenic protein (dairy allergy) or as directed by the physician. They come in a variety of flavors.

Rice protein in the form of K-Pax, LifeCore, or InflammaCORE (all by OrthoMolecular) may be substituted for the Whey Protein in any of the shakes above for those seeking hypoallergenic protein (dairy allergy) or as directed by the physician. They come in a variety of flavors.

GT's Kombucha can be purchased at Whole Foods or Fairway Markets, and in a growing number of food stores around the country.

Experiment with the recipes by adding flaxseed oil (Udo's or Barlean's), Pure Radiance Vitamin C, raw honey, Calcifood® Powder.

If a more complete meal replacement shake is desired, it is recommended that you use either PaleoMeal protein from Designs for

Health in place of Whey Cool *or* K-Pax Fuel of Life Protein Blend by OrthoMolecular.

Washing Instructions for Non-Organic Fruits and Vegetables:

Requirements: Food-Grade (30%) hydrogen peroxide *or* regular chlorine bleach

Instructions: Place vegetables and fruits in sink, and fill with filtered water. For every gallon of water, add two teaspoons of peroxide or bleach (so if you fill your sink with five gallons of filtered water, you would add 10 teaspoons of peroxide or bleach. Allow thick skinned fruits and vegetables to soak for 15 minutes; leafy greens, thin-skinned fruits and vegetables for 10 minutes. Once soaked for appropriate time, drain water and refill sink with clean filtered water. Allow fruits and vegetables to soak for 10-15 minutes in clean water. You may then remove them from the water and consume as needed.

*Do not confuse 3% Peroxide with Food Grade, 30% peroxide. They are **not** the same. 30% Food-Grade peroxide is concentrated and can burn you!! Under **no** circumstance should you consume this (unless properly diluted in water) nor should you use as a mouth rinse or gargle. Seek immediate emergency care if consumed.* **Keep out of reach of children.**

Gallbladder and Pancreas Diet

Here is a list of important recommendations concerning proper diet with regard to pancreatitis.

1. First, *avoid all alcohol, including beer and wine.* Alcohol aggravates the pancreas. The pancreas and gallbladder are the two crucial digestive organs targeted by this diet.

2. Second, and *equally important is maintaining balanced blood sugar levels.* Insulin is produced by the pancreas, and any large spikes in your blood sugar will result in further strain on the pancreas to produce insulin. Avoid foods containing added refined sugars including corn syrup, high fructose corn syrup, dextrose, cane juice.

3. You will then have to familiarize yourself with the Glycemic Index. This index tells you which carbohydrates elevate your blood sugar and which will not. Carbohydrates are given a glycemic value which reflects the amount they raise your blood sugar and

in return strain the pancreas. *The New Glucose Revolution: The Authoritative Guide to the Glycemic Index* by Jennie Brand-Miller, PhD, et al. provides a chart of all of the most common carbs we come into contact with and their impact on your blood sugar.

4. No gluten or gluten-containing foods. This includes wheat, barley, and rye among others (grain protein aggravates this condition as well as many others). Ask the doctor for a complete list if you know you are gluten sensitive.

5. Finally, limit "bad fats." Therefore, no fried foods and no hydrogenated oils including those containing trans fats. Avoid all liquid vegetable oils like soybean, vegetable blend, corn, canola, safflower, sunflower and rapeseed as well as margarines, shortenings and other "frankenfats" (man-made). Use extra virgin olive oil, flaxseed oil and coconut oil in moderate amounts. To guide you, the doctor has a list of specific fats to avoid as listed on product labels. Limit dairy using only lower fat raw milk or 1% milk fat.

Basic Supplements: You will need to take the following supplements to aid the pancreas and gallbladder:

1. A-F Betafood® used primarily for gallbladder problems. It gets the bile moving thus aiding in the digestion of fats.
2. Digestive Enzyme which must contain pancreatin, ox bile, and betaine HCL. Two good enzymes are Ortho Digestzyme by Ortho Molecular Products and Bio-Gest® by Thorne.
3. Pancreatrophin PMG® (optional, doctor will decide). This is a protomorphogen extract of the nucleic acids from the nucleus of the cell which control the function of the cell. This is crucial in rebuilding glandular function in more severe cases.

The following sample diet is advisable. Remember, this is just a sample and can be expanded with other fruits and vegetables according to the glycemic index and the list of fruits and vegetables given to you by the doctor.

Breakfast

1. Fresh fruit – choose from amongst the lower glycemic fruits as in this book. Some examples are grapefruit, pear, etc. Spread the fruit out throughout the morning according to what satisfies you.

2. Eggs – *(you may use one yolk, but the rest **must** be egg whites)* scrambled over easy, or made into a vegetable omelet. Make use of the different green and non-starchy vegetables according to the glycemic index: spinach, mushrooms, onions, zucchini, etc.

3. Steel Cut Oatmeal or Millet – these cereals, since they have to be cooked and are not processed, are slower-burning carbohydrates and therefore do not raise your blood sugar the way processed cereals do. However, they must be soaked overnight prior to eating, and are best purchased soaked in their whole form and freshly ground at home. Contact *To Your Health Sprouted Flour Company* (Appendix D p. 357 #18) to purchase. Add cinnamon, a dash of salt, and some berries to flavor. See the directions for soaking in Appendix C pp. 344-346.

Lunch
1. Sardines or any fish you like with two green vegetables and/or a side salad. Bake, broil or grill the fish. You may use herbs, pepper, or seasonings as long as they are not sugar sweetened. An excellent one is 365 Organic's Cajun Seasoning available at Whole Foods.
2. Baked sweet potato with a side mixed green or mesculin salad or two green vegetables. For the dressing on salads you may use olive oil, organic apple cider vinegar, Celtic brand sea salt, fresh lemon juice and black pepper. Ask the doctor for additional recipes.
3. Mixed green vegetable salad with raw cottage cheese. (See above for dressings).

Dinner
1. Chicken, fish, lean beef, veal or turkey – baked, broiled, boiled, grilled, or stir fried (low heat) with any combination of green or low glycemic vegetables you wish. A small mixed greens salad to start with. Use dressings as described above.

Guide to Knowing Your Fats

Important facts about real fats:
All **traditional fats** are good for you - no exceptions.
Regarding **animal fats**, the animal's food matters for our health. Remember, **grass is good.**
With **vegetable oils**, processing oil damages the nutrients. Plant oils should be **cold pressed.**

Real animal fats are good for us:
   Fat from grass-fed cattle, sheep, bison and other game
   Butter and cream from grass-fed cows
   Lard from pastured pigs fed a natural diet
   Poultry from pastured chickens, ducks and geese
   Fish oil (preferably wild), especially cod liver oil

Real vegetable oils are good too:
   Cold-pressed, extra-virgin olive oil
   Cold-pressed, unrefined flaxseed oil
   Unrefined coconut oil
   Cold-pressed, unrefined macadamia nut, walnut and sesame seed oils

The problem with industrial fats:

The industrial diet contains too many omega-6 fats from corn and soybean oil, and too few omega-3 fats from the above list. This leads to obesity, diabetes, heart disease and cancer. Trans fats cause inflammation, obesity, diabetes, heart disease and infertility. Do not eat hydrogenated and partially hydrogenated oils, including margarine and vegetable oil or interesterified fats— vegetable oils made solid but free of trans fats. This includes corn, safflower, sunflower, and soybean oils, especially when refined or heated.

Refined Sugars List **"The Forgettable Forty"**

The following is a fairly comprehensive list of refined sugars to be avoided at all cost. Many of these sugars are marketed as "healthy" or "healthier" choices. However, that is a marketing ploy. None of these sugars should be consumed with any regularity.

1. Brown rice syrup
2. Fruit juice concentrate
3. Fruit juice
4. Sugar
5. Invert sugar
6. Cane sugar
7. Cane juice
8. Evaporated cane juice
9. Raw cane sugar
10. Brown sugar
11. Beet sugar
21. Dextrose
22. Maltodextrin
23. Glucose
24. Glucose solids
25. Fructose
26. Sucrose
27. Maltose
28. Lactose
29. Galactose
30. Honey
31. Maple syrup

12. Palm sugar
13. Date sugar
14. Coconut sugar
15. Barley malt
16. Malt syrup
17. Rice bran syrup
18. Corn syrup
19. Corn syrup solids
20. High fructose corn syrup
32. Agave
33. Muscovado sugar
34. Turbinado sugar
35. Sucanat
36. Rapadura
37. Molasses
38. Caramel
39. Sorghum syrup
40. Almost anything with "syrup" in the name

APPENDIX D
Important Resources

1. A Campaign for Real Milk – www.realmilk.com – Serves to inform people regarding the facts, health, safety, and other pertinent information regarding raw milk. Helps you to locate fresh, clean, organic sources of raw milk and herdshares in your state/area.

2. The Weston A. Price Foundation – www.westonaprice.org – An important resource for learning about the work of Weston A. Price regarding traditional cultures and their diets. It provides honest research, nutrition news, abc's of health, and important information on all types of health topics and conditions.

3. Radiant Life Company – www.radiantlifecatalog.com – A wonderful research source for purchasing alternative health care products, water filters, supplements, and much more.

4. Green Pasture™ Products – www.greenpasture.org – A source for the highest quality, unprocessed, high-vitamin cod liver oil and butter oil.

5. The Center for Personal Rights – www.centerforpersonalrights.org – Provides resources for parents and individuals to help them make the best choices for themselves and their families regarding vaccines; includes information on vaccine injury compensation and the science, ethics, and politics of vaccine mandates.

6. The National Conference on State Legislatures – www.NCSL.org – Offers a summary of state laws regarding vaccinations. Type "School Immunization" in the search box and click on the link "School Immunization Exemption State Laws".

7. True Activist- www.trueactivist.com – Provides a PDF of a Physician's Warranty of Vaccine Safety Form which can be downloaded for free to give to your physician to sign regarding vaccinations. This can be used if you are pressured by any physician to vaccinate.

8. Sample Exemption Letters for Vaccines – www.vaclib.org/pdf/exemption.htm

9. Resource for State Laws on vaccinations, side effects, reports showing lack of effectiveness of vaccines, and list of ingredients for every vaccine by manufacturer – www.novaccine.com.

10. Standard Process Company – www.standardprocess com – In my opinion, bar-none, the best supplement company in the world. I have used their products for over 50 years with wonderful success. Visit their website for more information.

11. The Synergy Company – www.thesynergycompany.com – Makers of high-quality, whole-food vitamins including: vitamin C (Pure Radiance C); Pure Synergy (Super-food Green Food Powder); Cell Protector and more. Read about founder Mitchell May's personal experience with healing and his miraculous recovery using non-traditional methods after a near-fatal auto accident.

12. Chris Masterjohn's website – www.cholesterol-and-health.com – dedicated to the real truth about cholesterol and more. A must-visit website for anyone looking for the real scientific facts about cholesterol and fats.

13. The Heritage Company (Castor Oil) – www.heritagestore.com.

14. Ocean's Lab – www.oceanslab.com – Source for MMS (Miracle Mineral Solution). Visit – www.jimhumble.org – for information.

15. Natural Immunogenics Corporation – www.natural-immunogenics.com – Makers of Argentyn 23 Silver Hydrosol. Visit their website for more information and on where to purchase locally.

16. Diagnos-Techs – www.diagnostechs.com – Performs salivary lab testing for male/female hormones, food allergies, adrenal function tests, and much more. Visit their website for more information.

17. Genova Diagnostics Labs – www.gdx.net – Lab tests for nutritional and metabolic function including IgG/IgE food allergy testing, Vitamin/Mineral deficiencies, Toxic Elements, and more.

18. To Your Health Sprouted Flour Company – www.organicsproutedflour.net – specializes in sprouted whole grains and whole grain flours to meet all your healthy cooking and baking needs. All of their grains and legumes are certified organic and kosher. The grains are sprouted, dried, and milled at low temperatures (65-110°) to maintain enzymes, vitamins and minerals

19. Jupiter Grain Mill (Schnitzer Getreidemuhlen) – www.perfektegesundheit.de. – Recommended by Sally Fallon Morell in *Nourishing Traditions.* Product available $150 cheaper by ordering from German company named Perfekte Gesundheit Shop. Click on the British Flag in the top righthand margin of the webpage to translate the site to English. No problems ordering from this mill to my New Jersey home. Delivery takes about 10 days. There are two versions with many different adapters depending on whether you want to make your own cereal (a flaker adapter), etc. One is a hand crank model and the other has an electric motor. Both have natural stone as the grinding surface which is important. Both are suitable. You will need a $25 outlet transformer.

20. Enema Kits – Using either www.enemakit.com *or* www.amazon.com and type in enema kit. You should not have to spend more than $25 for a good quality product.

21. The Heritage Store - to purchase Glycothymoline - available online at www.theheritagestore.com.

22. Raw Honey - although many good brands are available, we use Really Raw Honey, from Fairway Markets. However, any local, unheated and unfiltered honey found in your area is best. We also recommend using the Weston A. Price Shopper's Guide for the best choices.

23. Progressive Labs – www.progressivelabs.com– 1-800-527-9512 – Texas-based lab makes excellent digestive enzyme called Digestin.

24. Flax Seed Oil Brands – Barlean's, Udo's Oil or Omega Nutrition. Can be purchased at Vitamin Shoppe and other local health food stores as well as online.

25. The Holistic Dental Association – http://www.holisticdental.org.

26. Artemis Itch Calm Cream available through their website – http://international.artemis.co.nz/itch-calm-cream.html.

27. Raw (unpasteurized) organic apple cider vinegar – I recommend Bragg's, available in most health food stores and Whole Foods; or Omega Nutrition's apple cider vinegar, available online at – www.healthalertstore.com.

28. Acid-Alkaline Food Chart – www.acidalkalinediet.com/Alkaline-Foods-Chart.htm – Use this color-coded chart as guide in choosing more alkaline-forming foods to balance your body's pH.

29. Foot Levelers – footlevelers.com or call 800-553-4860.

APPENDIX E
Recommended Reading

1. *Nutrition and Physical Degeneration* by Weston A. Price, DDS. A classic study of isolated populations and their native diets. The book catalogs the disastrous effects of processed foods on native, isolated populations all over the world.
2. *The Untold Story of Milk* by Ron Schmid, ND. Details the history of milk in this country, including the push for pasteurization, politics, and the conspiracy to remove healthy raw milk from the market.
3. *Nourishing Traditions* by Sally Fallon. A book to study and use as a resource for cooking, preparing and enjoying traditional, healthy, unprocessed foods. This masterpiece is a must-have teaching tool for learning about food and nutrition.
4. *The Nourishing Traditions Book of Baby and Child Care* by Sally Fallon and Thomas S. Cowan, MD. Important for parents, from planning to conceive, throughout pregnancy and childhood. The book pro-vides holistic advice for pregnancy and newborn interventions, vaccinations, breast-feeding and child development, as well as a compendium of natural treatments for childhood illnesses, from autism to whooping cough.
5. *Real Food Fermentation* by Alex Lewin. Make your own lacto-fermented foods like sauerkraut and others. Excellent instructions and explanations on the benefits of fermented foods.
6. *Beyond Broccoli* by Susan Schenck. All-around book on the dangers of veganism; the truth about nutrition and health; and helpful on many of today's debated issues, including cholesterol.
7. *Breaking the Vicious Cycle* by Elaine Gottschall. Contains the Specific Carbohydrate Diet (precursor of the GAPS diet by Natasha Campbell McBride), important for anyone suffering from IBS/Crohn's Disease or other inflammatory bowel conditions as well as other degenerative conditions.
8. *Gut and Psychology Syndrome* by Natasha Campbell-McBride and includes *The Gaps Guide* by Baden Lashkov. Important for anyone with digestive illness and resulting mental illness including ADHD, schizophrenia, depression and more. Explains how

destruction of the gastrointestinal lining can lead to mental illness and bowel diseases, and how to restore health through wholesome, traditional foods and supplementation.
9. *The Great Cholesterol Con: Why Everything You've Been Told About Cholesterol and Heart Disease is Wrong* by Anthony Colpo. Book covers facts and flaws regarding the major studies used to support the cholesterol hypothesis. Colpo presents the real facts and lays out his 12 commandments for a healthy heart, none of which involve lowering cholesterol.
10. *The Great Cholesterol Con: The Truth About What Really Causes Heart Disease and How to Avoid It* by Malcolm Kendrick, MD Insightful, occasionally humorous book on cholesterol and heart disease. Kendrick exposes the real causes of heart disease and why cholesterol is not to blame.
11. *The Vegetarian Myth* by Lierre Keith. Keith, like Susan Schenck, a vegan for over 20 years before acknowledging the shortcomings it created in her health, lays down a moral, political, environmental and nutritional foundation for why veganism did not work for her and is not a healthy diet for anyone to follow for any extended period of time. She dispels the myth that veganism is morally superior, better for the environment, and better for health.
12. *Cure Tooth Decay: Heal & Prevent Cavities with Nutrition* by Ramiel Nagel. By urging the reader back to a traditional diet rich in bone broths, cod liver oil, and free from industrially processed foods, Nagel explains how tooth decay can be stopped and even reversed. He offers insight into the much debated topics of root canal, implants and more.
13. *Cows Save the Planet* by Judith Schwartz. The author discusses desertification (the loss of carbon and nutrients in our soil to form vast deserts) created by modern farming methods like mono-cropping, and how intensive grazing can restore these deserts back to fertile land. Managed intensive grazing puts carbon back into the earth, thus rebuilding the soil. As Schwartz explains, plants provide a two-way transfer of nutrients: the plant brings minerals up from the soil and into the stems, leaves and fruit, and also carries carbon from the air down to the roots.
14. *Folks, This Ain't Normal* by Joel Salatin. A report on the ignorance of modern Americans regarding farming and the food we eat,

how this makes us vulnerable to the processed food industry, and ways for all of us to improve the quality of our health through the quality of our food while reconnecting to our agrarian roots.
15. *The World According to Monsanto.* Marie-Monique Robin discloses how Monsanto has single-handedly been responsible for destruction to the environment and our food supply by products like Agent Orange, dioxins, Round-up, GMO seeds, etc.
16. *Seeds of Deception* by Jeffrey Smith. Focuses on health hazards posed by genetically modified seeds.
17. *Pottenger's Prophecy: How Food Resets Genes for Wellness or Illness* by Gray Graham. Takes on the emerging field of epigenetics and reveals the foods that guide your genes on a path toward illness, as well as the diet that can activate genes that promote healing and good health.
18. *Clean, Green & Lean: Get Rid of the Toxins That Make You Fat.* Walter Crinnion's excellent guide to removing toxins from you life and home, while shedding unwanted pounds and detoxifying your body.
19. *What Your Doctor Won't Tell You: The Complete Guide to the Latest in Alterntive Medicine* by Jane Heimlich. An objective sourcebook on important alternative approaches to health.
20. *The Meat Fix* by John Nicholson. Story of a man whose journey through vegetarianism/veganism brought him to a long battle with irritable bowel syndrome and deteriorating health, only to find that the "fix" to his health problems was to return to eating meat.
21. *Eat Fat Lose Fat* by Mary G. Enig, PhD and Sally Fallon. Explains how to lose weight effectively by eating traditional foods including healthy fats like coconut oil, all while improving your health.
22. *Vaccine Epidemic: How Corporate Greed, Biased Science, and Coercive Government Threaten Our Human Rights, Our Health, and Our Children* by Louise Kuo Habakus, MA and Mary Holland, JD Exposes problematic issues about vaccine policy, harmful vaccine ingredients, and the basic human right to decide for oneself what goes into our bodies.
23. *Why We Get Fat.* Gary Taubes reveals the poor nutritional science of the past century and what really determines whether we gain

weight or not. He discloses that the old "calories-in, calories-out" approach is wrong and clarifies what foods make us fat, and pro-vides excellent information on nutrition and weight management.
24. *Put Your Heart in Your Mouth* by Natasha Campbell-McBride MD, M.MedSci (Neurology), M.MedSci (Nutrition). Important for anyone with heart disease or looking for the real truth about heart disease and nutrition.
25. *The Gall Bladder Survival Guide* by Jeremy Bernal. An important book for anyone diagnosed with gallbladder disease or who has already had their gallbladder removed.
26. *Rethinking Pasteur's Germ Theory: How to Maintain Your Optimal Health* by Nancy Appleton. A reader-friendly guide to maintaining good health.
27. *Béchamp or Pasteur?: A Lost Chapter in the History of Biology* by Ethel D. Hume. Discover the politics behind the Germ Theory and what really causes disease.

APPENDIX F
Appliances

1. **Cuno Water Filters** – http://www.freshwatersystems.com
2. **Water Filters** – http://www.radiantlifecatalog.com
3. **The Jupiter Grain Mill** – www.perfektegesundheit.de. – Click on the British Flag in the top righthand margin of the webpage to translate the site to English.
4. **Cervico 2000 Manual Traction Collar** – www.meditrac.co.il – Ask your physician for more information. Partially to fully reimbursable through most insurance plans including Medicare.

APPENDIX G
Charts and Illustrations

Food Combining Chart .... p. 24
New Food Pyramid .... p. 31
Traditional Wisdom Food Pyramid .... p. 32
Structure of the Ear .... p. 63
Hiatal Hernia and Stomach .... p. 96
Gall Bladder .... p. 113
Herniated Cervical Vertebrae .... p. 147
Vertebral Disc Anatomy .... p. 151
Balanced and Unbalanced Stance .... p. 156
Kyphotic Lordotic Posture .... p. 157
Nitric Oxide Biochemistry in ED .... p. 168
Male Reproductive System .... p. 173
Micronutrient Intakes in Traditional Diets .... p. 204
Evolution of Sugar Consumption .... p. 214
Hyper/Hypo Glycemia .... p. 227
Achilles Tendon .... p. 335
Exercise for the Prostate .... p. 337
Vertebral Subluxation and Nerve Chart .... p. 364
The Balance Beam of Holistic Health .... p. 365
Carbohydrates in Fruits/Nuts and Seeds .... p. 366
Carbohydrates in Vegetables .... p. 367
Acid/Alkaline Foods .... p. 368

A Legacy of Healing

VERTEBRAL SUBLUXATION AND NERVE CHART

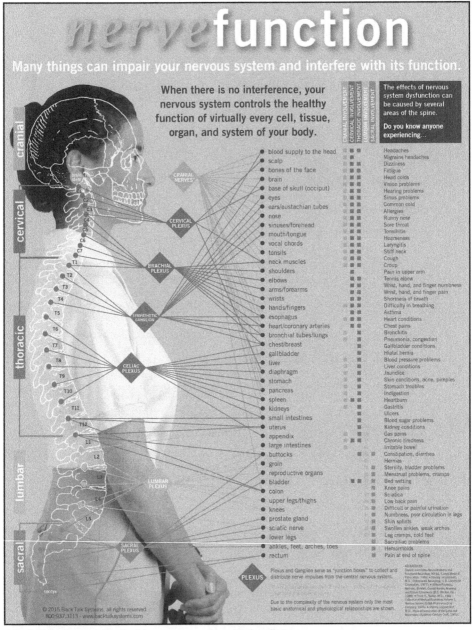

©Back Talk Systems. Used with permission from Back Talk Systems.

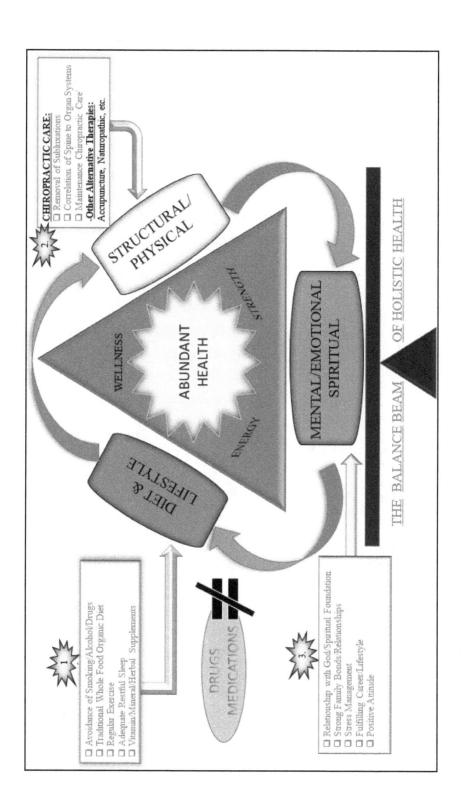

Carbohydrates in Fruits/Nuts and Seeds

Low-Carb Fruits (Allowed sparingly)
A few fruit types may be incorporated into the diet if eaten sparingly. Berries have the lowest carbohydrate content of all fruits.

Avocado (7.4g/cup) ®
Boysenberries (16g/cup) ®
Guava (4.8g in 1 med pc) ®
Raspberries (6.7g/cup) ®
Blueberries (17.5g/cup)®
Blackberries (6g/cup) ®
Lemon (4.0g in 1 med pc) ®
Strawberries (8.6g/cup) ®
Cranberries (unsweetened) (8.3g/cup) ®
Gooseberries (9g/cup) ®
Lime (5.1g/cup) ®

High-Carb Fruits (Avoid)
® All values given are for raw fruit

Apple (18g in 1 med)
Currants
Grapefruit (17g/med pc)
Kumquat
Orange (12g/med pc)
Pear (16g/med pc)
Prune (5g/pc)
Apricot (3.2g in 1 pc)
Dates (5.5g in 1 pc)
Grapes(14.2g/cup)
Mango (31g in 1 pc)
Papaya (24g/med pc)
Persimmon(25g/pc)
Raisins (54g/1/2cup)
Banana(24g/1 med pc)
Papaya (24g/med pc)
Raisins (54g/1/2cup)
Mulberries (13g/cup)
Passion Fruit (2.3 in 1 pc)
Pineapple (17.4 in 1 pc)
Melons (11-16g/wedge)
Cherries (1g/med pc)
Figs (8g in 1 med pc)
Kiwi (9g in med pc)
Nectarine (12g in 1 pc)
Peach (12g in 1 lg pc)
Plum (6.6g in 1 pc)
Watermelon (20g/wedge)

Low-Carb Nuts and Seeds

Almond (1g/10 pcs)
Brazil Nuts (7g/cup)
Hazelnut (2g/ ¼ cup)
Pecan (1.2g/oz)
Black Walnut (1g/4 pcs)
Coconut (24g/whole pc)
Macadamia Nut (7g/cup)

High-Carb Nuts and Seeds (Avoid/Limit)

Cashew (7.6g/oz)
Pine Nuts (3g/ ¼ cup)
Pumpkin Seed(1.2g/tbsp)
Soy Nuts
Peanut (2.1g/oz)
Pistachio (5g/oz)
Sesame Seed(0.84g/tbsp.)
Sunflower Seed (0.8g/tbsp.)

Carbohydrates in Vegetables

Low- Carb/Preferred Vegetables (Less than 8 grams per cup/8 ozs)
(® Denotes Raw Value; © Denotes Cooked Value)

Artichoke (2g in 4 pcs)	Avocado (4.8g) ®	Asparagus (4.8g)	Bamboo Shoots
Bean Sprouts (4.2g)	Beet Greens (2.4g) ®	Bok Choy (1.5g) ®	Broccoli (8.0g)
Brussels Sprouts (9.4g)	Cabbage (2.2g) ®	Carrots (7g)	Cauliflower (4.0g)
Celery (6.0g)	Celery Root/Celeriac (2.4g)®	Chard (1.3g)	Chives (0.1 in 1Tbsp.) ®
Collard Greens (4.0g)	Cucumber (8.0g) ®	Daikon Radish	Eggplant (8.0g)
Endive (0.4g) ®	Fennel(6.0g) ®	Green Beans (5.8g)	Herbs & Spices
Jicama (5.0g) ®	Kale (4.2g) ®	Lettuce (all types- 0.5g)	Mushrooms (3-5g) ®
Napa Cabbage (2.2g)	Okra (7.6g) ®	Peppers (all- 7.0g) ®	Radish(3.9g) ®
Rhubarb (3.4g) ®	Sauerkraut (4.2g)	Scallions (7.0g) ®	Seaweed (nori, etc)
Sprouts	Sorrel (4.3g) ®	Spinach (0.2g) ®	Snow Peas (6.7g) ©
Summer Squash(5.0g)	Tomatillos (7.8g) ®	Tomato (6.4g) ®	Turnips (4.6g)
Watercress (6.4g) ®	Wax Beans (5.8g) ©	Zucchini (5.0g) ©	

Medium-Carb Vegetables (between 8-25 grams per cup)

Beets (13g ®, 8g ©)	Yams (30g)©	Chickpeas (garbanzo) 35g©	Corn (organic only) (17.2g) ©
Kohlrabi	Leeks (13g) ®	Onion (10-15g)®	Parsnip (24g)©
Peas (13.5) ©	Rutabaga (8.5g)©	Spaghetti Squash(15g)	Dry Beans (black, ,kidney,etc) (24g)©
Jerusalem Artichoke	Lima Beans (26g)©	Lentils (22g) ©	Potato (30g) ©
Pumpkin (9.2g)	Sweet Potato (30g)©	Water Chestnuts (20g)®	Winter Squash (acorn, butternut, (24g)

A Legacy of Healing

ALKALINE/ACID FOODS

Alkaline Foods		Neutral/Moderately Acidic Foods		Acidic Foods	
Grains, Cereals & Breads	**Diary & Meat**	**Grains, Cereals & Breads**	Carbonated & Unfiltered Water	**Grains, Cereals & Breads**	**Drinks**
Amaranth	None	Brown Rice	Pasteurised Fruit & Tomato Juice	Barley	Alcohol
Buckwheat		Bulgar Wheat	Kombucha Tea	Bran, oat	Black Tea
Kamut	**Condiments & Spices**	Home Made / Minimally		Bran, wheat	Cocoa
Millet	(Unfermented Soy)	Processed Breads	**Diary & Meat**	Bread	Coffee
Quinoa	Almond Butter	Oats	Quorn (meat substitute)	Corn	Energy Drinks
Spelt	Bee Pollen	Wholegrain Pasta	Tofu	Corn Chips	Milk
Sprouted Breads	Bragg Aminos		Whey (Raw)	Cornstarch	Soda
Sprouted Tortillas	Chili Pepper	**Sweets & Desserts**	Yogurt (Organic Fresh)	Crackers	
Yeast-Free Breads	Cinnamon	Agave		Flour	**Dairy & Meat**
Dehydrated flax seed crackers	Curry Powders	Honey	**Condiments & Spices**	Granola	ALL products – including chicken, beef, pork, lamb, fish, cheese, milk, yoghurt, eggs
	Ginger	Lo Han Guo	Apple Cider Vinegar	Noodles	
Sweets & Desserts	Guacamole (fresh made)	Stevia	Miso	Pasta	
None	Herbs (all)		Tahini	Processed Grains	
	Houmous	**Beans & Legumes**	Spices (hot)	Rice Cakes	
Beans & Legumes	Lemon Juice	Black Beans		Rye	**Condiments & Spices**
All moderately acidic	Lime Juice	Canned Beans (Chick Peas)		Spaghetti	Fermented Sauces
	Sea Salt	Garbanzo Beans		Wheat Germ	Jams & Preserves
	Spices (most)	Kidney Beans		White Rice	Mayonnaise
Drinks		Lentils		Wheat	Soy Sauce
Alkaline Water	**Oriental Vegetables**	Lima Beans		Cous Cous	Sweet Chilli Sauce
Barley Grass Juice	Daikon	Mung Beans			Tomato Ketchup
Coconut Water	Kombu	Navy Beans		**Sweets & Desserts**	Vinegar
Fresh Lemon & Lime Water	Maitake	Pinto Beans		ALL Sugar, Sugar Products & Artificial Sweeteners	
Fresh Veg Juices	Nori	Red Beans			
Green Drinks	Reishi	Soy Beans			
Green Tea	Sea Vegetables	White Beans		**Beans & Legumes**	
Herbal Tea	Shitake			All moderately acidic	
Wheatgrass Juice	Umeboshi	**Nuts & Seeds**			
	Wakame	Almond Butter		**Nuts & Seeds**	
		Almonds		All salted are moderately acidic	
		Brazil Nuts			
		Carraway Seeds			
		Cashews			
		Cumin Seeds			
		Fennel Seeds			
		Hazel Nuts			
		Hemp Seeds			
		Peanuts			
		Pumpkin Seeds			
		Sesame Seeds			
		Sunflower Seeds			
		Walnuts			
		Drinks			
		Tap, Bottled.			

APPENDIX H
Acronyms

ABA	Applied behavioral analysis
ADA	American Dental Association
ADHD	Attention-deficit/hyperactivity disorder
AHA	American Heart Association
BCP	Birth control pills
CAFO	Concentrated animal feeding operation
CVD	Cardiovascular disease
CDC	Center for Disease Control
CDSA	Complete digestive stool analysis
CHF	Congestive heart failure
DDD	Degenerative disc disorder
DGL	Deglycyrrhizinated Licorice Root
DM	Diabetes mellitus
ED	Erectile dysfunction
EWG	Environmental Working Group
GAG	Glycosaminoglycans
GAPS	Gut and psychology syndrome
GERD	Gastroesophageal reflux disease
GMO	Genetically modified organism
GSE	Grapefruit seed extract
HCL	Hydrochloric acid
HFCS	High fructose corn syrup
HRT	Hormone replacement therapy
HSO	Homeostatic soil organisms
HTN	Hypertension
HVLAT	High velocity low amplitude thrust
IDDM	Insulin-dependent diabetes mellitus
INR	International normalized ratio
JAMA	The Journal of the American Medical Association
MCHC	Mean corpuscular hemoglobin concentration
MMS	Miracle Mineral Supplement
MSG	Monosodium glutamate
NIDDM	Noninsulin-dependent diabetes melllitus
NSAID	Nonsteroidal anti-inflammatory medications
PUFA	Polyunsaturated fatty acids
SAD	Standard american diet
SCD	Specific carbohydrate diet
USDA	United States Department of Agriculture
UTI	Urinary tract infection
VLDL	Very low density lipoprotein
WAPF	Weston A. Price Foundation

INDEX

A
Acne 250–51,340
Activator technique 145
Activator X 134,138, 145,185
ADD/ADHD
  -4Rs protocol for 72,78,291–301
  -chiropractic treatment 291
  -GAPS diet 291
  -implicated in in-vitro pregnancy 262
  -importance of saturated fat/cholesterol 293
  -Ω6:Ω3 ratio 293
  -sugar consumption, relation to 297
Allergies 53,58–61
Angular Stomatitis 77
Ankle, sprained 119
Applied Behavioral Analysis (ABA) 141
Argentyn 23 Silver Hydrosol 53–58,65,80–84,253–54,323,357
  -First Aid Gel 254,255
Arthritis 27,116–18,136–44
  -adult 136–40
  -juvenile 140,141
  -menopausal 141–44

B
Baroody, James 27,138,158,245
Back pain 144–54
Béchamp, Antoine 89–91,362
Bennett Technique 76
Bernal, Jeremy 111-113,361
Berry, Wendell 10
Birth Control Pill 145,164,184–88
  -nutrients depleted 187
  -thyroid damage 186
  -adrenal damage 183, 194
Bisphosphonate Drugs 163
Bitters/Bitter Reflex 112,300

Bleeding gums 72, 222
Blended diet 96–98
Boil treatment 252
Bone broth 42,81,96–100,108,149,281
BPH 170-76
  -case studies176-79
  -chiropractic treatment 173, 178
  -diet for 177
  -exercises for 337
  -zinc, role in 173, 176
  -vitamin B6, role in 173
Breaking the vicious cycle 104
Brogan, Kelly MD 85
Bronchitis 84–88
Bruxism 71
Buhner, Stephen 126
Burns 255–56
Bursitis 122–25
Burzynski, Stanislaw MD 317–19

C
Cancer 311–22
Calcium 164–65
Campbell-McBride, Natasha MD 78,101,104,140,206,220, 237,308,361
Candida infection/candidiasis 57, 72–75,78,190,243,251,298
Carpal tunnel syndrome (CTS) 114–15
Castor oil 53,64,67,192,254,256,324
Celtic sea salt 54,97,139,281,302
Cervical disc syndrome 144–50
Cervical traction 149
Cholesterol 198–210
  -vitamin D, deficiency in 201
  -Framingham Study 201
Cold laser therapy 115
Colonics -see Enema
Colpo, Anthony 199,219
Common cold 88–92
  -prevention of 91

Concentrated animal feeding
    operation(CAFO) 28,35
Congestive heart failure(CHF)
    232–337
    -protocol 235–36
Conjunctivitis 67–68
Constipation 88,106,108–09
Cowan, Thomas MD 202–206,262
Crinnion, Walter 21,36, 210,361
Crook, William G. MD 73,243
Crohn's Disease 102
Cystitis 196
    -chiropractic treatment 197
    -reflexology for 197

D
D-arabinitol Test for Yeast 104
Dairy 38–40
    -pasteurization effects 38,39
    -homogenization effects 38,39
Davis, William MD 7,220,225
Dechlorinator 27
Degenerative Disc Disease 150–53
Diabetes 224–226
    -protocol 217–22
    -juvenile 229–32
Digestion 17–18
Dr. Scholl's 14
Dust Bowl 9
Dyspareunia 184–87

E
Earache 65
Ear Conditions 61–67
    -chiropractic treatment 64
    -otitis media 62–65
    -tinnitus 65–66
Eczema 243–44
Enema 3,274–75,281–83,304,305,331
Enig, Mary 39,200–08,219–20,228,
    230,277,291,294,361
Environmental Working Group
    (EWG) 21–22,241,252
Erasmus, Udo 206,294

Erectile dysfunction (ED) 165–170
    -blood pressure drugs as cause
        168-69
    -thyroid involvement in 174
Eucalyptus oil 83,86
Eustachian tube 61-62
Exercise with oxygen therapy
    (EWOT) 236-37

F
Fallon-Morell, Sally 19,33,38,81,97,
    102,131,137,149,160,182,200,
    219,220,230,259,267-73,302,344
Fibroids 142, 188–90
Flatulence 100–02
Floaters 69–71,
Flu shot 85,86,238
Food combining chart 24
Food combining, proper 23–26,41
Food pyramid, traditional 32
Food pyramid, USDA 31,35
Food quality 18–21
Foot Levelers 14–15,117,157,358

G
Gallbladder disease 35,76–77,109–13
Gallstones 77,109,111,123,322
Gastritis (GERD) 6,16,25,41,50,78,
    93–99,108,156
Gedgaudas, Nora 212
Gelatin 41,141,150–51,155,162
Genova Labs
    57,60,71,104,125,133,167,175,
    180,238,241,248,280,297,357
Glaucoma 69–71
Glaxo Smith Kline 44
Glossitis/glossodynia 75–77
Glutathione 40,160
Gluten/gliadin 37,239
Glycosaminoglycans(GAGs) 151
Glycosylated hemoglobin
    (HbA1c) 166
GMO Labeling 30

Gokhale, Esther 153
-exercise for the spine 153
Gonzalez, Nicholas MD 313–321
Gormley, James J. 9–10
Gottschall, Elaine 106,232,293,362
Gut and Psychology Syndrome (GAPS) 79,102,106,142,232,310

H
Habba Syndrome 111
Halitosis 99–-100
Harvard, corruption 5–6
Headaches 47–55
-behind the eyes/sinus 53
-crown 47
-frontal 49–50
-general type 54–55
-occipital 51
-temporal 48
Helicobacter pylori 50,94
Herxheimer reaction 101
Hiatal hernia 94–99
-Chiropractic adjustment for 99
High fructose corn syrup 37,38,105
Hives 245–46
Homeostatic soil organisms 18
Huggins, Hal 239
Hydrogenated oils 34,38,43,131,352
Hypoglycemia 22,213–15

I
Infant Care 258–90
-breast feeding 271–73,277
-chiropractic care 280
-colicky baby 275–76
-fever treatment 273-74
-fevers 280–83
-formulas, homemade 277-80
-introducing solid foods 279
-picky eaters 289–90
-Poya Baby Shampoo 270
-soy dangers 278
-supplements 268
-vaccines 283–88
Inositol Hexaphosphate (IP-6) 183,189,278
Irritable bowel syndrome (IBS) 102–108,299,359
Itch Calm Cream 244,358

J
Joint pain 126,132–36
-older children 134–36
-younger children 132–34

K
Kelley, William Donald 310–11,318
Kendrick, Malcolm MD 200–202, 219
Keys, Ancel 33,199,205-207,219
Knee problems
-arthritis 117–18
-pain 118
-sprains/strains 115–16

L
Lacto-fermented foods 28,33,42,52, 81,102–109,196,248,262,307
Leaky gut syndrome 42,103–04,140, 209,243,292,297
Leptin 171
Lewin, Alex 33,102,248,262,369
Lung, disorders of 83–88
Lyme disease 125–132

M
Mann, George 200
Masai Tribe 200
Masterjohn, Chris 36,39,202,263-67, 295-966–69,356
McCully, Kilmer MD 222
McGee, Charles T. MD 223
Meinig, George 239
Menopausal bleeding 187-88
-chiropractic treatment of 188

Metchnikoff, Elie 292
Milk 19,20
Monounsaturated oils 34
Moritz, Andreas 49,77,111,122,188, 247,251,322
Morning sickness 262,271
Multiple sclerosis 238–240,341
Mustard plaster 86,326–27
Myogenic Theory of Heart Disease 202–03

N
Naessans, Gaston 90
Nail fungus 242-44
Neck pain 144–155
Nourishing Traditions 19,33,38,41,92, 97,102,105,106,130,134,137,150, 153,160,181,226,230
Nourishing Traditions Book of Child and Baby Care 259–65, 268, 270–272,358
Novartis 44
Nutrition and physical degeneration 108

O
Omnivore's Dilemma 20
Oral contraceptive
   -see Birth control pill
Oregano tea (for ear) 64
Orthotics (Foot Levelers) 14–15, 117,122,154
Osteoporosis/Osteopenia 27,156–164
Otitis Media (middle ear infection)
   - see Ear conditions
Ovarian cysts (PCOS) 179–186
   -adrenal dysfunction in 180
   -diet for 180-182
   -testing, hormones 186
   -thyroid disease in 179

P
Pagano, John DC 247–250,291
Painful intercourse
   -see dyspareunia
Pao d'arco 74-76,336
Patient assessment, holistic 11–17
Peanut oil 34,118–19
Pes planus (flat foot) 13
Pfizer 43
pH 26–29,59–61
Phytates 37, 138–39,161
Pink eye -see Conjunctivitis
Plantar fasciitis 119-122
Pollan, Michael
   -see *Ominovore's Dilemma*
Polyunsaturated oils/fats 34,203
Pregnancy/Infant Care 258–90
   -Choline, importance of 267,279
   -Cod Liver Oil, importance of 235,265-272,280,332,333
   -DHA (Docosahexanoic Acid) 235,266–68,293
   -folate, importance of 187,222,264
   -preconception diet 264,265
   -soy, dangers of 275,277-78
   -ultrasound during 259
   -vitamin A, role in 265
   -vitamin D, role in 266
   -vitamin E, role in 265
   -vitamin K, role in 266
Price, Weston A. 20-211,107,154,209, 232,260,263,266,289,291,307,355
Probiotics 33,51
Protomorphogens 142
Psoriasis 247–250

R
Ravnskov, Uffe MD 199–203
Recombinant Bovine Somatotropin (rBST) 38
Reverse Osmosis Water Filter 27,43
Review of findings 11,16
Round-Up 37

S

Salatin, Joel 7–10,18,234,260
Saturated Fats, benefits 221,293-297
Savory, Allan 10,18
Schmid, Ron 20,39,40,45,58, 105,163
Sciatica 150–155
Semmelweis, Ignaz 289–90
Shamsuddin, Abulkalam MD 176,183
Shiva, Vandana 10
Sinus infection/sinusitis 55–58
Skin cancer 161,241,246-47,
Slow-Burn Exercises 169,236,237
Soil depletion 7–10,231
Sore throat 77-81,323
Specific carbohydrate diet (SCD) 104,239
Standard Process 46
Statin drugs 200-203,218-19,223,294
Styes 68
Subluxation, defined 13,15-16,150
Sunscreen 241,246,252,266
Sun tanning 246-47
Sweet oil 64
Syndrome X 211,217,226
Systems Survey Form 11

T

Taheebo tea 74
Thrush 72–75
Thyroid disease 160
Tinnitus 65–67
 -chiropractic treatment 66–67
Tongue, conditions of 75–78
 -fissured 78
 -geographic 78
 -painful 75–77
Toxicity Questionnaire 11–12
Trowbridge, John MD 73,196,243

U

Unilever 44
Urinary tract infection 195-97
 -chiropractic treatment 197
 -reflexology for 197
 -yeast involvement 195–97

V

V7–3D scanner (Foot Levelers) 14,117,122,154
Vagus nerve 15,50,66,229
Vitamin C 68,72,91,106,130,151–52, 185–87,196,212,222,224,249-257,265,282,300
Vitamin K_2 125,134,138,185
Voisin, Andre 7

W

West, Bruce DC 2218,220,234,243
West, Stanley MD 187-189
Weston A. Price 4,7,18,20,33
 -Foundation (WAPF) 43,112,133, 201-02,209-10,223,295-98
 -Shopper's Guide 21,42,107,139
Williams, Louisa 239
Wound healing 253-257
Wright, Jonathan V. MD 25,50,94,187
Wulzen Factor 185
Wulzen, Rosalind 185

Y

Yeast -see Candida
Yeast fighters 74

Z

Zyflamend 115–17,121,124,150
Zypan test 49–50,157,343-44

CPSIA information can be obtained
at www.ICGtesting.com
Printed in the USA
FSHW011921071221
86693FS

9 781524 645854